Monographs on Endocrinology

Volume 25

The Pituitary and Testis

Clinical and Experimental Studies

Edited by
D.M. de Kretser, H.G. Burger, B. Hudson

With 92 Figures and 17 Tables

Springer-Verlag
Berlin Heidelberg New York Tokyo
1983

David M. de Kretser

Department of Anatomy, Monash University
Clayton, Victoria 3168/Australia

Henry G. Burger

Medical Research Center, Prince Henry's Hospital
St. Kilda Road, Melbourne, Victoria 3004/Australia

Bryan Hudson

Howard Florey Institute of Experimental
Physiology and Medicine, University of Melbourne
Parkville, Victoria 3052/Australia

ISBN-13:978-3-642-81914-8 e-ISBN-13:978-3-642-81912-4
DOI: 10.1007/978-3-642-81912-4

Library of Congress Cataloging in Publication Data
Main entry under title: The pituitary and testis.
(Monographs on endocrinology; v. 25)
Includes bibliographical references and index.
Contents: Patterns of secretion and metabolism of the gonadotrophic hormones – Control of FSH and LH secretion – Pituitary testicular axis during pubertal development – Changes in the pituitary-testicular axis with age – [etc.]
1. Pituitary hormones. 2. Testis. I. De Kretser, David. II. Burger, Henry. III. Hudson, Bryan.
IV. Series. [DNLM: 1. Pituitary gland – Physiology. 2. Testis – Physiology.
WI MO57 v. 25 / WK 502 P962]
QP 572.P52P57 1983 612'.492 82–19185
ISBN-13:978-3-642-81914-8 (U.S.)

Softcover reprint of the hardcover 1st edition 1983

2127/3020-543210

List of Contributors

H.W.G. Baker, Howard Florey Institute of Experimental Physiology and Medicine, Melbourne, Australia

W.J. Bremner, Division of Endocrinology and Metabolism, Veterans Administration Medical Centre, Seattle, Washington, U.S.A.

H.G. Burger, Medical Research Centre, Prince Henry's Hospital, Melbourne, Australia

Y.M. Hodgson, Department of Anatomy, Monash University, Melbourne, Australia

B. Hudson, Howard Florey Institute of Experimental Physiology and Medicine, Melbourne, Australia

J.B. Kerr, Department of Anatomy, Monash University, Melbourne, Australia

D.M. de Kretser, Department of Anatomy, Monash University, Melbourne, Australia

V.W.K. Lee, Medical Research Centre, Prince Henry's Hospital, Melbourne, Australia

K.A. Rich, Department of Anatomy, Monash University, Melbourne, Australia

Preface

This monograph brings together our work concerning the relationships between the hypothalamus, pituitary and testis. The studies span approximately a decade of collaborative work. Over this period our contributions and those of many others have advanced greatly our understanding of many aspects of male reproductive biology. This monograph attempts to survey these developments and to highlight many unresolved issues. It also provides an opportunity to demonstrate the value of investigations which relate biochemical to structural parameters and to illustrate the importance of animal studies in elucidating biological principles with clinical applications. The reverse is also important since the pathophysiology of human disorders often provides insight into hitherto unsuspected basic mechanisms.

In any rapidly expanding field it is difficult to stop revising and extending a manuscript. It is equally difficult to quote every reference in the field but we trust that those of significance have not been omitted. Some of our former students have collaborated with us as co-authors in producing this monograph. It is equally important to recognise the contributions of our other former students and colleagues who have physically participated in the studies and without whose intellectual contributions a number of concepts would not have been elucidated. Their work is acknowledged in the text of the monograph and the extensive list of references.

David de Kretser
Henry Burger
Bryan Hudson

Acknowledgements

In reviewing the contributions of our laboratories over a decade, it is difficult to acknowledge in person the personnel involved in the studies at the scientific, technical, illustrative and secretarial stages. We have been particularly fortunate to have enjoyed working with many excellent technicians, secretaries and illustrators and we hope that the preparation of this volume does justice to their work.

No scientific study is possible without money and we wish to acknowledge the support of the National Health and Medical Research Council of Australia, the Ford Foundation, the National Institutes of Health in the United States and the Expanded Programme of Research in Reproduction of the World Health Organisation. The support of our institutions, Monash University, the Medical Research Centre, Prince Henry's Hospital and the Howard Florey Institute of Physiology and Experimental Medicine was vital in the work described.

It is also important to acknowledge the participation of numerous patients in the studies described. Without their help, clinical research would not be possible and quite often their misfortune prompted a new study or helped to elucidate a novel concept.

Finally, and perhaps of greatest importance, we would like to acknowledge the part played by our wives, Jan, Jenny and Norma, who provided a stable home environment, enabling us to concentrate our endeavours, often too greatly, on our research, teaching and patient care. Without their sacrifice and that of our families, our contributions to this field would have been considerably smaller.

David de Kretser
Henry Burger
Bryan Hudson

Contents

1	**Patterns of Secretion and Metabolism of the Gonadotrophic Hormones** (H.G. Burger and V.W.K. Lee)	1
1.1	Assay Methods	1
1.1.1	Human FSH, LH and Prolactin	1
1.1.2	Animal Gonadotrophins	2
1.2	Patterns of LH and FSH Secretion in Normal Men	3
1.3	Metabolic Clearance and Gonadotrophin Secretion Rates in Normal Men	6
1.3.1	MCR and Production Rate of LH	6
1.3.2	MCR and Production Rate of FSH	9
1.3.3	Initial Clearance of Gonadotrophin Subunits	11
1.3.4	Effect of Renal Disease on MCR	11
1.4	Summary	11
2	**Control of FSH and LH Secretion** (D.M. de Kretser, H.G. Burger and W.J. Bremner)	12
2.1	Sites of Production of FSH and LH	12
2.2	Hypothalamic Influences on FSH and LH Secretion	13
2.3	Influence of Testicular Feedback	23
2.3.1	Feedback Control of LH	23
2.3.2	Feedback Control of FSH	25
2.4	Assays for Inhibin	28
2.4.1	Modified Steelman-Pohley Bioassay	28
2.4.2	Bioassays Using Castrate Rams	29
2.4.3	Bioassays In Vivo Using Rodents	30
2.4.4	In Vitro Bioassays for Inhibin	31
2.5	Assay Specificity	32
2.6	Sources of Inhibin	34
2.7	Evidence for Inhibin from Immunisation Studies	40
2.8	Characteristics and Mode of Action of Inhibin	41
2.9	Physiological Implications of Inhibin	42
2.10	Summary	43
3	**Pituitary Testicular Axis During Pubertal Development** (V.W.K. Lee and H.G. Burger)	44
3.1	Studies in Men	44

3.1.1 Changes During Fetal Life 44
3.1.2 Changes in the Newborn 45
3.1.3 Changes During Childhood and Adolescence 45
3.1.4 Pituitary Responses to LHRH 48
3.2 Studies in Rats 53
3.2.1 Changes in LH, FSH and Testosterone Concentrations with Age 53
3.2.2 Relationship Between Age and Hormonal Levels 56
3.2.3 Changes in Testicular Histology with Age 56
3.2.4 Significance of Hormonal Changes in the Developing Rat . . 57
3.3 Studies in Rams 60
3.3.1 Changes in FSH, LH, Prolactin and Testosterone Concentrations with Age 61
3.3.2 LH, FSH and Testosterone Responses to LHRH with Age . . 63
3.3.3 Changes in Testicular Histology with Age 65
3.3.4 Significance of Hormonal Changes 66
3.4 Overall Comments 69

4 **Changes in the Pituitary-Testicular Axis with Age** (H.W.G. Baker and B. Hudson) 71

4.1 Introduction 71
4.2 Methods 72
4.2.1 Testing the Pituitary-Testicular Axis 72
4.2.2 Selection of Subjects 73
4.2.3 Statistical Methods 73
4.3 Summary of Results 74
4.3.1 Virility, Testicular Size and Histology 74
4.3.2 Gonadotrophin and Sex Hormone Levels 76
4.3.3 Metabolic Clearance and Production Rates of Sex Steroids . 76
4.3.4 Dynamic Tests of Gonadotrophin and Testosterone Secretion 79
4.4 Significance of Senescent Testicular Degeneration 80
4.4.1 Mechanism of Hormone Changes with Age 80
4.4.2 Further Studies 81
4.4.3 Aetiology of Testicular Damage 81
4.5 Clinical Relevance 82
4.6 Summary 82

5 **Spermatogenesis and the Sertoli Cell** (K.A. Rich and D.M. de Kretser) 84

5.1 Spermatogenesis 84
5.1.1 The Spermatogenic Cycle 85
5.1.2 Kinetics of the Spermatogenic Process 87
5.1.3 Duration of Spermatogenesis 88
5.1.4 Requirements for Quantitation of Spermatogenesis 88
5.2 The Sertoli Cell 89

5.2.1 Morphological Characteristics 89
5.2.2 Nucleus 90
5.2.3 Cytoplasm 91
5.2.4 Inter-Sertoli Cell Junctions 93
5.2.5 Sertoli Cell Maturation 95
5.2.6 Secretory Products 96
5.2.6.1 Seminiferous Tubule Fluid 96
5.2.6.2 Androgen-Binding Protein 97
5.2.6.3 Inhibin 99
5.2.6.4 Plasminogen Activator 99
5.2.6.5 Other Secretory Products 99
5.2.7 Steroidogenic Activity 100
5.2.8 Hormonal Regulation of Sertoli Cell Function 101
5.2.9 Actions of FSH on the Sertoli Cell 102
5.2.10 Effects of Androgen on the Sertoli Cell 103
5.2.11 Biochemical Changes Associated with Sertoli Cell Maturation 104

6 **Leydig Cell Function** (Y. Hodgson and B. Hudson) 107

6.1 Introduction 107
6.2 Morphology of the Leydig Cell 108
6.3 Steroid Biosynthesis and Secretion 115
6.4 Regulation of Leydig Cell Function 118
6.5 Hormonal Regulation of LH Receptors 121
6.5.1 LHRH and Leydig Cell Function 125
6.6 Leydig Cells and Spermatogenesis 126
6.7 Androgens in Blood 127
6.8 Abnormalities of Leydig Cell Function 128
6.8.1 Congenital Disorders 128
6.8.2 Acquired Disorders 130
6.8.2.1 Cirrhosis of the Liver 131
6.8.2.2 Chronic Renal Failure 131
6.8.2.3 Age 131
6.8.3 Testicular Disorders 132

7 **The Effect of Testicular Damage on Sertoli and Leydig Cell Function** (D.M. de Kretser and J.B. Kerr) 133

7.1 Introduction 133
7.2 Spermatogenic Damage and the Control of FSH Secretion . 133
7.3 Sertoli Cell Function and Testicular Damage 135
7.4 Luteinising Hormone, Testosterone and Spermatogenic Damage 142
7.5 Leydig Cell Structure and Spermatogenic Damage 147
7.6 Leydig Cell Function and Testicular Damage 150

References 155

Subject Index 185

1 Patterns of Secretion and Metabolism of the Gonadotrophic Hormones

H.G. Burger and V.W.K. Lee

The dominance of the female as an object of study in the science of reproductive biology is nowhere more clearly emphasised than in the introduction to a chapter on the secretion and metabolism of the gonadotrophic hormones, as these relate to the pituitary-testicular axis: the commonly accepted names of these hormones refer to their functions in female reproduction! Luteinising hormone (LH) is also called by a little-used name relevant to the male (interstitial cell-stimulating hormone, ICSH) but there is no counterpart for follicle-stimulating hormone (FSH) or prolactin (Prl). In this chapter, the methods of gonadotrophin assay used in our laboratories are described and the results are reviewed of their application to studies of their patterns of secretion and metabolism.

1.1 Assay Methods

1.1.1 Human FSH, LH and Prolactin

The basic concepts regarding secretion of gonadotrophins were established by application of bioassay procedures long before the advent of radioimmunoassay. It has generally been held that gonadotrophin secretion commences at puberty and there is evidence that gonadotrophin levels are lowered by pituitary lesions and elevated in primary testicular disorders. The development of radioimmunoassays for pituitary hormones began with human growth hormone (Greenwood 1962; Utiger et al. 1962; Roth et al. 1963) and was soon followed by assays for LH (Midgley 1965, 1966; Bagshawe et al. 1966; Franchimont 1966a,b,c) and for FSH (Franchimont 1966a,b; Faiman and Ryan 1967). Results obtained with these assays quickly confirmed some of these concepts, but have led to a greatly increased understanding of gonadotrophin secretion and to the generation of new concepts not previously anticipated.

We developed our first gonadotrophin assay for LH, using paper chromato-electrophoresis as the separation method for bound and free hormone; this development was dependent on the generous gift of highly purified LH from Dr. Anne Stockell-Hartree, of the Department of Biochemistry, Cambridge University, U.K. (Burger et al. 1968). A method for LH using antibody-coated tubes to immobilise the antibody and thus the bound hormone was developed at about the same time (Catt et al. 1968).

More recently we have used double antibody radioimmunoassays, which have been adopted routinely for human FSH, LH and prolactin (Alford et al. 1973b; Healy et al. 1977). Since these assays have been utilised for the studies described in this monograph, their characteristics will be described in some detail below.

Reagents and Standards. The standard used for both FSH and LH has been a clinical grade crude pituitary gonadotrophin powder, similar in characteristics to the widely used standard distributed by the U.S. National Institutes of Health (NIH), LER 907. As assessed by specific bioassays (ovarian ascorbic acid depletion and ovarian augmentation) the potency of our standard is 144 IU/mg LH and 40 IU/mg FSH. Reagents for FSH have been supplied throughout by the NIH, and have included various batches of purified FSH for labelling, and of anti-FSH antisera. LH supplied by Hartree has been used for radio-iodination and an anti-LH serum has been prepared in our laboratory, using highly purified LH made according to the technique of Stockell-Hartree (1966). Assay results have been expressed in mIU/ml with reference to the pituitary standard. Current normal ranges for young adult males for FSH are: mean 2.1, range 0.5–4.2 mIU/ml; and for LH: mean 1.9, range 0.6–3.6 mIU/ml.

For prolactin, reagents including standards have again been supplied generously by NIH; the normal values for serum prolactin in young adult males are 12.8 (mean), with a range between 6.4 and 19.2 ng/ml.

It is important to emphasise that for all three hormones there are substantial differences in the values reported as normal between laboratories; for both FSH and LH our figures are considerably lower than those from many other sources (Franchimont and Burger 1975). The reasons for such discrepancies may include differences in reagents and separation techniques, but some of the differences are inexplicable (Bangham et al. 1973). The observation of differences between laboratories in normal ranges requires that every laboratory undertaking gonadotrophin assays, whether for clinical or physiological studies, must establish its own normal range. In the authors' laboratory, particular care has been taken to establish a normal range in young adult men which is derived from a population known to be clinically free of testicular disease, and to have normal semen analyses. The specificity of each of the assays has been checked carefully, and there is no significant cross-reactivity with other pituitary hormones or plasma constituents.

The laboratory has also undertaken a limited number of studies using the immunoassay of urinary gonadotrophins. Reagents for these assays are as described above except that the second international reference preparation for human menopausal gonadotrophins (2nd IRP HMG) has been used as the standard. Urinary gonadotrophins are prepared for assay by acetone or ethanol precipitation, as described for LH by Baghdassarian et al. (1970). Normal ranges for urinary FSH and LH are 3–30 IU and 15–58 IU per day respectively.

1.1.2 Animal Gonadotrophins

Ovine Gonadotrophins. Ovine FSH and LH have been measured using heterologous double-antibody radioimmunoassays (Salamonsen et al. 1973; Lee et al. 1976a). For FSH, the reference standard is NIH-FSH-S6, which has a biological potency of 1.24 × NIH-FSH-S1 in the hCG augmentation assay, and contains 0.0045 U/mg LH measured by ovarian ascorbic acid depletion. A preparation generously donated by Dr. H. Papkoff (G4-150C) is used for iodination, and a rabbit antibody against human FSH as the first antibody. The preparation NIH-LH-S9 (biological activity 1.07 × NIH-LH-S1) is used as the standard for ovine LH, while a Papkoff antigen is used for iodination (G3-222B or 14-28BP). The first antibody has been prepared in rabbits, using bovine LH (NIH-LH-B5). Both assays are highly specific for their respective gonadotrophins.

Rat Gonadotrophins. Reagents for the rat gonadotrophin assays have been supplied by the NIH. Purified rat LH (NIAMDD rat LH-I1, biological activity 1.0 × NIH-LH-S1) is used for radio-iodination and as a standard, while the antiserum is NIAMDD-A-Rat LH-S1. Purified rat FSH (NIAMDD-rat FSH-I1) is iodinated for use as tracer in the rat FSH assay, the reference preparation being NIAMDD-rat FSH-RP1 (biological activity 2.1 × NIH-FSH-S1), and the antisera being NIAMDD-A-rat FSH-S4 (AF4) and NIAMDD-A-rat FSH-S-6 (AF6).

1.2 Patterns of LH and FSH Secretion in Normal Men

A striking advance in knowledge regarding the normal pattern of gonadotrophin secretion has resulted from the application of two techniques – gonadotrophin radioimmunoassay, which allows measurements to be made on small single blood samples, and repetitive blood sampling at short time intervals. As a consequence, it has been recognised that both gonadotrophins are normally secreted episodically (Nankin and Troen 1971; Naftolin et al. 1972; Boyar et al. 1972). The phenomenon is more marked for LH, for which pulses of 100%–300% increments occur at intervals of 60–100 min, whereas for FSH oscillations are 10%–50%, not always synchronised with LH (Naftolin et al. 1973). We have used a continuous blood sampling technique to confirm these findings (Alford et al. 1973a). The results in one subject in whom continuous sampling, with blood collections broken up into 40-min intervals, was made over a 48-h period are shown in Fig. 1.1. A detailed study of the phenomenon of episodic secretion has been made by Santen and Bardin (1973), who have shown that in normal men the mean pulse amplitude is 68 ± 12% (range 20%–400%) above the preceding nadir, and the secretory spike interval is 3.7 times per 6 h. Serial measurements of LH, whether at daily, hourly, 20- or 10-min intervals, are extremely variable (coefficient of variation 21–435). With regard to the clinical interpretation of LH levels, these authors conclude that a single LH measurement in a normal man allows an estimate of his mean LH value with an accuracy of 50%, whereas sampling every 20 min for 6 h reduces the inaccuracy to ± 12%. Although a single sample is usually sufficient to distinguish normal subjects from those with levels elevated as a consequence of primary gonadal failure, multiple sampling is required in order to detect minor to moderate changes in LH.

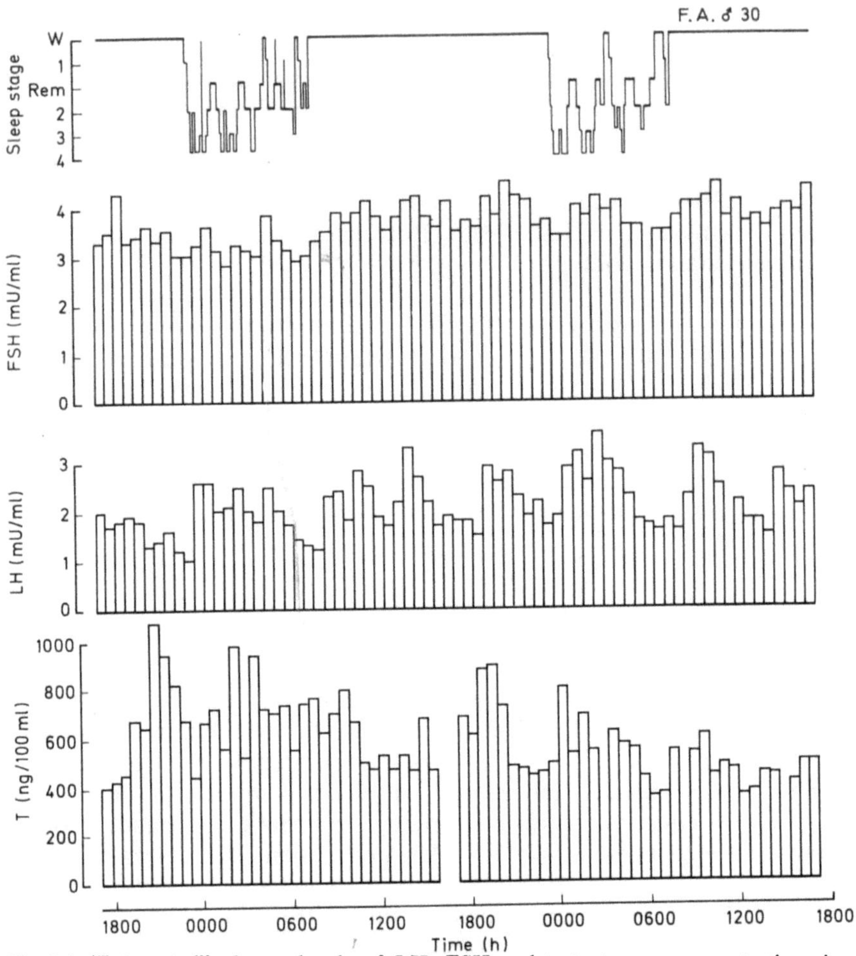

Fig. 1.1. "Integrated" plasma levels of LH, FSH and testosterone concentrations in a normal young man. Blood was collected continuously for 48 h through a specially designed indwelling catheter into a fraction collector, the fractions being of 40-min duration. Each *vertical block* thus represents the mean or "integrated" hormone concentration during the 40-min period of collection. Sleep stages are depicted at the top of the figure (Alford et al. 1973a)

In order to determine the degree of correlation between single and multiple estimates of gonadotrophin concentrations in serum, we studied 15 normal men and 31 patients with oligo- or azoospermia, from whom blood samples were drawn at 15-min intervals for 3 h. Marked fluctuations in the levels of LH and FSH occurred in some patients, while in others there were no oscillations. It was not possible to identify a single pattern of episodic secretion. These results are shown in Figs. 1.2 and 1.3. Mean levels of FSH are above the normal range in 10 of these 31 patients, in whom individual levels were all greater than normal so that a single estimate would have given a correct result in these patients. In the remaining 20, the mean values are in the normal range, but in five the FSH levels in individual samples are greater than our upper limit of normal, while in two they were less than the lower

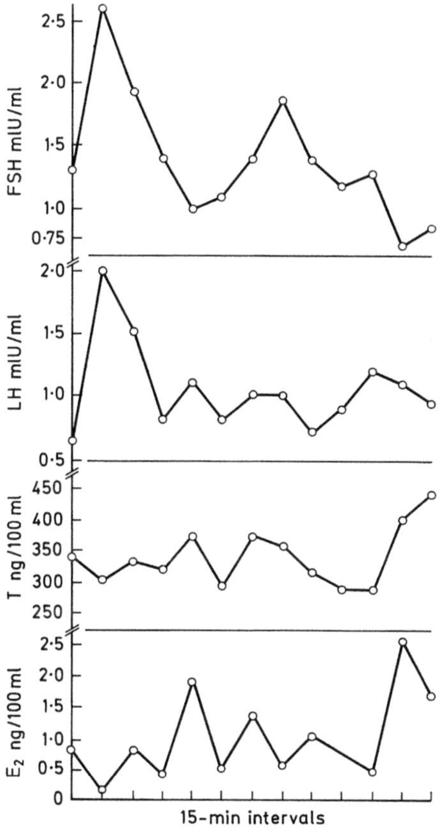

Fig. 1.2

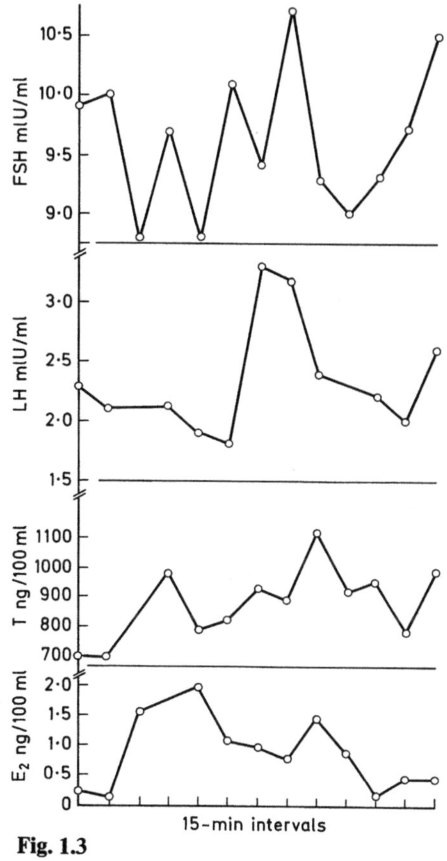

Fig. 1.3

Fig. 1.2. The fluctuations of FSH, LH, testosterone and oestradiol in serum and plasma are shown over a 3-h period during which sampling was performed at 15-min intervals in a patient with hypospermatogenesis

Fig. 1.3. The fluctuations of FSH, LH, testosterone and oestradiol in serum and plasma are shown over a 3-h period during which sampling was performed at 15-min intervals in a patient with Sertoli cell syndrome

limit of normal. This indicates the degree to which misclassification can occur if we rely on individual blood samples. Similar misclassification also occurs for LH with single blood samples.

The same comment applies to normal individuals, and we stress that classification of any individual's gonadotrophic status is open to error if only a single estimate is made, particularly when these values are at the extremes of the normal range. We now regard a value of serum FSH of 6.0 mIU/ml or greater in the presence of azoospermia to indicate irreversible damage to the seminiferous epithelium.

1.3 Metabolic Clearance and Gonadotrophin Secretion Rates in Normal Men

Estimates of the daily production rates of gonadotrophins are made by measuring the metabolic clearance rate (MCR) and the mean blood concentration; the production rate is the product of these two values. The MCR is measured either by the technique of constant infusion to reach a steady state equilibrium, or by integrating the area under the disappearance curve of the hormone following a single intravenous injection. We have used the former method to measure the MCRs of FSH and LH in normal men, and in one man with germinal cell aplasia (Pepperell et al. 1975). We have shown that there is no significant difference between estimates of MCR made by the infusion of labelled or non-labelled hormone (Table 1.1).

Table 1.1. Metabolic clearance rates of LH in two normal men. Two different gonadotrophin preparations were given by constant infusion

LH preparation infused	Basal plasma LH level (mIU/ml)	Infusion rate	Plateau level	MCR (ml/min ± SD)
Subject 1				
LER-1533-B 76–93[a]	0.80	73704 ± 271 cpm/min	1612 ± 65 cpm/ml	45.7 ± 1.9
LER-1533-B 76–93	0.95	211.9 ± 15.6 mIU/min	5.3 ± 0.3 mIU/ml	48.4 ± 5.3
HPG-025	0.60	381.5 ± 32.6 mIU/min	8.4 ± 0.2 mIU/ml	48.9 ± 4.4
Subject 2				
LER-1533-B 76–93[a]	0.75	52900 ± 182 cpm/min	1118 ± 36 cpm/ml	47.3 ± 1.5
HPG-025	0.75	614 ± 65 mIU/min	13.1 ± 0.5 mIU/ml	49.7 ± 5.6

[a] ^{125}I-labelled

1.3.1 MCR and Production Rate of LH

We tested three LH preparations of varying purity to determine their suitability for these measurements, and showed that the metabolism of these was the same, so that it was not necessary to use highly purified LH for this purpose (Table 1.2). A crucial factor in the methodology is the use of highly specific

Table 1.2. Half-times of three LH preparations

LH preparation	LH half-time (min)
LER-1533-B 76–93	42.8
LER-1533-B 76–93 ^{125}I	43.6
HPG-025	42.1

antisera for the immunoprecipitation of the infused hormone, and determination of hormone concentrations. We prepared such antisera using LH purified by the method of Stockell-Hartree (1966) and obtained identical results for MCR in the same subject with each of the three antisera prepared in this way.

In ten normal men we found the MCR to be 43.9 ± 8.5 (SD) ml/min (25.6 ± 3.6 ml/min/m²). These values are significantly higher than the value of 19.2 ml/min/m² found in three normal women in the mid-follicular phase, and of 17.4 ± 1.9 ml/min/m² in four post-menopausal women. Our values for these women are higher than those reported by Kohler et al. (1968). These results are shown in detail in Table 1.3.

The mean production rate of LH in the normal men was 85.1 IU/day, and the mean urinary excretion rate of LH on the day prior to the production rate study, 35.0 ± 21.3 IU/day. A male with germinal cell aplasia had an MCR similar to those of the normal men (39.6 ml/min) despite endogenous LH levels more than twice those of the normal men. The production rate was 166.5 IU/day. Taken together with the findings that MCR was the same in pre- and post-menopausal subjects, that is in women with varying levels of endogenous LH, the findings indicate that MCR of LH is probably independent of endogenous LH concentration, and that, providing renal and hepatic function are normal, differences in plasma LH levels in various conditions represent differences in pituitary secretion rates. We do not understand why there should be a sex difference in the MCR of LH.

A major problem in comparing our data with other reports concerns the choice of the appropriate standard to be used to express the units of LH secretion. Kohler et al. (1968) expressed the plasma concentration of LH in terms of the 2nd IRP-HMG and used the figures derived for the secretion rate to conclude that the pituitary content of LH is turned over once each day. It is now recognised that a pituitary standard should be used to estimate the potency of pituitary preparations since the use of a urinary standard, such as the 2nd IRP-HMG, will give a potency estimate (by radioimmunoassay) between 5 and 6 times higher than that obtained by bioassay, using the same urinary standard.

It has been a matter of controversy as to which standard should be used to estimate plasma concentrations (Albert et al. 1968). In these studies we used a pituitary standard in view of the general tendency over recent years to employ such standards, and we have expressed our units as the biological potency when assayed against the 2nd IRP-HMG. Because of this our ranges of values differ significantly from those of Kohler et al. (1968), who calculated production rates of LH of 734 ± 170 mU/min, equivalent to 1060 ± 245 IU/day, for normal women, and 2400 mU/min (3456 IU/day) for post-menopausal women. These are striking differences which can be attributed almost entirely to the differences in the estimates of endogenous LH concentrations, differences which result from the use of different standards and different immunoassays. Comparable difficulties arise in the interpretation of values for the urinary excretion of LH.

We would stress that because of the differences in standards and immunoassays which result in widely divergent values in the estimation of production

Table 1.3. Results of constant infusion studies in men to measure MCR and PR of HLH

Patient	Age (years)	Radioactive studies		Non-radioactive studies		MCR (ml/min	Endogenous plasma LH (mIU/ml)[a]	PR (IU/24 h)	Urinary LH[b] excretion (IU/24 h)
		Precipitable cpm infused (cpm/min)	Plasma level at equilibrium (cpm/ml SD)	Hormone infused (mIU/min)	Plasma level at equilibrium (mIU/ml SD)				
Normal men									
1	20	42411	844 ± 18	–		50.2	1.70	122.9	–
2	29	73682	1612 ± 65			45.7	0.95	64.4	28.4
				211.9	5.3 ± 0.3	48.5			
						mean 47.1			
3	30	52917	1118 ± 36			47.3	0.75	52.4	29.4
				614.0	13.1 ± 0.5	49.7			
						mean 48.5			
4	33	90134	1419 ± 37	–	–	63.5	1.12	102.4	–
5	19	114900	2720 ± 132	–	–	42.2	1.69	102.7	–
6	22	13598	373 ± 10	–	–	36.5	1.71	89.9	12.2
7	19	169485	3938 ± 124	–	–	43.0	1.60	99.1	76.7
8	45	88077	2267 ± 41			38.9	1.32	71.7	11.3
				1078.0	30.8 ± 1.4	36.5			
						mean 37.7			
9	20	226038	6088 ± 232	–	–	37.1	1.10	58.8	51.3
10	52	166532	5055 ± 139	–	–	32.9	1.82	86.2	35.8
Mean ± SD						43.9 ± 8.5	1.38 ± 0.36	85.1 ± 21.5	35.0 ± 21.2

[a] In terms of HPG units
[b] In terms of the Second International Reference Preparation of Human Gonadotrophin

rates, each laboratory can only use its own data to compare the production rates in different reproductive states.

1.3.2 MCR and Production Rate of FSH

We used two different preparations of human pituitary FSH in the study of six normal men aged between 22 and 60 years. One preparation was highly purified (LER 1563) and had immunological potencies of 2580 IU FSH and 240 IU LH/mg and bioassay potencies of 2900 IU FSH/mg (Steelman-Pohley Assay) and 310 IU LH/mg (ovarian ascorbic acid depletion), assayed in terms of the 2nd IRP-HMG. The second preparation was the clinical grade FSH that we used for the determination of LH clearance rates. This was used only in its unlabelled form. The highly purified FSH was used both unlabelled and labelled following chloramine-T iodination with ^{125}I to a specific activity of 100–150 mCi/mg. With this and the other unlabelled preparations we showed that there were no differences in the initial half-times of disappearance from plasma, nor in the MCR in one man in whom all the preparations were used for this measurement (Tables 1.4, 1.5).

Production rates for FSH were measured from the product of the MCR and the mean plasma level of hormone. We collected blood samples every 15 min for between 1 and 3 h prior to commencing the constant infusion of FSH, and subtracted the endogenous FSH levels from the plateau levels achieved during infusion.

Infused FSH reached plateau levels in four men after 5–6 h, but did not plateau for 10 h in one man and not at all in another in whom the infusion continued for 16 h. We do not understand why equilibrium was not achieved, but we found that the same phenomenon occurred in four of eight anovulatory women who were studied at the same time.

The mean production rate of FSH in three normal men was 29.6 IU/24 h (Table 1.6). The mean urinary excretion of FSH was 11.8 IU/24 h and the percentage excretion ranged from 28% to 45% of the infused dose. There were no sex differences in the MCR of FSH: 9.5 ± 1.0 (SD) ml/min for men; 8.7 ml/min for the normal; and 7.8 ± 1.5 ml/min for four anovulatory females. These figures are somewhat lower than those of 14.25 ± 1.1 (SEM) for seven pre-menopausal women and 12.6 ± 1.1 ml/min in six post-menopausal women reported by Coble et al. (1969).

In these studies we employed a pituitary standard (as for LH) and the units were those of biological potency in terms of the 2nd IRP-HMG. As a result the values obtained for the production rate of FSH are significantly lower than those obtained by Coble et al. (1969). These authors found a production rate of 146 ± 28 mU/min (equivalent to 210 ± 39 IU/day) compared to the levels of 34.5 IU/day and 24.3 IU/day we found in our studies. These striking differences can be attributed mainly to differences in the estimated plasma concentrations of endogenous FSH which result from the use of different standards in two different immunoassays.

Table 1.4. Half-times of three FSH preparations

FSH preparation	FSH half-lives (min)
LER-1563	194.1
LER-1563-^{125}I	193.1
HPG-025	189.2

Table 1.5. Metabolic clearance rate of FSH determined by two different techniques in a normal male subject

FSH preparation	Technique used	MCR (ml/min ± SD)
LER-1563-^{125}I	Constant infusion	10.5 ± 0.4
	Disappearance curve	8.0 ± 0.5
LER-1563	Constant infusion	8.5 ± 0.5
HPG-025	Constant infusion	8.4 ± 0.5

Table 1.6. Results of constant infusion studies with FSH-^{125}I to measure MCR and PR of hFSH

Patient	Age (years)	MCR (ml/min)	Endogenous plasma FSH (mIU/ml)[a]	PR (IU/24 h)[a]	Urinary FSH[b] (IU/24 h)	Percentage of PR excreted in the urine
Normal men						
1	45	10.5	1.22	18.4	5.7	31.0%
2	41	8.1	5.06	59.0	26.6	45.0%
3	22	9.9	0.80	11.4	3.2	28%
Mean ± SD		9.5 ± 1.0	2.36 ± 2.34	29.6 ± 25.7	11.8 ± 12.8	

[a] In terms of HPG units
[b] In terms of the Second International Reference Preparation of Human Gonadotrophin

1.3.3 Initial Clearance of Gonadotrophin Subunits

We measured the initial half times of the α- and β-subunits of LH labelled with ^{125}I in two normal men. Values of 14–17 min were obtained, as compared with 31–43.6 min for the intact hormone in the same subject. The subunits thus have initial half times of disappearance which are about 50% of those for LH.

1.3.4 Effect of Renal Disease on MCR

We had previously shown that the MCR of growth hormone is significantly lowered in patients with chronic hepatic or renal failure. We had also demonstrated that in men with chronic renal failure treated by haemodialysis there is disordered spermatogenesis, and that some disorder of the pituitary-testicular axis was likely. In many, but not all, of the 29 men we studied LH and FSH were elevated (LH 5.1 ± 0.6 vs. 1.3 ± 0.04 mIU/ml; FSH 4.2 ± 0.5 vs. 1.7 ± 0.09 mIU/ml) and testosterone was low (12.5 ± 1.3 vs. 21.5 ± 0.7 nmol/litre). The mean increment in the levels of plasma testosterone following hCG stimulation was significantly less than normal and the rises in plasma gonadotrophins in response to LHRH were also abnormal. Although the initial rise was normal, the return to basal levels was much slower than normal. Because of these responses we measured the MCR of LH in nine patients with chronic renal failure, and found the mean MCR to be significantly reduced: 7.8 ± 1.1 as compared to 25.6 ± 1.2 ml/min for normal men. Production rates of LH were significantly elevated in five of these men: 108 ± 12.6 vs. 85.1 ± 8.1 IU/day.

There is other evidence which indicates that the kidney plays a role in the metabolism of LH. de Kretser et al. (1969) showed that ^{125}I-LH is localised to the proximal convoluted tubule of the kidney, and that nephrectomy in sheep leads to a prolongation of the half time of disappearance of LH. In the kidney LH degradation appears to take place by endocytosis, followed by lysosomal catabolism (Ascoli et al. 1976).

The overall results show that in chronic renal failure there is a severe disturbance of both the steroidogenic and spermatogenic functions of the testis. Although LH production and LH levels are increased, pituitary function is intact and the high FSH levels almost certainly reflect the severe disruption of spermatogenesis. Although not measured, it seems likely that FSH clearance would be significantly reduced.

1.4 Summary

Gonadotrophin and testosterone secretion in adult males is episodic in nature, a characteristic which develops at the time of puberty. The metabolic clearance rate of LH is between three and four times greater than that of FSH, and is impaired in chronic renal failure, suggesting a role for the kidney in LH clearance.

2 Control of FSH and LH Secretion

D.M. de Kretser, H.G. Burger and W.J. Bremner

Central to any discussion of the interrelationship between the pituitary and testis is a consideration of factors controlling the secretion of FSH and LH by the pituitary gland. These factors can be broadly subdivided into two groups (a) hypothalamic and (b) gonadal. The effects of the interaction of these two groups of factors on the synthesis and release of FSH and LH by the gonadotropes is the likely determinant of the ratio of FSH and LH secreted by the pituitary gland. In this chapter, the cellular site of production of FSH and LH is considered and the relative role of hypothalamic and gonadal factors influencing gonadotrophic hormone secretion is discussed.

2.1 Sites of Production of FSH and LH

Numerous studies have attempted to identify and classify the cells responsible for FSH and LH secretion by the pituitary gland according to the tinctorial properties resulting from differing staining techniques (see review by Baker 1974). The synonymous terms applied to these cells have been summarised by Phifer et al. (1973), who attempted to relate these tinctorial properties to cells identified as gonadotrophin secretors on the basis of immunocytochemistry. The major unresolved question is whether FSH and LH are produced by the same cell or whether each hormone is produced by a specific cell. The data presented by Phifer et al. (1973) and others (Nakane 1970; Robyn et al. 1973) suggest that both FSH and LH are present in the same cells, which they have termed gonadotropes. Ultrastructural studies have demonstrated that cells with the light microscopic characteristics of gonadotropes can be subdivided broadly into two categories, those containing a single type of secretory granule (200 nm) and those containing two types (200 nm and 700 nm) (Yoshimura and Harumiya 1965; Kurosumi and Oota 1968; Tougard et al. 1971). However, the observation that many intermediate forms exist has prompted the view that the cellular differences represent different phases of a secretory cycle rather than two distinct cell types which may secrete different hormones.

The fact that FSH and LH share a common polypeptide subunit *(α)* has no doubt led to difficulties in the identification of specific secretory cell types. With the purification and subsequent sequencing of the structure of FSH and LH, antisera to the entire hormone or its α- and β-subunits have been developed and used in immunocytochemical tests (Baker et al. 1972; Phifer et al. 1973; Herbert 1975). Studies of the site of localisation of labelled antisera against the β-subunit of FSH or LH have shown that both antisera bind to the same cell type within the pituitary (Herbert 1975, 1976), confirming results of earlier studies using antisera to intact FSH and LH (Nakane 1970; Phifer et al. 1973; Robyn et al. 1973; Bugnon et al. 1974). These observations support the concept that FSH and LH can be identified in the same population of cells in the pituitary gland.

Alternative evidence has, however, been presented by Steinberger (1975), who showed that pituitary cell populations derived in culture by cloning techniques could produce either FSH or LH or both hormones, thereby suggesting that cells could be limited to the production of one hormone. It is possible that the secretory process in these pituitary cells may have been modified by dedifferentiation in culture, but alternatively the immunochemical evidence could be criticised from the view that enough common antigenic determinants could be shared on β-FSH and β-LH to render cross-reacivity possible at the relatively high concentrations of antisera used. More recent studies with antisera to the β-subunits of FSH and LH have shown in the rat and in man that 10% of the gonadotropes are stained with an antiserum against β-FSH only whereas the remaining cells stain with antisera to β-LH and β-FSH (Purandare et al. 1978; Pelletier et al. 1976). The resolution of these differing views must await further studies. Should both FSH and LH be produced by the same cell, the biochemical control mechanisms responsible for altering secretory ratios of the two hormones must be complex in view of the likely possibility that only one releasing hormone exists.

2.2 Hypothalamic Influences on FSH and LH Secretion

The concept that the hypothalamus controls reproductive status by the production of humoral factors secreted into the pituitary portal system was conclusively established by the isolation, characterisation and synthesis of a decapeptide which stimulated both LH and FSH secretion and the anterior pituitary (Schally et al. 1971; Amoss et al. 1971). This releasing factor or hormone has been termed luteinising hormone releasing hormone (LHRH) but in view of its property to cause the secretion of both FSH and LH it has also been called "gonadotrophin-releasing hormone". Although some circumstantial evidence suggests that a separate FSH-releasing hormone may exist, to date no isolation of such a substance has been achieved (Bowers et al. 1973).

The absence of a specific FSH-releasing factor poses the difficult question of trying to explain the disproportionately large increase of FSH that occurs in certain states such as in severe seminiferous tubule damage (Fig. 2.1). However, a review of the available data concerning the action of LHRH on FSH and LH secretion in differing physiological and pathological reproductive states allows a hypothesis, considered below, to be proposed as a possible mechanism for relatively independent FSH secretion under certain conditions.

The infusion of LHRH into the peripheral circulation and notably into the hypophyseal portal system results in granule extrusion from the gonado-

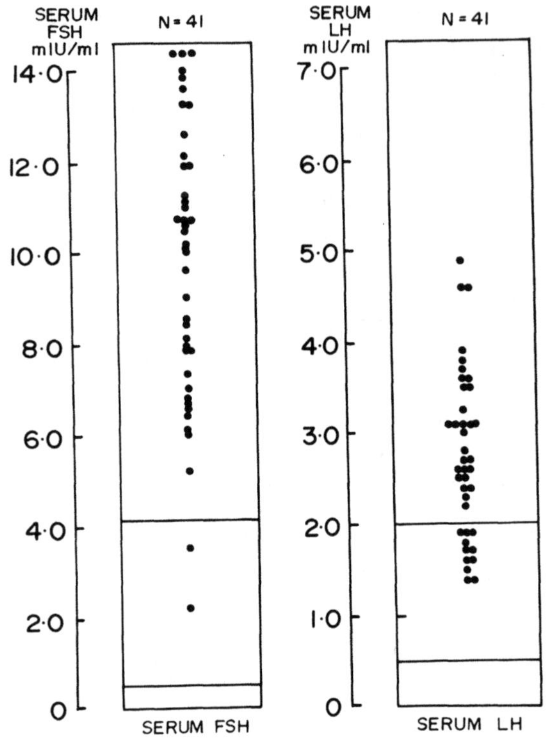

Fig. 2.1. The serum FSH and LH levels from a group of men with Sertoli cell only syndrome (germ cell aplasia). The *horizontal lines* indicate upper and lower limits of normal male range

tropes within the pituitary gland and a rapid increase in the secretion of FSH and particularly LH (Shino et al. 1972; Luborsky-Moore et al. 1975). This finding is in keeping with the results of numerous physiological studies demonstrating that a single injection of LHRH causes a dose-dependent, rapid increase in serum LH levels and to a lesser extent in serum FSH levels (Besser et al. 1972; Rebar et al. 1973; Wollesen et al. 1976). In all species evaluated to date, in the normal adult, the LHRH-stimulated rise in LH is greater than that of FSH and the recent demonstration that LHRH is secreted into the hypophyseal portal system in a pulsatile manner (Carmel et al. 1976) makes it the likely reason for the episodic secretory spikes for LH and FSH.

In normal men, Wollesen et al. (1976) have demonstrated a dose-dependent rise of LH and FSH to LHRH administered in doses from 1 to 3000 μg, particularly if the total secretory area under the response curve is considered, since at the highest doses the peak level reached does not alter extensively but the duration of the response is lengthened. The extension of the secretory reponse to LHRH in high dose is probably akin to the gonadotrophin rise evoked by continuous prolonged infusions of LHRH (Bremner and Paulsen 1974; de Kretser et al. 1975a). During the prolonged infusion of LHRH in men at doses of 0.2–1.0 μg/min, a biphasic pattern of LH secretion results, the pattern showing an initial peak occurring between 15 and 45 min, with a plateau between 60 and 90 min and a secondary rise subsequently until the termination of the infusion at 4h (Bremner and Paulsen 1974; de Kretser et al. 1975a). Bremner and Paulsen (1974) interpreted the biphasic pattern of LH secretion as evidence for the existence of two pools of pituitary LH, one acutely releasable and the other requiring longer LHRH stimulation in analogy with similar postulates for insulin and glucagon (Iversen 1971; Grodsky 1972).

The existence of a biphasic pattern of LH release to LHRH has been demonstrated in both normal adult men and women at different phases of the mentrual cycle except for a short interval around ovulation where the pattern is that of a large LH discharge in the first phase (de Kretser et al. 1976; Wang et al. 1976; de Kretser 1978). Hoff et al. (1977) have extended the concept of the two pool compartmentalisation of LH by proposing that the magnitude of the initial phase of secretion represents an index of the sensitivity of the pituitary and the second phase represents an assessment of the reserve of the gonadotropes of the pituitary gland. The concept that the biphasic pattern is representative of two pools, however, requires closer scrutiny since the acutely releasable pool during LHRH infusions probably represents that LH released by a single intravenous injection of LHRH and many studies have shown that the amount of LH secreted is dependent on the dose of LHRH, i.e. there is no finite limit to the amount of LH releasable (Wollesen et al. 1976). This can be clearly illustrated if, in addition to the commencement of the LHRH infusion, a loading dose of LHRH is given, a regimen which results in an augmented secretion of LH in the first phase (Fig. 2.2). Consequently, it is clear that a finite first pool size does not exist and that the extent of secretion is dependent on processes mobilised to differing degrees by the differing doses of LHRH. This LHRH dose de-

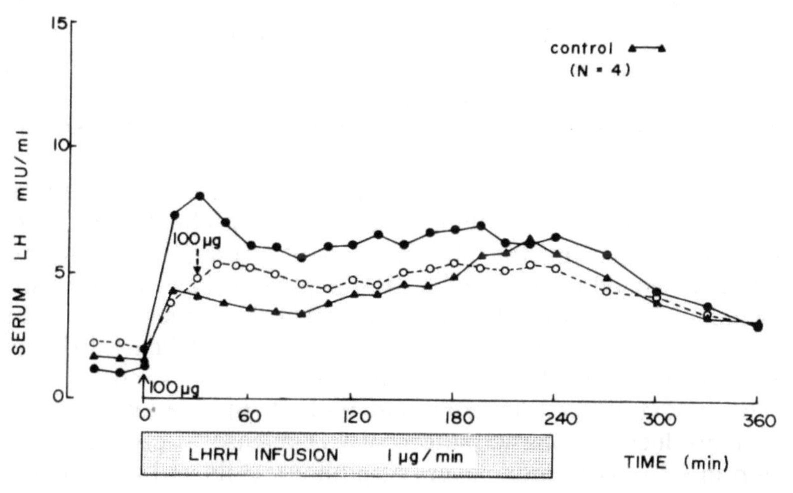

Fig. 2.2. Mean serum LH response during a 4-h LHRH infusion in normal men (▲—▲). The pattern of LH secretion when a loading intravenous injection of LHRH is combined with the infusion is shown (●—●) as well as that resulting from an intravenous injection given during the plateau phase (O---O)

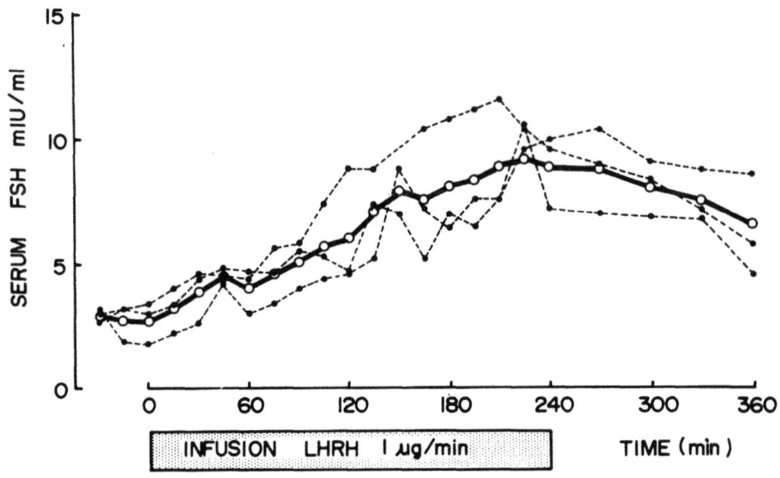

Fig. 2.3. Serum FSH response to an LHRH infusion in normal women on day 4 of the menstrual cycle, demonstrating a biphasic response

pendent pattern of the first phase of LH secretion could be explained by differing thresholds of pituitary gonadotropes to LHRH stimulation, the larger LHRH doses recruiting gonadotropes that are "less sensitive" into the secretory response.

To date, no satisfactory explanation has been adduced for the plateau phase of LH secretion. The augmentation of LHRH levels by a further injection at the start of the plateau does not result in increased secretion of LH, indicating that the pituitary is in a refractory state to LHRH (Fig. 2.3). This concept is in keeping with the studies of Schneider and Dahlen (1975), who noted that if the interval between two intravenous injections of LHRH was shorter than 2 h, there was no LH response to the second injection. The cellular mechanism responsible for refractoriness still remains to be explored.

The secondary rise of LH which has been equated with a second pool and the concept of pituitary LH reserve probably result from the same mechanism causing the phenomenon of priming whereby the response of LH to a second injection of LHRH is greater than the first (Aiyer et al. 1974; Wang et al. 1976). The priming effect has been demonstrated in vitro using isolated rat pituitaries (Edwardson and Gilbert 1975) and studies in vitro and in vivo have established that protein synthesis is necessary for the priming effect (Pickering and Fink 1976). Hopkins (1977) has been able to reproduce a biphasic pattern of LH release to prolonged LHRH stimulation in vitro using monolayers of pituitary cells and has provided a means of exploring the cellular phenomena involved in producing this response. Protein synthesis is also required for the secondary rise of LH during LHRH stimulation both in vivo and in vitro as indicated from studies using chemical inhibition of protein synthesis (Vilchez-Martinex et al. 1976; de Koning et al.

1976). Whether the synthesised protein represents LH or a protein involved in the secretory response is yet to be determined. That LHRH can increase the stores of LH has been demonstrated by direct and circumstantial evidence in vivo and in vitro (Taleisnik and McCann 1961; Evans and Nikotovich-Winer 1969; Mittler et al. 1970; Redding et al. 1972). They have shown that in the absence of LHRH, pituitary LH content declines and can be restored by exogenous LHRH administration. Further evidence supporting the likelihood of protein synthesis being involved in the secondary phase is the change in the ratio of bioactivity to immunoactivity of LH secreted after LHRH stimulation (Dufau et al. 1976). Immediately after a single 100-μg injection of LHRH in normal women, the ratio of LH bioactivity to immunoactivity is approximately 1.0. However, by 1 h and later, this ratio increases to as much as 4.1.

The secretory pattern of response of FSH has been less dramatic. Studies in men during prolonged LHRH infusions could not demonstrate a biphasic pattern of FSH secretion, but instead a slow, progressive increase was noted plateauing at about 4 h (Bremner and Paulsen 1974; de Kretser et al. 1975a). However, in women in the follicular phase, a biphasic pattern of FSH release is discernible (Fig. 2.3). The reasons for the lack of a definitive biphasic pattern of FSH release remain unclear. It is possible that the longer half-life of FSH may obscure any drop following the initial response especially when combined with the relatively sluggish initial response and its low magnitude. Recently, Koninckx et al. (1976) proposed that if the longer half-life of FSH is taken into account by a mathematical manœuvre, the actual secretion of FSH is biphasic with a time course similar to LH.

Though the cellular events responsible for the biphasic pattern of secretion in response to continuous LHRH stimulation remain to be established, there is evidence that steroid secretion by the gonads can modulate the magnitude and pattern of response. In women, the follicular phase rise in oestradiol is most likely the responsible factor, converting a biphasic into an essentially monophasic initial phase of secretion of great magnitude, immediately preceding ovulation (de Kretser et al. 1976, 1978; Hoff et al. 1977). The results in normal men (Bremner and Paulsen 1974) and in patients with Klinefelter's syndrome (de Kretser et al. 1975a) indicate that exogenous testosterone administration exerts a greater suppressive effect on LH secretion from the first pool than from the second. Similar results have been obtained from studies of rams during LHRH infusions where high-dose chronic testosterone administration significantly decreased both phases of LH secretion but particularly the first. Short-term infusions of testosterone cause no change in the pattern and the response of long-term castrated rams to LHRH results in an augmentation of the initial phase of LH secretion with little change in the second phase, again suggesting that the effect of testosterone is predominantly on the first phase of secretion (Bremner et al. 1980).

The studies in rams also demonstrate an unusual phenomenon in that the LH response to LHRH could not be maintained beyond the 3rd hour of stimulation (Bremner et al. 1976). Though the testes produce a rapid rise in plasma testosterone to the LHRH-induced LH secretion, this steroid

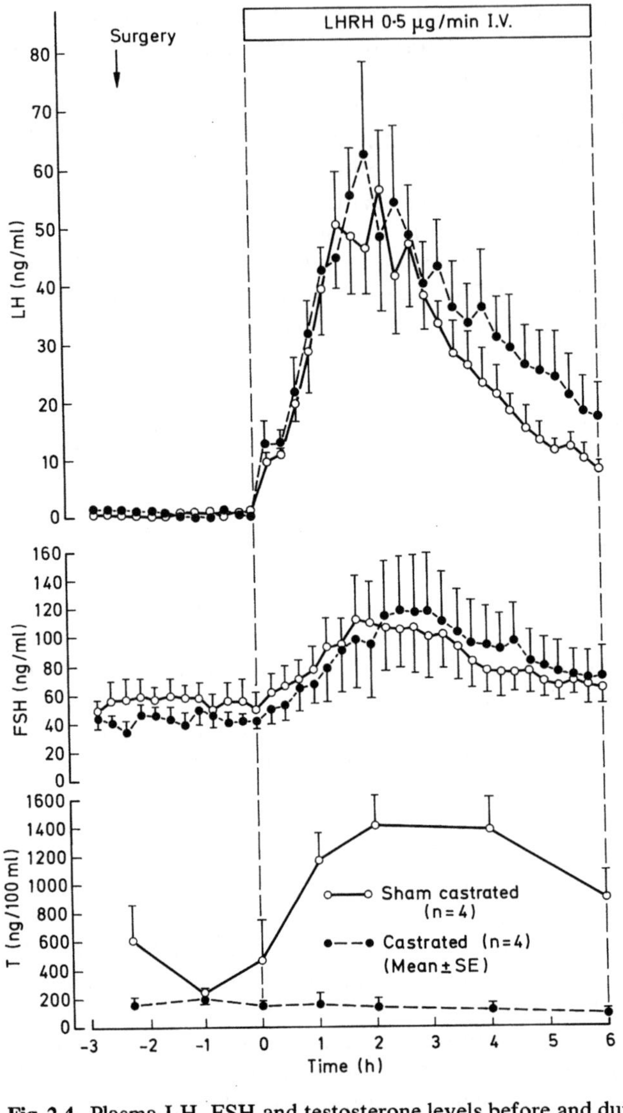

Fig. 2.4. Plasma LH, FSH and testosterone levels before and during LHRH infusions (0.5 μg/min for 6 h) into short-term castrated and sham-castrated rams. Surgery was performed 2–2.5 h prior to the onset of the infusions. (Bremner et al. 1980)

does not cause pituitary refractoriness to LHRH since the same phenomenon is seen following castration (Fig. 2.4). This pattern of LH secretion in the ram is dissimilar to man since 18-h infusions of LHRH evoke continuously elevated LH levels in normal men (Bremner and Paulsen 1977). The major factor that could contribute to this difference is the fact that LHRH evoked a 100-fold rise in LH in the ram but only a threefold rise in man. Administration of LHRH in higher dosage or for longer times may also induce refractoriness in man. However, studies in ewes have shown that pituitary LH stores are not exhausted during this declining phase of LHRH-induced LH secretion (Rippell et al. 1974). The reason for this refractoriness remains unclear, but the demonstration that exposure of hormone receptors to high levels of the hormone may result in loss of its receptors and modulation of its secretory responses (Sharpe 1976).

In both normal adult men and women, the response of FSH is always of lesser magnitude than LH during LHRH stimulation. However, this pattern is reversed in pre-pubertal children (Reiter et al. 1976b) (Fig. 2.5) in whom the LH response to an infusion of LHRH is of low magnitude,

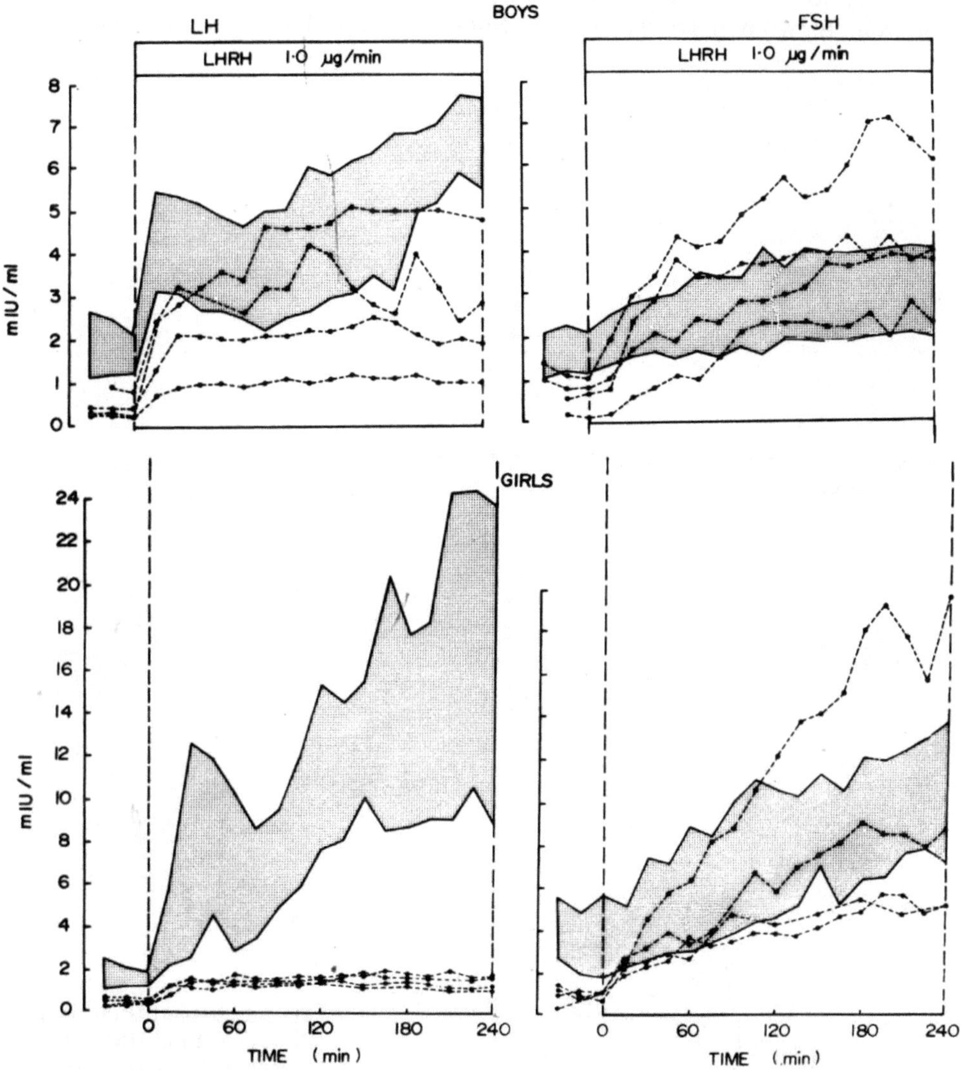

Fig. 2.5. Serum LH and FSH levels in normal pre-pubertal boys and girls before and during LHRH infusions of 1.0 µg/min for 4 h. *Shaded areas* represent ranges of hormone levels found during similar studies in normal men and women

monophasic in type and less than the FSH response. As children pass through puberty, reversion to the adult pattern is seen. Studies in pre-pubertal males with hypogonadotrophic hypogonadism also show a response of FSH and LH to LHRH which is identical to the response seen in pre-pubertal children in the majority of cases, a few patients showing very poor responsiveness of both FSH and LH (Fig. 2.6a,b). This confirms the results of studies by Bremner et al. (1977), who also demonstrated that treatment of some of these men with LHRH over 4 days could convert the "pre-pubertal type" of response into one resembling that seen in adults.

The results of our studies in women with anorexia nervosa show a marked similarity to those in hypogonadotrophic hypogonadism and in pre-pubertal children. In women whose body weight was less than 90% of ideal body

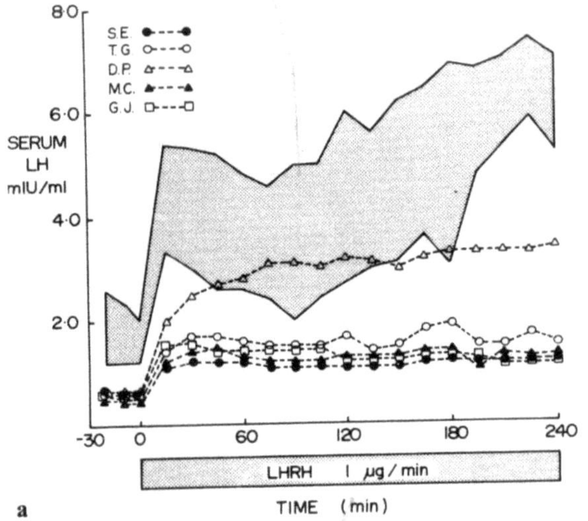

a

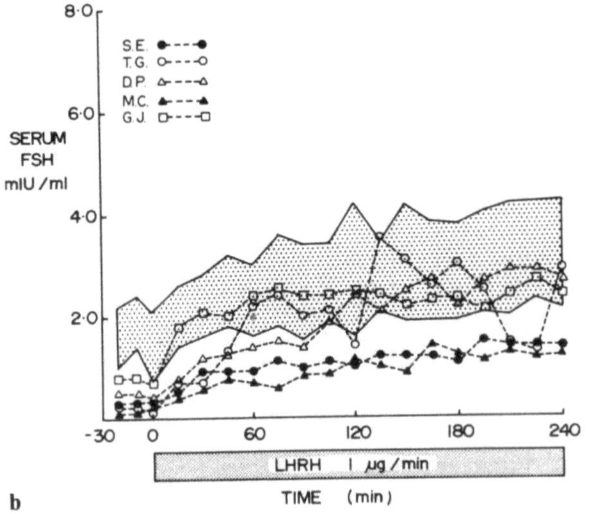

b

Fig. 2.6. Serum LH (**a**) and FSH (**b**) response to LHRH infusions in men with hypogonadotrophic hypogonadism. *Shaded areas* represent responses in normal men weight, two response patterns to LHRH infusions were noted. One pattern consisted of normal or hyper-responsive FSH secretion with an attenuated monophasic rise of LH while the other demonstrated poor responsiveness of both FSH and LH. Again, treatment for 3–4 days with LHRH could convert the FSH and LH responses into a more adult type pattern. A similar reversion to an adult type of response was also evident following restoration of body weight (Fig. 2.7) as has been reported by others using single injections of LHRH (Palmer et al. 1975; Warren et al. 1975; Sherman et al. 1975; Beaumont et al. 1976).

The remarkable similarity of the patterns of FSH and LH release to LHRH stimulation in pre-pubertal children, men with hypogonadotrophic hypogonadism and women with severe weight loss (anorexia nervosa) suggest a common mechanism since these three states also exhibit loss of episodic LH secretion and are non-responsive to clomiphene (Santen et al. 1971; Boyar et al. 1972). It is possible that endogenous LHRH deficiency may be

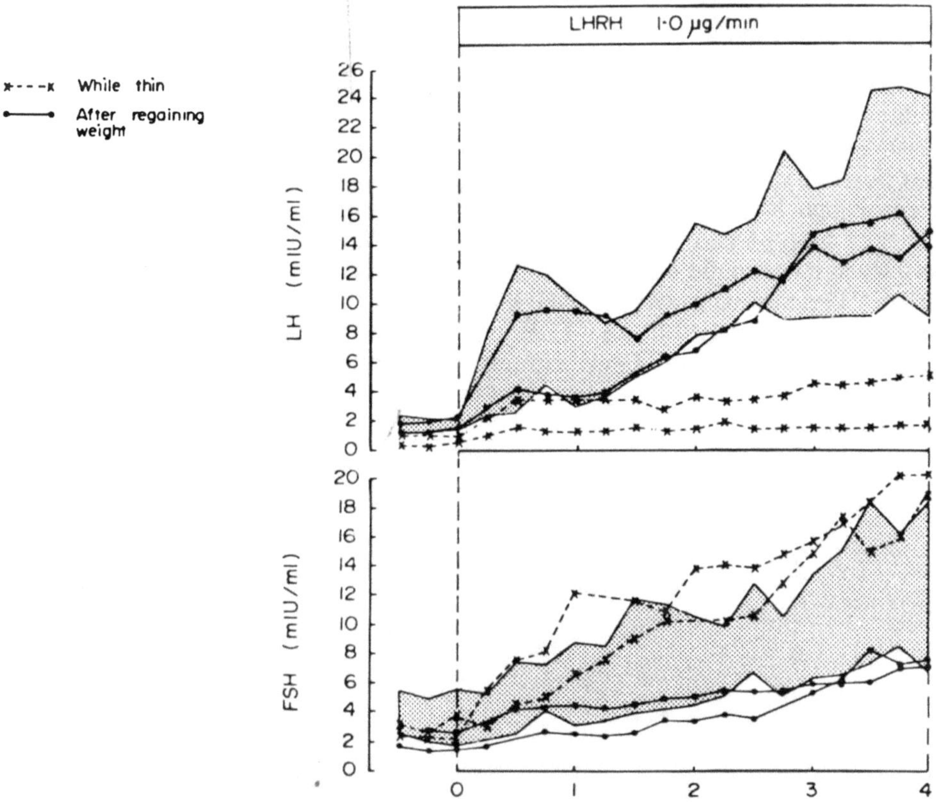

Fig. 2.7. Serum LH and FSH levels in two patients with anorexia nervosa before and during two LHRH infusions (1.0 μg/min for 4 h). For each patient, one infusion was administered while she was thin and amenorrheic and the second infusion was administered after she had gained weight and normal menstrual function. *Shaded areas* represent normal ranges found during similar infusions in normal women (Bremner 1977)

the common factor linking these three states. In normal pubertal maturation, it is assumed but not proven that the secretion of FSH and LH in the early phases of puberty occurs in response to hypothalamic changes mediated by increasing endogenous LHRH secretion, presumably of episodic nature (Carmel et al. 1976). From the studies of patients with hypogonadotrophic hypogonadism at post-mortem, the concept has arisen that the basic defect is hypothalamic with consequent failure of endogenous LHRH secretion (Bremner et al. 1977). Since body weight and sexual maturity have been closely linked in animals and man (Watson et al. 1956; Frisch 1974) the loss of weight associated with anorexia nervosa may be considered to have reduced women to a "prepubertal state" associated with endogenous LHRH deficiency.

The concept that the loss of LH responsiveness and augmented FSH secretion to LHRH is the result of endogenous LHRH deficiency is supported by the demonstration that LHRH treatment of patients with anorexia nervosa or hypogonadotrophic hypogonadism in whom with further LHRH stimulation there is a further increase of LH responses over FSH results in the adult type of pattern.

Support for this concept can be drawn from the studies of Arimura et al. (1973) and Debeljuk et al. (1973b), who transplanted pituitaries under the kidney capsule of hypophysectomised rats and allowed the grafts to regress. With exogenous LHRH in the doses used, they were able to restore FSH but not LH secretion to normal, perhaps due to the failure to achieve sufficiently high levels of LHRH necessary to produce normal LH responses. Further support can be obtained from our studies of a normal female who sustained a traumatic stalk section from a car accident, resulting in hypopituitarism. When infused with LHRH 3 weeks after injury, LH responded poorly and monophasically but the FSH pattern was normal (Fig. 2.8). However, when studied 9 months later without any treatment to restore reproductive

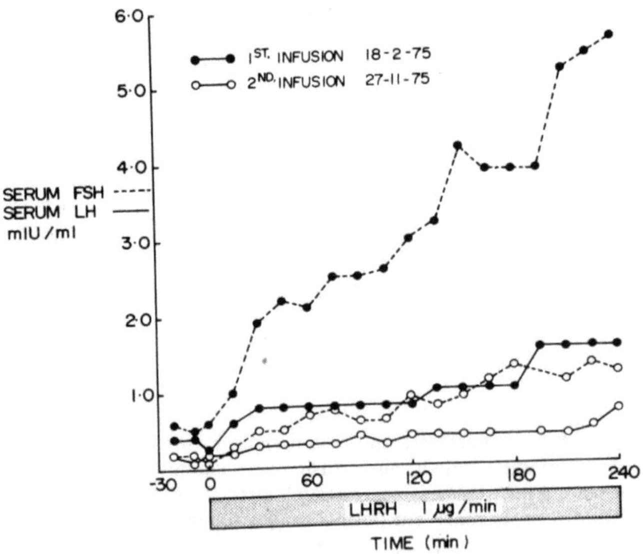

Fig. 2.8. Serum FSH and LH responses to two LHRH infusions in a female patient with a traumatic stalk section of her pituitary gland. The first infusion (●---●) was performed 21 days after the injury and the second was carried out 9 months later (○---○)

function, the response of both FSH and LH was now poor. The demonstration by Reitano et al. (1975) that repetitive administration of LHRH for 1 week to six men with isolated gonadotrophin deficiency resulted in a greater restoration of FSH secretion than LH further supports this concept.

From the evidence presented, LHRH is responsible for both the secretion and synthesis of both LH and FSH. It is also likely that the degree of endogenous LHRH stimulation can be responsible for altering the ratio of LH to FSH secreted by the gonadotroph. The interaction of this factor with the feedback signals emanating from the gonad forms the subject of the next section.

2.3 Influence of Testicular Feedback

With the development of techniques to measure gonadotrophin excretion in urine by bioassay, elevated levels were detected in the castrate state, indicating a feedback influence of the gonad in controlling pituitary secretion (Nelson 1952; Heller et al. 1952). These early studies have been confirmed by measurements of both FSH and LH using more specific and sensitive radioimmunoassay techniques which have allowed the changes following castration to be monitored sequentially (Swerdloff et al. 1971). Such observations indicate that the testis exerts a controlling influence on the secretion of both LH and FSH and this section is devoted to the mechanisms involved, in particular, whether independent and different control systems exist for each gonadotrophic hormone.

2.3.1 Feedback Control of LH

Testosterone and Oestradiol. It is well established that LH is localised to the interstitial cells and stimulates steroidogenesis therein, resulting in the secretion of testosterone (de Kretser et al. 1971; Eik-Nes 1975). The results of early studies demonstrated suppression of LH following injections of testosterone but very minor, if any, changes in FSH levels (Petersen et al. 1968; Swerdloff and Odell 1968; Franchimont 1972). However, our own results (Fig. 2.9) and those of P. A. Lee et al. (1972) demonstrate that testosterone injections given to normal men result in suppression of both LH and FSH levels. More detailed studies involving the infusion of testosterone at levels equivalent to or double the daily production rate also produce decreases in both LH and FSH levels (Stewart-Bentley et al. 1974; Sherins and Loriaux 1973).

While it is well accepted that testosterone exerts a negative influence on LH secretion by the pituitary the mechanism by which this control is exerted is still an area of controversy. Numerous investigations have shown that oestradiol in microgram quantities is capable of suppressing both LH and FSH (Kulin and Reiter 1972; Sherins and Loriaux 1973; Stewart-Bentley et al. 1974), whereas milligram quantities of testosterone are required. A number of studies have shown that testosterone may be aromatised to oestradiol in the hypothalamus, limbic system and pituitary gland (Naftolin et al. 1971a,b;

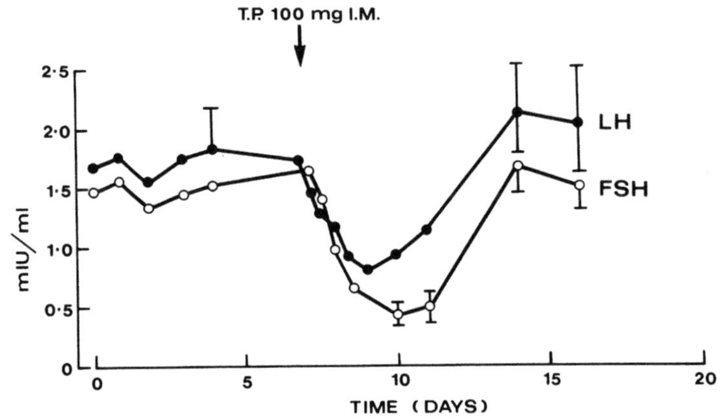

Fig. 2.9. The response of serum LH and FSH in six normal men to a single injection of testosterone propionate. (Baker 1974)

Naftolin et al. 1972; Ryan et al. 1972; Reddy et al. 1973). Since oestradiol can mediate a negative influence on LH secretion, it was postulated that the suppression of LH by testosterone is exerted by its aromatisation to oestradiol. However, in a detailed study, Santen (1975) demonstrated convincingly that testosterone and oestradiol exert different effects on LH secretion. Six-hour infusions of testosterone at double the production rate caused

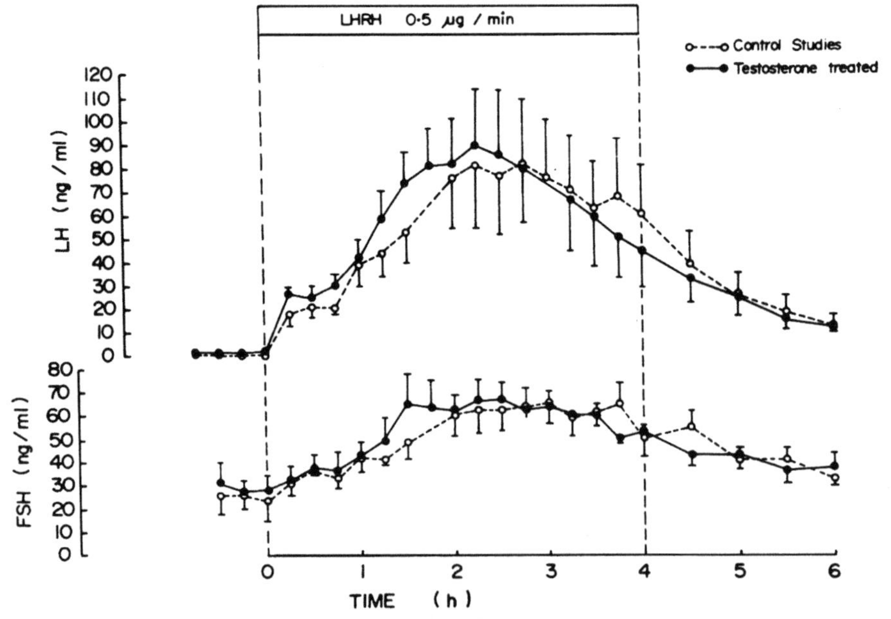

Fig. 2.10. Plasma LH and FSH levels in three normal rams before, during and after two LHRH infusions separated by 2 weeks. For 4 h before and during the second LHRH infusion the animals received testosterone by the intravenous infusion at a dose of 83 µg/min (Bremner et al. 1980)

a decrease in the mean LH levels by decreasing the frequency of the episodic secretory spikes but in fact increasing the amplitude. Oestradiol, however, decreased the amplitude of the secretory episodes with no significant effect on their frequency (Santen 1975). Furthermore, an acute infusion of testosterone causes no change in the LH reponse to LHRH both in men and rams (Fig. 2.10) whereas oestradiol causes a decrease in the secretion of LH to LHRH (Santen 1975). Santen (1975) concluded that both steroids exert suppressive effects on LH secretion by independent mechanisms.

A number of studies have also demonstrated that treatment with non-aromatisable androgens such as dihydrotestosterone, mesterolone, fluoxymesterone, danazol and 2-methyl-DHT suppress LH levels (Bardin et al. 1967; Sherins et al. 1971; Stewart-Bentley et al. 1974; Wang et al. 1974). The evidence therefore exists that testosterone can exert a direct effect on LH secretion without invoking aromatisation to oestradiol. However, since at least 50% of the daily production rate of oestradiol is derived from peripheral conversion of testosterone, the total suppressive action of the testosterone secreted by the testis is mediated by both direct and indirect mechanisms.

The majority of studies confirm that both oestradiol and testosterone suppress both LH and FSH without discernible selectivity (see p. 27). However, investigations in castrate rats using $3\beta,5\alpha$-androstanediol have shown selective suppression of LH without changes in FSH levels (Swerdloff et al. 1973; Zanisi et al. 1973). Enzymatic mechanisms for the conversion of testosterone to this metabolite exist in the hypothalamus and further studies are necessary to elucidate its role in the normal control of LH secretion.

2.3.2 Feedback Control of FSH

The concept that a separate feedback control exists for FSH arose from the observation of Mottram and Cramer (1923) that castration cells appeared in the pituitary gland of animals with severe destruction of the seminiferous tubules and normal interstitial cells. The subsequent measurement of FSH levels by specific radioimmunoassays has provided direct evidence that FSH can vary independently of LH, usually resulting in disproportionate increases in FSH with significant alterations in the FSH to LH ratio. Such changes are evident in the early follicular phase of the menstrual cycle and following damage to the ovary or testis (de Kretser et al. 1972; Franchimont and Burger 1975).

The original observations of Mottram and Cramer (1923) were supported by the early measurements of gonadotrophins in urine by bioassay techniques. A number of studies detected elevated gonadotrophin levels in men with severe testicular damage (Klinefelter et al. 1942; Heller and Nelson 1945; del Castillo et al. 1947; Howard et al. 1950; McCullagh et al. 1950). The more specific radioimmunoassay techniques have confirmed that the levels of FSH are increased in men with severe damage to the seminiferous tubules resulting in the biopsy appearance of severe hypospermatogenesis, germ cell arrest, Sertoli cell only syndrome or seminiferous tubule hyalinisation (Fig. 2.11). In general, the more severe the degree of germ cell loss, the greater the proportion of men showing elevated levels of FSH regardless

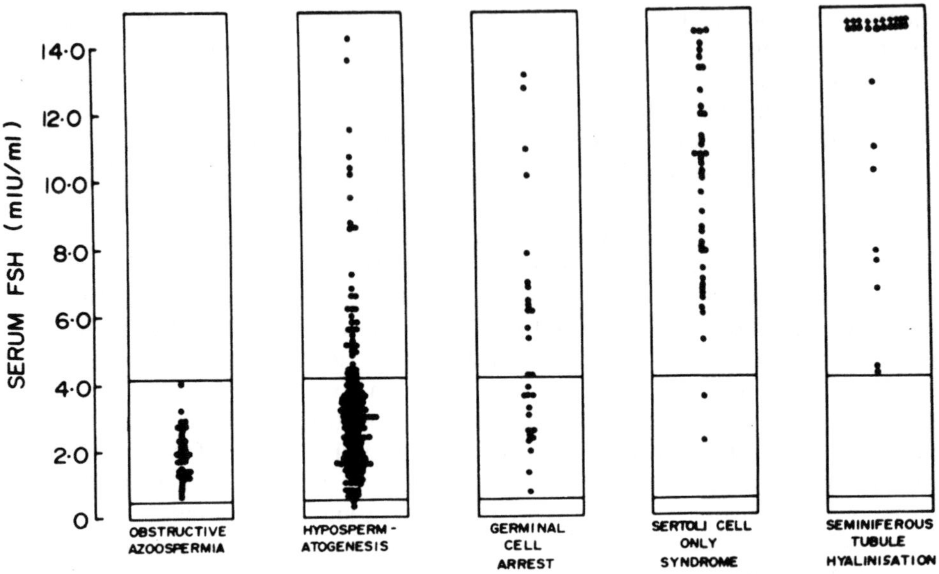

Fig. 2.11. Serum FSH levels in men with infertility divided into categories according to their testicular biopsy appearance. The upper and lower limits of the normal male range are indicated by the *horizontal lines*

of whether the aetiological factor was cryptorchidism, varicocele, irradiation, Klinefelter's syndrome or treatment with cytotoxic drugs (Paulsen et al. 1968; Johnsen 1970; Rosen and Weintraub 1971; de Kretser et al. 1972; Leonard et al. 1972; Van Thiel et al. 1972; Kjessler and Wide 1973).

The association of severe damage to the seminiferous epithelium and elevated levels of FSH has been also noted in rats following a variety of experimental procedures such as cryptorchidism, irradiation, heat treatment and the use of cadmium and antispermatogenic drugs (Amatayakul et al. 1971; Swerdloff et al. 1971; Debeljuk et al. 1973a; Verjans and Eik-Nes 1976; Rich and de Kretser 1977b). It is important to note that in these rats the rise in FSH is often accompanied by a rise in LH, suggesting that complete dissociation of control of the gonadotrophins is not possible. Similar observations have been made in a number of men with severe destruction of the seminiferous epithelium (see Figs. 7.13–7.15), again suggesting that the lack of the FSH feedback signal may also influence LH secretion. However, in these men and in the rodent models of damaged spermatogenesis, defects of interstitial cell function have been demonstrated and may provide the explanation for the elevated LH levels (discussed more fully in Chap. 7).

Two hypotheses have been advanced for the control of FSH secretion: the first proposes that testosterone controls both FSH and LH while the second advocates a separate control of FSH by an unidentified steroidal substance or a non-steroidal compound.

Evidence for the Control of FSH by Steroids. As indicated earlier, testosterone is capable of causing suppression of FSH levels when administered in amounts equivalent to or greater than the production rate (Lee et al. 1972; Sherins and Loriaux 1973; Stewart-Bentley et al. 1974; Santen 1975). In all of these studies the extent of FSH suppression is the same or less than LH and occurs over an almost identical time frame. It is consequently difficult to conceive the circumstances whereby a fall in testosterone could account for the large rises of FSH seen following germ cell damage. Furthermore, some investigators using large doses of testosterone esters administered parenterally have claimed to show no effect on FSH levels (Heller et al. 1970) for reasons that are not obvious. Steinberger and Chowdhury (1974) provided data in cryptorchid and castrated rats which suggest that testosterone controls the release and not the synthesis of FSH and consequently proposed that testosterone and an intratubular factor modulate FSH secretion.

The possibility that a steroid other than testosterone is the feedback signal for FSH is supported by ultrastructural studies of Sertoli cells which show significant amounts of smooth endoplasmic reticulum, mitochondria with tubular cristae and lipid inclusions, all features found in steroid-producing cells (Brokelmann 1963; Christensen 1965; Fawcett 1975). Further support is derived from the demonstration that the seminiferous tubules can metabolise progesterone and pregnenolone but not cholesterol to androgens (Christensen and Mason 1965; Hall et al. 1969). More recently, Dorrington and Armstrong (1975) provided direct evidence that Sertoli cell cultures can convert androstenedione and testosterone to oestradiol under the influence of FSH.

The prospect that oestradiol may be a selective inhibitor of FSH secretion has been raised by the results of two studies which demonstrated that FSH was suppressed selectively at lower doses of oestradiol than LH (Kulin and Reiter 1972; Legros et al. 1972). However, the infusion of oestradiol at a rate equivalent to its normal daily production or at twice this rate to normal men did not cause suppression of both FSH and LH (Sherins and Loriaux 1973; Stewart-Bentley et al. 1974; Santen 1975). Also Walsh et al. (1973b) showed parallel suppression of both LH and FSH in elderly castrate men given ethinyl oestradiol. Furthermore, active immunisation of rabbits with oestradiol produced an increase in LH but not FSH, providing additional evidence that oestradiol is not involved in the selective control of FSH secretion (Nieschlag et al. 1975).

A number of other C_{18}, C_{19} and C_{21} steroids have been tested in castrate rats to determine their ability to cause selective suppression of FSH (Swerdloff et al. 1973). While many were capable of suppressing FSH levels, they also caused parallel inhibition of LH. Thus the majority of the evidence available does not support the existence of a steroid capable of specifically suppressing FSH levels.

The relative contributions of inhibin and the sex steroids to the control of FSH remain an area of controversy. Studies in the rhesus monkey and the rat demonstrate that silastic implants of testosterone suppress FSH levels into the normal range and argue that the contribution of inhibin must be small (Plant et al. 1978; Decker et al. 1981). However, the delivery of testosterone in a tonic rather than an episodic manner may complicate the issue. Additionally, while FSH levels in castrate rats could be restored to the normal range by 2.5 cm silastic implants containing testosterone, further suppression of FSH could not be achieved despite implant lengths of up to 40 cm.

Evidence for Non-steroidal Control of FSH. The concept that the seminiferous tubules produced a non-steroidal inhibitor of FSH secretion was based on the experiments of McCullagh and co-workers (McCullagh 1932; McCullagh and Schneider 1940), who claimed that such a material prepared from water-soluble extracts of testes could prevent the appearance of castration cells within the pituitary gland. McCullagh (1932) termed this material inhibin and despite the lack of direct evidence for an effect of this substance on FSH secretion, this name has remained as the usual term to refer to a selective inhibitor of FSH secretion. Despite supportive circumstantial evidence from the studies of FSH levels in men with seminiferous tubule damage (Howard et al. 1950; de Kretser et al. 1972), until recent years no direct re-examination of the experimental observations of McCullagh (1932) had been undertaken using specific radioimmunoassay measurements of FSH.

Our own studies commenced with an attempt to prepare extracts of bovine testes according to the regimen proposed by McCullagh and Schneider (1940) and to test their ability to selectively influence FSH levels in castrate rams. The extracts so prepared were infused for periods of up 48 h into these animals but in no experiment was an effect found on either FSH or LH levels.

Despite the failure to demonstrate that extracts prepared according to McCullagh's (1932) method could suppress FSH levels, a considerable amount of evidence has now accumulated to indicate that a non-steroidal inhibitor of FSH exists. This evidence is now reviewed from the viewpoint of the assay used to measure inhibin and the sources from which it can be extracted. It complements the recent review published on this topic by Franchimont et al. (1979).

2.4 Assays for Inhibin

Since Setchell and Sirinathsinghji (1972) produced evidence that inhibin activity could be found in concentrated rete testes fluid of the ram or boar, a number of bioassays for inhibin have been proposed but none has proved easy to reproduce or rapid to perform. Furthermore, many assays have been poorly validated and have not incorporated dose-response curves, use of a standard or parallel line design.

2.4.1 Modified Steelman-Pohley Bioassay

In their original studies, Setchell and Sirinathsinghji (1972) detected inhibin activity of rete testis fluid (RTE) by its ability to prevent the rise in uterine weight produced by an injection of hCG, the uterine weight response being assumed to be due to a rise in endogenous FSH levels. This assay provides only indirect evidence for the action of the extract on FSH levels, and in their later studies Setchell and co-workers have used alternative systems.

Chari et al. (1976) have also used a modified Steelman-Pohley assay, basing their assessment of inhibin on its ability to inhibit the increment of ovarian weight produced by hCG administration to immature female rats. The modification has proved difficult to reproduce and again provided indirect evidence of inhibin activity.

2.4.2 Bioassays Using Castrate Rams

Our original studies (Lee et al. 1974, 1976; Keogh et al. 1976) of inhibin activity in bovine testes extracts made use of castrate rams (wethers), into which infusions of extracts were given intravenously over a 24- to 48-h period during which numerous blood samples were collected for the measurement of FSH (Fig. 2.12). The multiple samples were necessary to take account of the variability caused by episodic secretory pulses of FSH in attempting to detect suppression. Using this model system, suppression of FSH levels occurred 12–25 h after the start of the infusion but the amount of material required, the time involved and the numerous assays generated made this impractical as a method by which to screen multiple column fractions during the further purification of inhibin.

Using cryptorchid rams, Blanc et al. (1978) developed an alternative system for an inhibin assay which necessitated the collection of multiple blood samples for 25 h with intravenous injections of the test substances

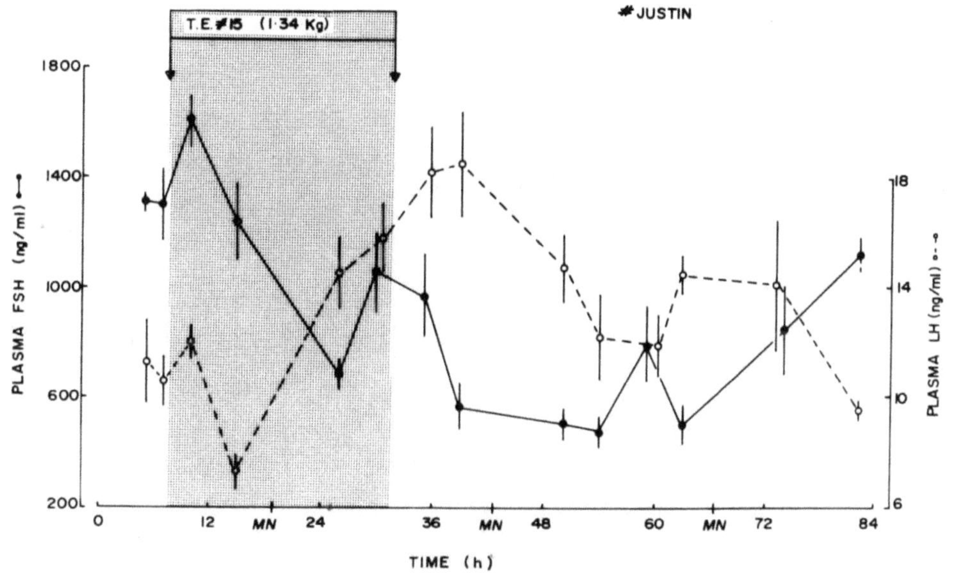

Fig. 2.12. Plasma FSH and LH responses in a castrate ram before, during and after an infusion of bovine testicular extract equivalent to 1.34 kg wet weight of bovine testis. Each *point* represents the mean ± SEM of the measurement of FSH and LH in three blood samples drawn at 10-min intervals around each time point. Extracts prepared according to schedule in Fig. 17

at the 5th and 6th hours. Using RTF, suppression of FSH occurred 8 h after the first injection and lasted for approximately 7 h while LH suppression occurred within 2 h of the first injection and lasted 3–5 h.

2.4.3 Bioassays In Vivo Using Rodents

A number of investigators have used adult male rats either intact or castrate, to assess the activity of inhibin extracts (Franchimont et al. 1975a; Baker et al. 1976a). While in some experiments a significant suppression of FSH could be achieved, these assays in our hands have not proved readily reproducible, most probably due to episodic secretion of FSH and the limited number of blood samples that can be collected to counter this variability. The studies of Nandini et al. (1976) suggest that the use of 35-day-old male rats approximately 24 h after castration could give reproducible results and they detected inhibin activity in extracts of ovine testes.

Similar results were obtained by Lee et al. (1977), who showed that if adult male mice were castrated and injected with test extracts at the time of castration and 20 h later, suppression of serum FSH levels could be detected 2 h after the second injection of active extracts (Fig. 2.13). This assay appears to be reasonably reproducible but the limited volume of blood that can be collected may lead to problems with the radioimmunoassay of FSH.

Immature female rats that have been hemicastrated show a rise in serum FSH which can be suppressed with inhibin extracts and thus can be used as a model system for that substance (de Jong et al. 1978). Using this model, inhibin activity has been identified in bovine follicular fluid (de Jong et al. 1978).

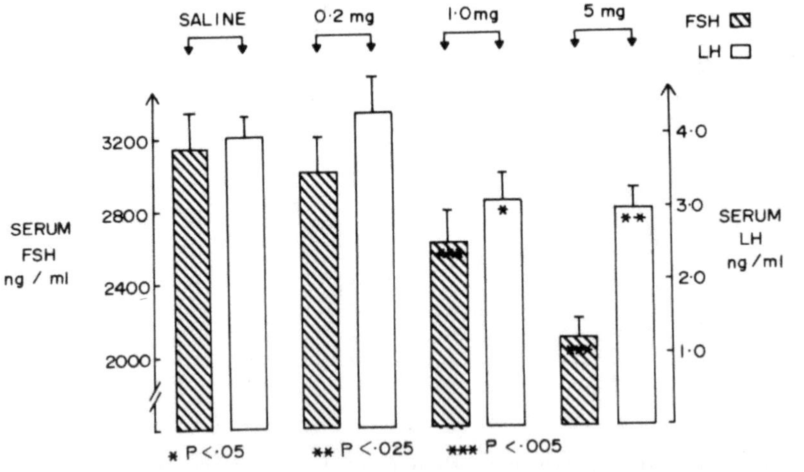

Fig. 2.13. Serum FSH levels in mice castrated 22 h earlier and given injections of bovine testis extract (INH 123) at the time of castration and 20 h later. Data represent the mean ± SEM per group. Extracts prepared according to schedule in Fig. 2.17

2.4.4 In Vitro Bioassays for Inhibin

Two systems have been described: (a) hemipituitaries and (b) monolayers of pituitary cells in culture. The incubation over 3–4 h of hemipituitaries from intact adult or 35-day-old rats with inhibin extracts has been used as an assay for inhibin by Main et al. (1978). The end-point is the measurement of FSH levels in the incubation medium which in the presence of active extracts is suppressed. The assay offers rapidity but in comparison with the pituitary cell culture assay, the use of hemipituitaries has proved to be less sensitive.

The most sensitive assay system for inhibin involves the use of monolayers of dispersed pituitary cells in culture. The effects of inhibin have been assessed either on LHRH-stimulated or on basal gonadotrophin levels. In the former system, pituitary cells are grown for 5 days in Dulbecco Modified Eagle's Minimum Essential Medium containing the inhibin extracts. The medium is then changed and the cells are incubated for a further 6 h with LHRH at a concentration of 10^{-8} M with or without test extracts in the medium (Baker et al. 1976a; Eddie et al. 1979). Active extracts suppress in

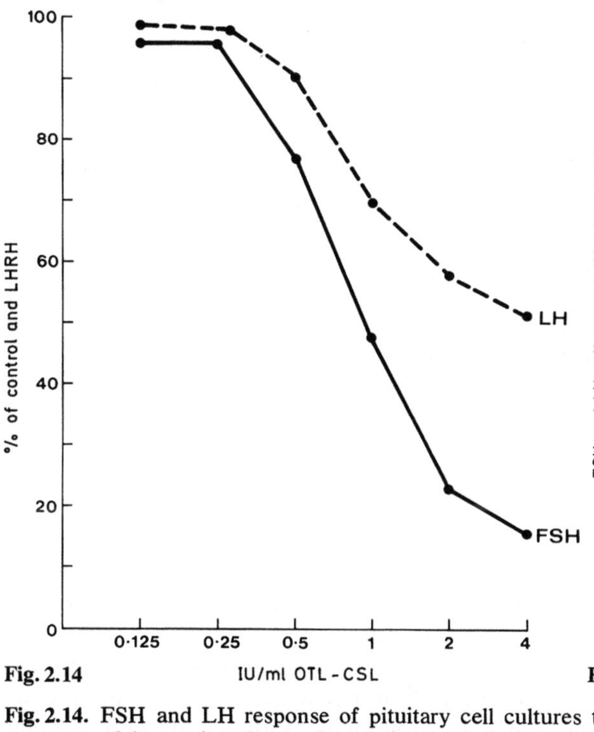

Fig. 2.14

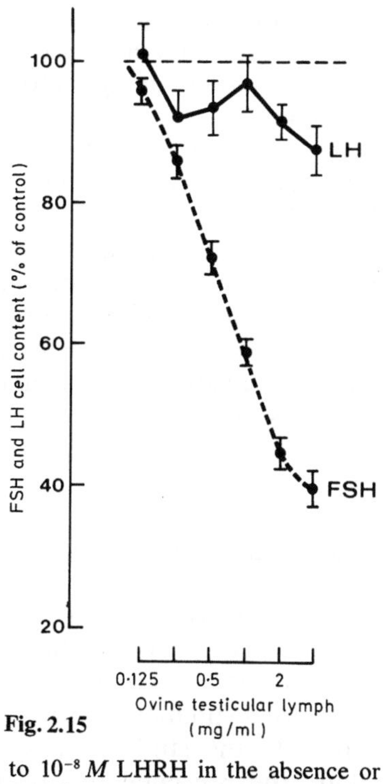

Fig. 2.15

Fig. 2.14. FSH and LH response of pituitary cell cultures to 10^{-8} *M* LHRH in the absence or presence of increasing doses of an ovine testis lymph preparation containing inhibin activity. One unit of inhibin activity is arbitrarily designated as that FSH suppressing activity contained in 1 mg of the ovine testes lymph preparation

Fig. 2.15. Changes in the FSH and LH pituitary cell content to increasing doses of an inhibin-containing preparation. Details of the assay are given in Scott et al. (1980)

Table 2.1. Comparison of the sensitivities (number of units required for detection) in different assay for inhibin (Hudson et al. 1979)

FSH suppression in rat	Inhibition of post-castration rise		Large animals		FSH augmentation		In vitro pituitary	
	Rat	Mouse	Sheep	Monkey	Ovarian wt	Uterine wt	Cells	Halves
$>5700^{a}$	150^{b}	$>2^{a}$	3500^{a}	ca 5000^{c}	$>70^{a}$	$100–1500^{d}$	0.5^{a}	1000^{a}

[a] This monograph
[b] Lee et al. (1977)
[c] E.J. Keogh (personal communication)
[d] N.R. Moudgal (personal communication)

a dose-dependent fashion the rise in FSH in the medium caused by LHRH (Fig. 2.14). LH levels are also suppressed but in a non-parallel fashion and at higher doses than those at which FSH suppression occurred. The sensitivity of this assay system is approximately 2000 times greater than the hemi-pituitary assay (Table 2.1). The principal disadvantage of the system is the 5-day interval required for growth of the cells before use, which together with the time taken for radioimmunoassay measurements usually indicates a 7- to 10-day delay before an estimate of the activity of an extract is available.

Recently, an alternative method of assay has been developed based on the effects of inhibin on the cell content of FSH and not involving LHRH stimulation (Scott et al. 1980). After a pre-incubation period of 18 h the cells are incubated for 72 h in the presence of inhibin preparations. The medium is then removed and the cells are lysed, releasing their intracellular hormones directly into radioimmunoassay buffer. Cell content of FSH is selectively reduced without change in LH, growth hormone or prolactin (Fig. 2.15). The assay is sensitive, precise and specific and can handle relatively large sample numbers. It has now been adopted for studies of inhibin purification and physiology.

2.5 Assay Specificity

One major issue which remains incompletely resolved is that of the specificity of assays for inhibin. Because an inhibitory effect is used as the end-point, there is a greater possibility of false positive results than for systems measuring stimulatory effects. The in vivo cell culture systems are particularly suited to the study of assay specificity. Criteria which may be applied include the presence or absence of morphological evidence of cell damage during incubation (cell detachment, increased cytoplasmic granulation, rounding and clumping of cells) and departure of dose-response lines from parallelism with the standard and effects on hormones other than FSH. In this regard, the cell content assays have been particularly useful, as inhibin extracts selectively reduce FSH content in the absence of toxic contaminants. Furthermore, a correlation has been found between the degree of morphological cell damage and the degree of inhibition of LH cell content. Failure to control for assay non-specificity may lead to incorrect conclusions regarding inhibin activity in biological fluids.

Another aspect of specificity is possible interference by steroid hormones. We have tested oestradiol, progesterone, 17α-hydroxyprogesterone, testosterone, dihydrotestosterone and androstenedione at concentrations of 10–100 nM. Testosterone and dihydrotestosterone were the most active steroids in causing stimulation of FSH content, whereas other steroids caused more modest effects (Fig. 2.16). None of these steroids caused a reduction in FSH cell content. A limited study was made of the interaction of steroids with an inhibin preparation and when cells were incubated with a steroid mix of oestradiol 10 nM, DHT 10 nM, testosterone 10 nM and progesterone 10 nM for 72 h in the presence of an inhibin preparation derived from ovine testicular lymph, the percentage inhibition of FSH cell content was unchanged as compared with an incubation carried out in the absence of steroids.

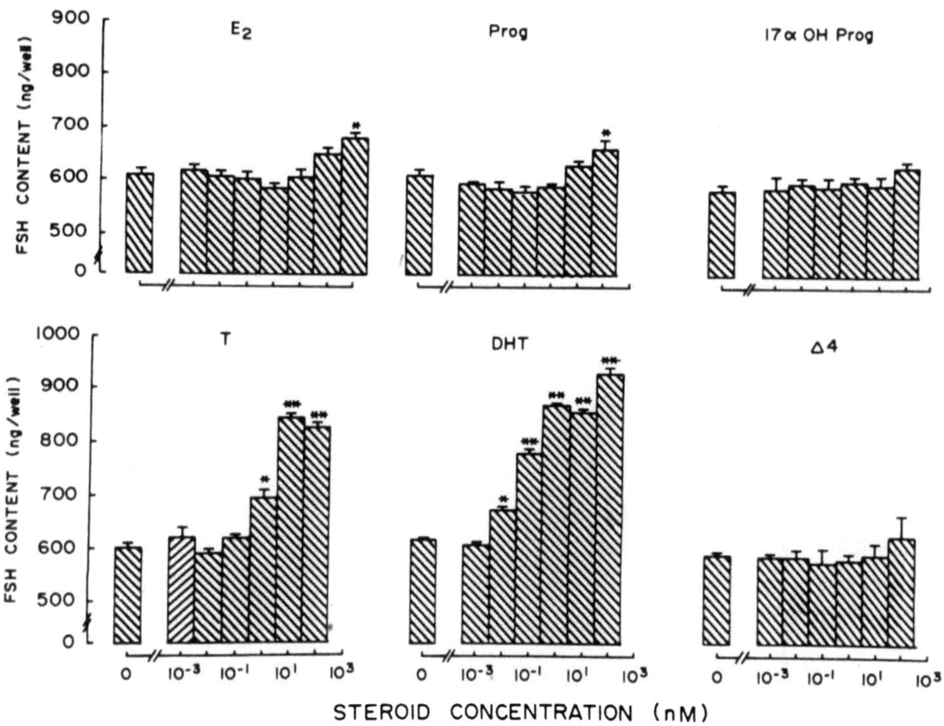

Fig. 2.16. After prior 72-h exposure of pituitary cell cultures to the steroids indicated, the medium was aspirated and the cells lysed into 500 μl tritron buffer (Scott et al. 1980). The changes in FSH cell content are shown. (Scott 1980)

2.6 Sources of Inhibin

Testis Extracts. Testis extracts from bulls (Lee et al. 1974, 1976; Keogh et al. 1976) and sheep (Nandini et al. 1976) have been shown to contain inhibin-like activity. The bovine testis extracts were prepared according to the scheme outlined in Fig. 2.17 and when infused into wethers cause selective suppression of FSH without significant alterations in LH (Fig. 2.12). The extracts did not elevate testosterone or oestradiol levels in the test animals and the inhibin activity could be destroyed by heat. Preliminary attempts to purify inhibin from these extracts on Sephadex G-100 resulted in the demonstration of activity in the fraction with a molecular weight range of 10000–70000 (0.1–0.7 kdaltons).

Seminiferous Tubule Cultures. Eddie et al. (1978) demonstrated that the media of cultures of seminiferous tubules from sexually mature rats contained a substance which suppressed LH-RH stimulated FSH secretion by cultured rat pituitary cells. The material did not alter the secretion of TSH but suppressed LH release to a lesser exent than FSH.

Sertoli Cell Cultures. In an important paper, Steinberger and Steinberger (1976) showed that the co-culture of Sertoli cells with pituitary monolayers resulted in the suppression of basal FSH secretion by the latter. They extended these observations by demonstrating that the culture media alone from Sertoli cell cultures were equally effective in suppressing the FSH levels from pituitary monolayers. Their observations therefore indicate that the Sertoli cells are capable of producing an inhibin-like material, supporting the circumstantial evidence available that the Sertoli cells are responsible

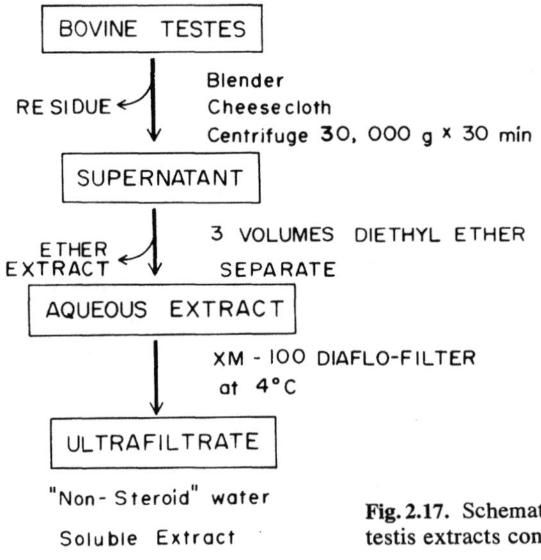

Fig. 2.17. Schematic outline of the preparation of bovine testis extracts containing inhibin

for secreting inhibin (Rich and de Kretser 1977b). More recent studies (De Jong et al. 1978, 1979; Labrie et al. 1978b) have confirmed this effect not only on basal FSH release but also on LH-RH stimulated FSH release. A lesser inhibition of LH release was also noted, but de Jong et al. (1978) showed that this inhibition was seen during LH-RH stimulation since the basal LH secretion in the presence of Sertoli cell culture medium actually increased.

Rete Testis Fluid. A number of investigators have demonstrated inhibin activity in rete testis fluid of sheep, using a number of different bioassay systems (Setchell and Sirinathsinghji 1972; Setchell and Jacks 1974; Franchimont et al. 1975a; Baker et al. 1976a). Crude rete testis fluid (RTF) following charcoal extraction causes a dose-related suppression of FSH levels in the pituitary cell culture assay system (Fig. 2.18). Different preparative steps have been utilised prior to bioassay which have included charcoal extraction to remove steroids, ethanol precipitation, concentration over amicon membranes, or gel filtration. These different preparative techniques have made it

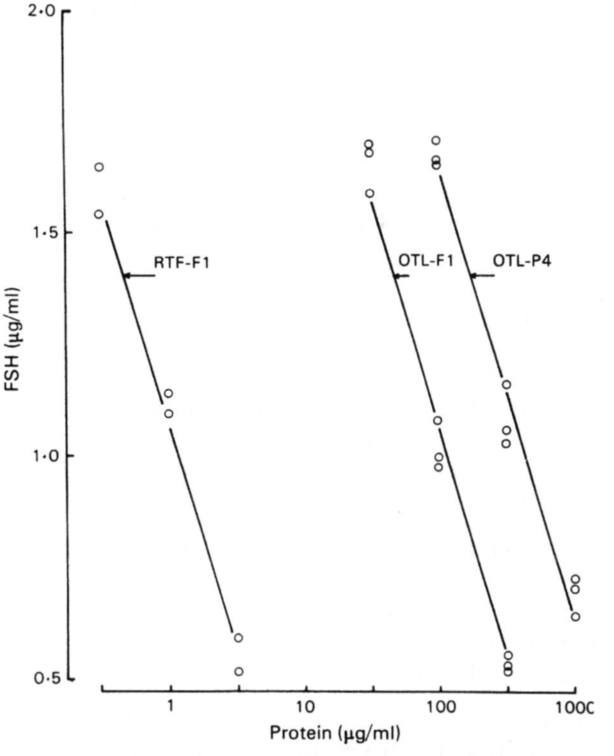

Fig. 2.18. Monolayer cultures of pituitary cells were exhibited to an inhibin standard (OTL-P_4) and test preparations from ovine testis lymph (OTL-F_1) or ovine rete testis fluid (RFT-F_1) for 3 days. The FSH concentration in each plate was measured after washing and exposure of the cells to fresh medium containing LHRH (10 n*M*) with or without test substances for 6 h. Protein was measured by absorbancy at 280 nM. Potencies and 95% confidence limits were OTL F_1, 3.8 (3.4–4.2) U/mg protein and RTF-F_1, 360 (320–410) U/mg protein. (Hudson et al. 1979)

difficult to compare the results between investigators. Preliminary results of gel filtration of rete testis fluid (Baker et al. 1976a) revealed four distinct peaks within inhibin, activity in peak *3* being demonstrated by prolonged infusions into castrate sheep with absence of activity in peaks *I* and *II*. More recently, Franchimont et al. (1978) have shown two active extracts prepared from ovine RTF which had been chromatographed on Sephadex G-100. One form consisted of a low molecular weight substance (5000 daltons) which appeared to be generated from the higher molecular weight species during column chromatography. They suggest that the higher molecular weight species may be a polymer of the lower molecular weight species or alternatively may represent a carrier substance or a precursor molecule for the smaller material. Davies et al. (1978) were also able to demonstrate heterogeneity of inhibin-like activity during gel filtration by finding three molecular weight species of 90000, 20000 and occasionally 5000.

Some investigators, including ourselves, have not been able to demonstrate a low molecular weight material with inhibin activity. This may have resulted from the use of charcoal to extract steroids from potential inhibin preparations. It is also likely that the recent demonstration that ovarian and testis extracts contain an LH-RH like material will further complicate the isolation of a low molecular weight inhibin preparation.

Data concerning the behaviour of the higher molecular weight species on inhibin during several biochemical procedures have been provided by Baker et al. (1978) using RTF and ovine testis lymph preparations. Both charcoal and ethanol extraction resulted in significant losses of inhibin activity but effectively removed steroids. Inhibin activity was concentrated in the precipitate obtained with 50%–80% ethanol whilst during ammonium sulphate precipitation activity was concentrated in the 35%–45% fractions. In a more recent report, Baker et al. (1980) concluded that inhibin was a moderate-sized protein (16000–20000 daltons) which exhibits the tendency to aggregate and elute at a higher molecular weight range. They were able to dissociate inhibin from its binding to other proteins by gel filtration in 1 M acetic acid. Their purification schedule, outlined in Fig. 2.19, resulted in a 30-fold purification, yielding a preparation with an activity of 6200 U/mg, where a unit is arbitrarily defined as the inhibin activity in 1 mg of an ovine testicular lymph protein preparation.

Ovine Testis Lymph. Lymph obtained by cannulation of the testicular lymphatics contains inhibin activity following removal of steroids by charcoal adsorption (Hudson et al. 1979). A dose-dependent suppression of FSH in the pituitary cell culture system can be seen, though its activity is considerably less than preparations of rete testis fluid.

Seminal Plasma. Investigations by Franchimont (1972) have shown that non-steroidal extracts of seminal plasma from bull or normal men have the capability of suppressing FSH levels in several bioassay systems (Franchimont et al. 1975b; Davies et al. 1978). Recently, Chari et al. (1978) claim to have isolated a protein with inhibin activity (mol. wt. 18000–20000) from bovine seminal plasma, using a modified Steelman-Pohley bioassay. This preparation also suppresses the post-castration FSH rise in rats but the

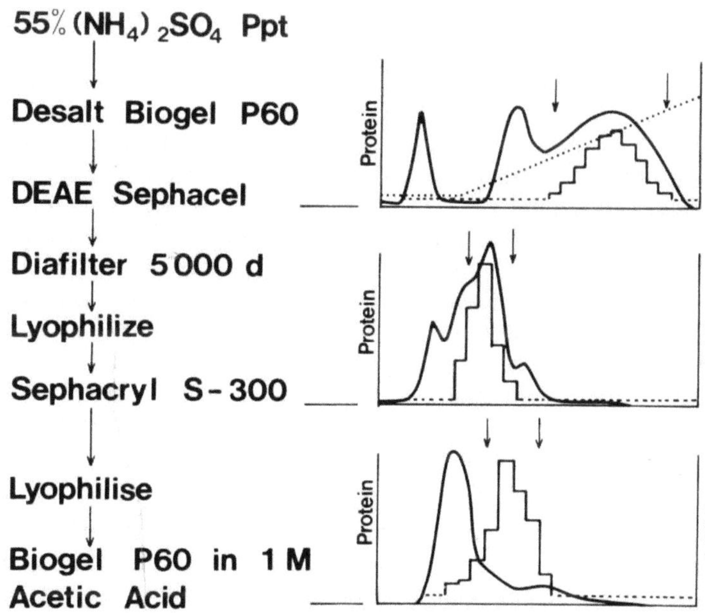

Fig. 2.19. Partial purification of inhibin from rete testis fluid commencing with the precipitation by 55% saturation of ammonium sulphate. The precipitate was dissolved in 0.1 *M* TRIS HCl, pH 8.75, desalted on Biogel P60 in 0.1 *M* TRIS HCl, pH 8.75, with 0.05 *M* NaCl and the void peak run directly onto DEAE Sephacel. The active fractions were pooled, diafiltered with a 5000-dalton hollow fibre cartridge and lyophilised. Subsequent gel filtration on Sephacryl S-300 in 0.1 *M* NH_4 HCO_3, pH 8.0, yielded an inhibin preparation with a molecular weight of approximately 90000. The active fractions were then gel filtered on Biogel P60 in 1 *M* acetic acid, yielding an inhibin preparation of an apparent molecular weight of 16000. (Baker et al. 1980)

yield of "inhibin" obtained from seminal plasma is surprisingly large. Franchimont et al. (1978) have also identified low molecular weight (5000 d) inhibin activity from human seminal plasma with features similar to the low molecular weight species obtained from ovine RTF.

Sperm Extracts. A number of papers from Lugaro, Fachini and co-workers (1963, 1969, 1973, 1974) have suggested that extracs of sperm possess inhibin-like activity. The extracts were of the "Nemasperm", the exact nature of which has not been defined in terms of the conventional terminology of spermatozoal structure and their findings have yet to be confirmed independently.

Sources of Inhibin in the Female. Steroid-free extracts of follicular fluid from bovine, porcine and human sources have been shown to have the capacity to suppress FSH secretion in a number of in vivo and in vitro bioassays (de Jong and Sharpe 1976; Hopkinson et al. 1977; Marder et al. 1977; Schwartz and Channing 1977; Daume et al. 1978; de Jong et al. 1979). Furthermore, the cellular source in the ovary would appear to be the granulosa cells since media from their cultures show inhibin activity (Erickson and Hsueh 1978). That this activity may result from the action of FSH on the follicle is supported by the finding that the inhibin activity is greater in fluid obtained from larger follicles.

Studies by de Jong et al. (1980) have shown that inhibin from bovine follicular fluid elutes with a molecular weight of 65 000; they describe the material as being relatively heat-stable and hydrophobic in nature. More recently, they have produced a lower molecular weight inhibin of approximately 23 000 daltons (Jansen et al. 1981), which is in reasonable agreement with the studies of Baker et al. (1980) using RTF as starting material.

Our own studies have confirmed that bovine follicular fluid (BFF) has inhibin activity as demonstrated with the in vitro pituitary cell culture assay system. Gel filtration of BFF on Sephacryl G-200 in ammonium acetate at pH 7 demonstrates several peaks of inhibin activity, the largest being consistent with a molecular weight in the range of 90 000 (Fig. 2.20). Gel filtration of this large molecular weight form in 1 M acetic acid yielded a lower molecular weight form of 20 000–25 000 daltons.

Cellular Source of Inhibin. The correlation between the elevation of FSH levels and the degree of germ cell loss has prompted some investigators to postulate that certain germ cell types, in particular the spermatid phase, are responsible for the elaboration of the feedback signal for FSH (Johnsen 1970; Franchimont et al. 1972). However, the techniques used in these studies were qualitative and depended on testicular damage, resulting in a sequential loss of germ cell populations, the most mature stage being lost first. Detailed quantitative studies of germ cell numbers from men with testicular damage have demonstrated that a proportion of men with total absence of spermatids maintain normal levels of FSH, thereby making untenable a direct link between this cell type (Fig. 2.21) and the production of the feedback signal for FSH (Leonard et al. 1972; de Kretser et al. 1974). Nevertheless, an inverse correlation could be found with each germ cell type and serum FSH levels

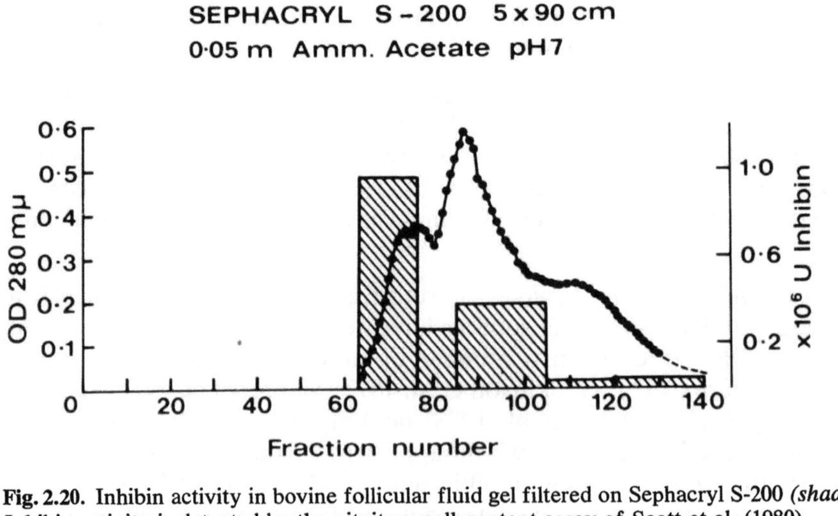

Fig. 2.20. Inhibin activity in bovine follicular fluid gel filtered on Sephacryl S-200 *(shaded areas)*. Inhibin activity is detected by the pituitary cell content assay of Scott et al. (1980)

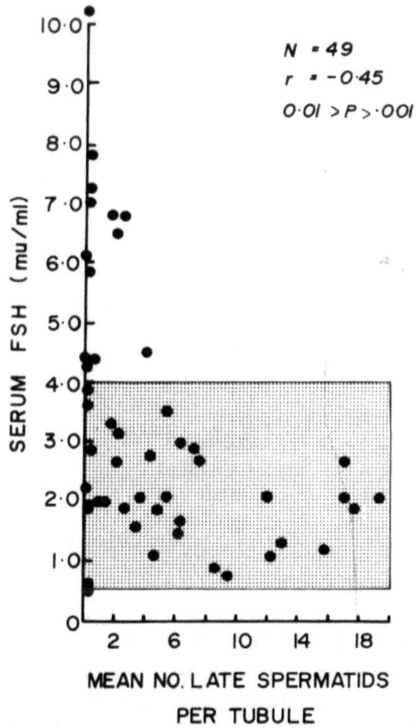

Fig. 2.21

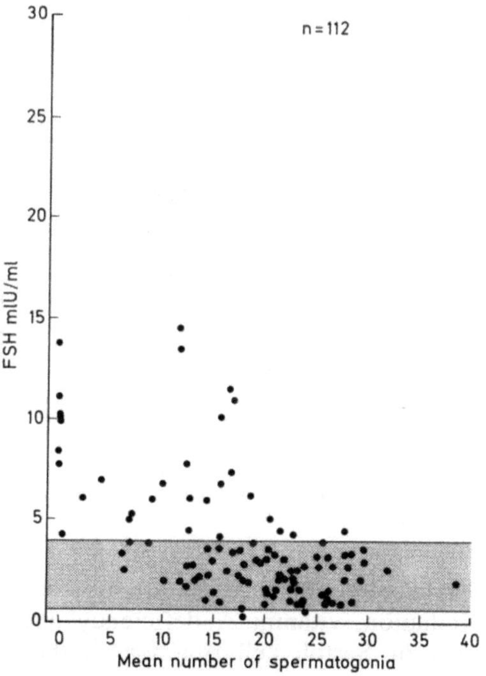

Fig. 2.22

Fig. 2.21. Mean number of spermatids (late) per tubule cross section obtained by counting the germ cells in 25 cross sections per patient and related to the serum FSH level in each man. The normal male range for serum FSH is *shaded.* (de Kretser et al. 1974)

Fig. 2.22. Mean number of spermatogonia per tubule cross section derived by counting germ cells in 25 cross sections per patient and related to the serum FSH level. The *shaded area* represents the normal male range for serum FSH. (de Kretser and Holstein 1976)

(Fig. 2.21), particularly with the number of spermatogonia (Fig. 2.22) such that if the mean spermatogonial number decreased below six per tubule cross section, FSH levels were elevated. However, the converse did not apply since some men with a normal spermatogonial complement demonstrated elevated FSH levels, severing any direct link between a specific germ cell type and the FSH feedback signal.

All of these studies failed to consider the Sertoli cell other than by number, since there is no correlation between the number of Sertoli cells and serum FSH levels (de Kretser et al. 1974). Sertoli cell function can be assessed by the measurement of androgen-binding protein (Hansson et al. 1974; Hagenas et al. 1975) and by the amount of seminiferous tubule fluid produced, as measured by the increment in testicular weight following unilateral efferent duct ligation (Smith 1962). Recently, Hagenas and Ritzen (1976) demonstrated that Sertoli cell function as measured by ABP production was impaired in rats following the induction of cryptorchidism. Similarly, Rich and de Kretser (1977b) have shown that ABP and fluid production

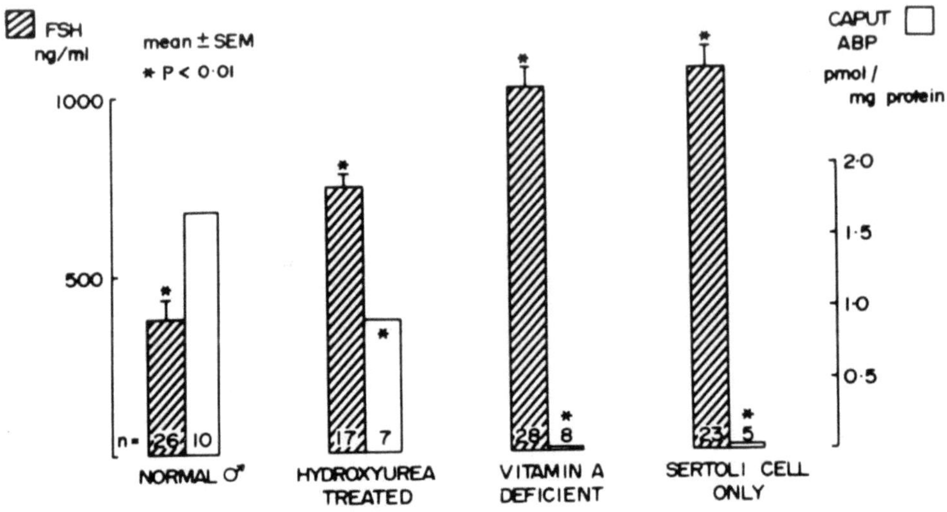

Fig. 2.23. Serum FSH levels and caput epididymal ABP concentration in rats with differing testicular disorders

are impaired in three models of spermatogenic damage induced by fetal irradiation, vitamin A deficiency and hydroxyurea treatment. The impairment of Sertoli cell function in these models correlates directly with the degree of spermatogenic damage and inversely with the level of FSH (Fig. 2.23). The observation of impaired Sertoli cell function in association with germ cell loss suggests that Sertoli cells could be the site of production of inhibin. This postulate has received support from the results of studies by Steinberger and Steinberger (1976), who showed that FSH production of monolayers of pituitary cells could be inhibited by co-cultures of Sertoli cells or the media from such cultures. The identity of this factor remains to be elucidated before its nature can be compared to those FSH-suppressing factors that can be detected from other sources.

2.7 Evidence for Inhibin from Immunisation Studies

Franchimont et al. (1975b) have raised antisera in rabbits to inhibin extracts from seminal plasma and ovine rete testis fluid. They have demonstrated that by passive immunisation using these antisera, the serum FSH levels of normal male rats can be elevated significantly. However, their passive immunisation experiments in immature female rats raised FSH levels to 8900 ng/ml, levels clearly above those seen after castration. It is difficult to envisage how, after the neutralisation of inhibin, the pituitary can secrete FSH to levels above those seen when total gonadal feedback is removed by castration. Caution must be exercised in such experiments involving passive immunisation with rabbit serum in which the hormone levels in recipient animals are measured by double antibody radioimmunoassay techniques using a second antibody raised against rabbit gamma globulin. The effect of passive immunisation is to raise the gamma globulin concentration of recipients to such an extent that insufficient anti-rabbit gamma globulin is present in titres of the second antibody used for precipitation of bound tracer FSH, thus falsely elevating FSH levels. This phenomenon may be the explanation for the elevation of FSH to levels above those seen following castration.

It is vital that this evidence should be confirmed since it would provide data to indicate that the extracts being purified are similar to those occurring naturally, and more importantly, that the natural material is involved in the control of FSH.

2.8 Characteristics and Mode of Action of Inhibin

From the foregoing discussion, considerable evidence exists that inhibin-like activity can be detected from a number of different sources. Whether this activity will be due to one compound or a series of materials cannot be answered at present and will depend on further purification. The possibility that the active extract from different sources may prove to be identical is supported by Franchimont's observation (1977) that crude follicular fluid is capable of neutralising the "anti-inhibin" activity of antisera raised against active fractions from ovine rete testis fluid (RTF). In all studies reported to date, inhibin extracts have been relatively steroid free and the inhibin activity can be destroyed by heat or digestion with proteolytic enzymes (Keogh et al. 1976; Baker et al. 1976a; Franchimont et al. 1975b), providing evidence that the activity is not due to a steroid. No consensus is available as yet regarding the molecular weight of inhibin.

It is evident that inhibin extracts can produce related suppression of FSH secretion in both in vivo and in vitro bioassay systems. Studies of the time course of action of inhibin on pituitary cell cultures indicate that an independent action on FSH synthesis and release can be shown (Scott and Burger 1981). A suppression of FSH release can be demonstrated within 6 h of exposure to inhibin-containing extracts (Fig. 2.24), and the suppression of FSH cell content, taken to imply an effect on sythesis, can be seen after 48 h and persists for up to 72 h after removal of the inhibin source. Further evidence for an effect on FSH synthesis has been provided by Chowdhury et al. (1978), who have shown that Sertoli cell culture fluid can inhibit the incorporation by pituitary cells of ^{3}H-leucine into FSH but not into LH.

Many investigators have shown that LH levels can also be suppressed by inhibin-containing extracts but to a lesser extent than FSH and at higher doses. However, the effects are variable and some studies have shown a stimulation of LH levels in response to inhibin extracts (Keogh et al. 1976; de Jong et al. 1979). In his review, de Jong (1979) suggests that different substances may be the reason for these variable effects on LH. It is of interest that the effect of the same inhibin on LH synthesis in pituitary cell cultures is negligible whereas the suppression on LHRH-stimulated LH release is more marked (Scott et al. 1980). No effect of inhibin extracts on TSH, GH or prolactin secretion could be demonstrated by Franchimont et al. (1977).

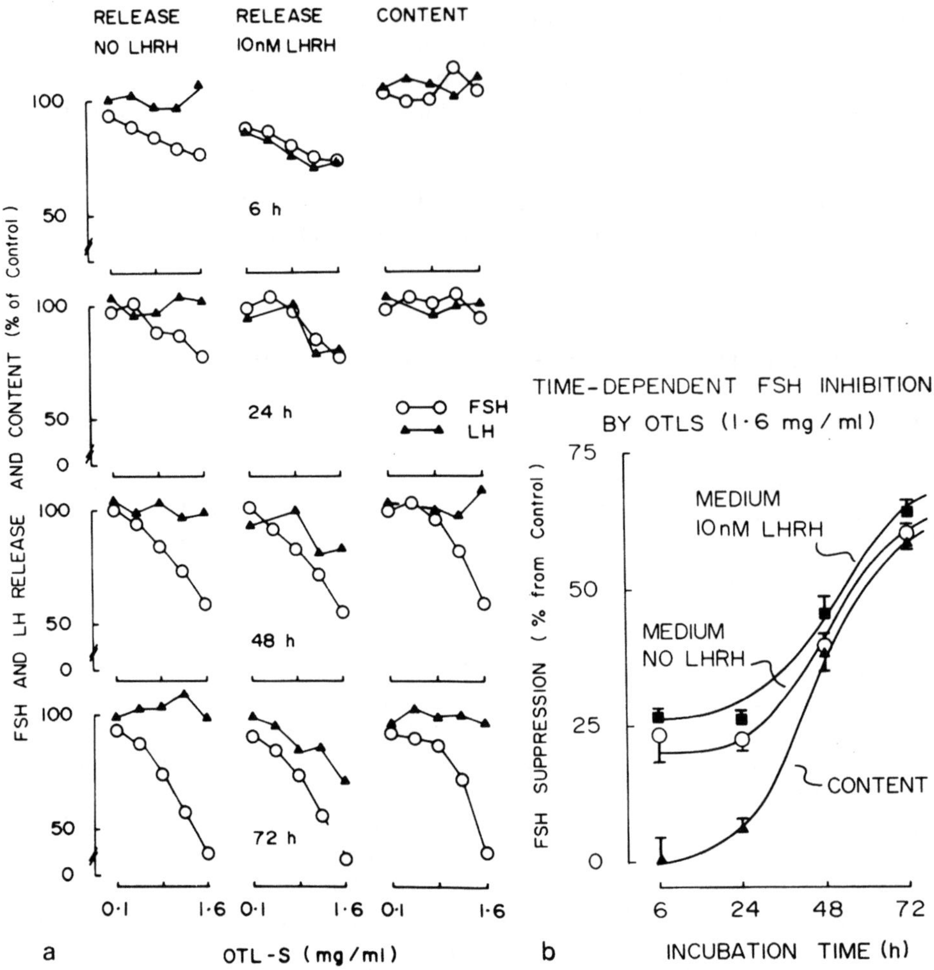

Fig. 2.24. a Pituitary cells were incubated with inhibin proteins for 6, 24, 48 and 72h before measuring stimulated release basal release and cell content of FSH and LH. All cells were 96h old when procedures of release and content were performed and the results represent means of quadruplicate wells expressed as percent of control (no inhibin protein). **b** Composite data for the figures given in **a** at the highest concentration of the ovine testis lymph standard (1.6mg/ml). (Scott and Burger 1981)

2.9 Physiological Implications of Inhibin

The physiological significance of inhibin in the male is still speculative. In adult intact male animals, the control of spermatogenesis by FSH has not been definitively demonstrated. If FSH is essential for sperm maturation, lack of inhibin during spermatogenic failure would assist in the recruitment of stem cells into the spermatogenic process. However, recent evidence concerning the role of FSH in spermatogenesis is controversial since in the rat it would seem that FSH is not required for the maintenance of spermatogenesis though it appears to be essential to initiate the process during puberty (Dym et al. 1979; Davies et al. 1979). However, in primates and sheep FSH does appear to be necessary for normal spermatogenesis (Murty et al. 1979; Courot et al. 1979).

In man, Scott and Burger (1980) have found low or undetectable levels of inhibin in seminal plasma of men with azoospermia and elevated levels of FSH. This confirms the earlier observation of Franchimont (1972) that a substance which diminishes FSH levels in castrated male rats is present in the seminal plasma of normal and oligospermic men but is absent from those with azoospermia caused by the inhibition of gametogenesis. Furthermore, a significant reciprocal relationship ($r = 0.736$, $P < 0.001$) between FSH levels and inhibin in seminal plasma has been shown for 32 normal men and 34 men with non-obstructive disorders of fertility (Scott and Burger 1980). This relationship supports the concept that inhibin is a physiologically important modulator of FSH secretion. Furthermore, men who had undergone vasectomy have seminal plasma inhibin levels approximately 50% of normal controls. These findings suggest that inhibin may gain access to seminal plasma both from rete testis fluid and from the secretion of the accessory organs.

2.10 Summary

The control of FSH and LH secretion by the pituitary gland is clearly multifactorial. The evidence that LHRH influences the release and stores of both FSH and LH is considerable, and equally well documented is the fact that testosterone and oestradiol will suppress the secretion not only of LH but also of FSH. Recently evidence points to the existence of inhibin which will suppress FSH secretion but which in higher doses will also decrease LH levels. It is therefore likely that the ratio of FSH to LH secreted by the gonadotrope is determined by the summation of the action of these factors on cellular mechanisms that remain to be determined.

3 Pituitary Testicular Axis During Pubertal Development

V.W.K. Lee and H.G. Burger

The sequence of events involved in the growth and maturation of the testes affords excellent opportunities for studying the pituitary-testicular axis and relationships between changes in structure and hormone levels. We have studied three species: man, rat and sheep. In man our studies have been confined to defining the hormonal changes that occur in the immediate prepubertal, pubertal and adult periods, whereas in the rat and sheep our studies have started at birth, and have included both hormonal and histological correlations.

3.1 Studies in Men

3.1.1 Changes During Fetal Life

The testis first becomes recognisable between the 7th and 8th weeks. Leydig cell differentiation commences during the 8th week, and by 12 weeks Leydig cells are disseminated throughout the testes and show a well-developed, smooth, agranular endoplasmic reticulum, consistent with a capacity for steroid biosynthesis. Growth of Leydig cells is maximal at 14 weeks when they occupy half the testicular volume. At 18 weeks Leydig cells start to degenerate, while the seminiferous epithelium becomes better defined. These changes in Leydig cell numbers are affected by the local (testicular) testosterone concentrations, which are maximal between 12 and 16 weeks. Blood levels of testosterone range between 0.5 and 6 ng/ml. There is a close temporal correlation between maternal serum and amniotic fluid and chorionic gonadotropin (hCG) levels, and maximal testosterone concentrations. By contrast, although LH is detectable in the fetal pituitary at 10 weeks, maximal circulating levels are not reached until about 18 weeks, decline to low levels by 30 weeks and remain low until term. FSH levels also rise between 12 and 20 weeks and decline during the last trimester. The transformation of primordial germ cells into spermatogonia, and the differentiation of Sertoli cells, coincide with the commencement of fetal gonadotrophin secretion. Hypothalamic levels of LHRH increase with fetal age in parallel with circulating FSH and LH levels. Reyes et al. (1976) have provided a useful review of fetal pituitary and testicular function.

3.1.2 Changes in the Newborn

Testosterone levels decline rapidly in the first five or six neonatal days, from about 2.5 ng/ml to less than 0.3 ng/ml, but increase again to reach levels of about 2.5 ng/ml between the 4th and 9th weeks of life. These levels again decline to low values between the 7th and 12th months, and remain low (less than 0.1 ng/ml) until the onset of puberty. Circulating gonadotrophin levels are increased during the early post-natal period, but by the 4th or 5th month decline to the low levels characteristic of childhood. The significance of this early post-natal androgen secretion in boys is unknown. This subject has been reviewed fully by Forest et al. (1976).

3.1.3 Changes During Childhood and Adolescence

There are several studies which describe changes in gonadal steroids and gonadotrophins in relation to pubertal development. These have been reviewed by Franchimont and Burger (1975). Our own studies have been described in several publications (Baker et al. 1976c; Bremner 1977; Bremner et al. 1978). Our findings are based on the examination of 31 pre-pubertal boys, 58 pubertal boys, and 104 mature adolescents, whose ages range from 14–21 years. In the children we assessed genital and pubic hair development by the method of Tanner (1962), and measured testicular volume with an orchidometer (Prader 1966). Most of the measurements of testosterone and oestradiol were by radioimmunoassay (Wang et al. 1974b) while a small number of the earlier steroid estimations were based on a competitive protein binding assay (Baker et al. 1973). There were no differences between the results of either assay. The sex hormone binding globulin (SHBG) capacity in free testosterone and oestradiol fractions were measured by an ammonium sulphate precipitation method (O'Connor et al. 1973).

Table 3.1 shows the data from our clinical observations. There is a progressive increase in pubic hair stage, testicular volume, height and weight, with successive stages of genital development. The correlations between all these measurements are highly significant. The levels of LH, FSH. testosterone

Table 3.1 Clinical measurements in children and adolescents (mean ± SD)

	State of genital development				
	I	II	III	IV	V
No.	31	21	19	54	120
Age (years)	8.5 ± 3.4	13.0 ± 1.0	14.4 ± 1.2	15.5 ± 1.3	16.6 ± 1.3
Stage of pubic hair development	1	1.2 ± 0.4	2.5 ± 0.9	4.4 ± 0.8	5.2 ± 0.7
Testicular volume (ml)	2.3 ± 0.8	5.2 ± 3.0	14.6 ± 3.8	18.6 ± 4.1	22.7 ± 3.3
Height (cm)	–	152.2 ± 5.3	162.3 ± 7.5	170.1 ± 7.4	174.3 ± 9.1
Weight (kg)	–	41.6 ± 6.8	50.1 ± 6.6	57.9 ± 7.6	64.9 ± 7.9

Table 3.2. Hormone levels in children and adolescents related to stage of genital development (Mean ± SD)[a]

	State of genital development				
	I	II	III	IV	V
LH (IU/litre)	0.5 ± 0.2 (21)	0.8 ± 0.5 (16)	1.2 ± 0.7 (13)	1.5 ± 0.5 (21)	1.6 ± 0.4 (102)
FSH (IU/litre)	0.5 ± 0.5 (21)	1.8 ± 1.2 (15)	1.2 ± 0.6 (13)	2.4 ± 1.3 (21)	2.2 ± 1.4 (102)
Testosterone (nmol/litre)	1.9 ± 1.0 (16)	6.5 ± 2.5 (10)	7.8 ± 3.5 (13)	13.6 ± 2.7 (13)	16.9 ± 6.3 (22)
Oestradiol (pmol/litre)	19.3 ± 11.5 (9)	19.3 ± 17.8 (6)	24.8 ± 18.9 (11)	33.0 ± 30.3 (12)	61.9 ± 38.1 (21)

[a] The numbers of subjects are shown in parentheses

and oestradiol are shown in Table 3.2, and are grouped according to the stage of genital development. Progressively higher mean levels of LH, testosterone and oestradiol were found with advancing genital development, while FSH levels increased more abruptly at the onset of puberty (stage II).

It is important to stress that pre-pubertal boys may have very low levels of FSH. In our series there were five young children (1.7–5 yrs) who had undetectable levels and ten pre-pubertal boys whose levels of FSH were at or below the detection limit of the FSH assay.

There are several points of interest in the group of adolescents between the ages of 14–20 who had achieved adult genital development. Five of this group had levels of FSH greater than 5.2 IU/litre; one had a level of 10.5 IU/litre. We confirmed four of these results in a second assay. These boys, who appeared to have no testicular abnormalities, all had testicular volumes between 18 and 25 ml. A comparison of the results of adolescents who had adult genital development with those of men aged between 21–50 years showed that the LH levels were significantly higher ($P < 0.01$) and the testosterone levels significantly lower ($P < 0.001$) in the younger subjects, whereas the FSH and oestradiol levels were not significantly different. The relationships

Table 3.3. Correlation coefficients for LH, FSH, testosterone and oestradiol levels and clinical measurements in children and adolescents

	LH	FSH	Testosterone	Oestradiol
FSH	0.70[c]			
Testosterone	0.44[b]	0.29[a]		
Oestradiol	0.12	0.13	0.50[c]	
Age	0.61[c]	0.65[c]	0.69[c]	0.40[b]
Stage of genital development	0.73[c]	0.59[c]	0.82[c]	0.43[b]
Stage of pubic hair development	0.72[c]	0.58[c]	0.81[c]	0.40
Testicular volume	0.53[c]	0.12	0.71[c]	0.38[a]
Height	0.45[c]	0.28[b]	0.63[c]	0.46[b]
Weight	0.44[c]	0.28[b]	0.63[c]	0.50[b]

[a] $P < 0.05$; [b] $P < 0.01$; [c] $P < 0.001$

between hormone levels and the clinical measurements are shown in Table 3.3. There are highly significant correlations between LH, FSH and testosterone levels of age, stage of genital development, stage of pubic hair development, height and weight. The correlations of the latter with oestradiol levels are less significant, and there is no correlation between testicular volume and FSH levels.

The binding capacities (q) of SHBG and the fraction of absolute free testosterone and oestradiol levels measured in the pre-pubertal boys, and in plasma pools from pubertal subjects, is shown in Table 3.4. Binding capacity was high in two pre-pubertal boys, and in the normal adult range after mid-puberty. The fractional and absolute free steroid levels were low in the pre-pubertal subjects and higher in samples from subjects with more advanced development.

The close relationships between genital and pubic hair development, testicular volumes and blood levels of testosterone LH and FSH found in this study generally confirmed the results of Winter and Faiman (1972) and of August et al. (1972). Blood levels of FSH and LH increase from undetectable or low levels at the age of 8 years prior to the onset of puberty. There is a progressive rise in LH, and a somewhat earlier, more abrupt rise in FSH levels during puberty. In a number of subjects with stage II – stage V genital development, and in more mature adolescents under the age of 20 years, LH levels are at or above the upper limit of the normal adult value.

Similar investigations of changes in gonadotrophin levels during childhood and adolescence have been reported (Root 1973; Kulin and Reiter 1973). There is general agreement that LH and FSH levels rise prior to the onset of and during puberty in boys, but the magnitude and timing of changes with respect to these stages of development are controversial. Thus, Burr et al. (1970) report that LH and FSH increases after the age of 9 years, and that LH rises before FSH, and the overall increase in FSH was greater than that of LH, whereas Winter and Faiman (1972) described significant rises in

Table 3.4. SHBG binding capacity *(q)* and free testosterone and oestradiol levels in boys before and during puberty. Stage I subjects aged 7 and 10 years, stages III and IV from plasma pools, stage V pools from subjects 14–16 and 17–19 years of age

	Stage of genital development				
	I	II	III	IV	V
$q(\times 10^{-8}\ M)$	15.0	–	6.2	4.5	5.4
	16.5				4.5
Free testosterone	0.22	–	0.93	1.60	1.51
(%)	0.32				1.39
(pmol/litre)	6.9		125	233	399
Free oestradiol	0.61	–	2.44	2.84	2.82
(%)	0.44				2.61
(pmol/litre)	0.22		0.26	0.85	2.41
	0.11				0.78

both LH and FSH after the age of 6 years, and a more abrupt and greater rise in LH during puberty.

It must be noted that the hormone levels of single daytime samples in pubertal subjects should be interpreted with caution, in view of the occurrence of noctural episodes of LH and testosterone secretion which occur at the onset of puberty (Boyar et al. 1972, 1974). This phenomenon does not, however, account for the high levels of LH and FSH in some pubertal boys and adolescents, and the higher mean levels in mature subjects under the age of 20, compared to adult levels (21–50 years). We have no obvious explanation for this finding.

Testosterone levels are in the adult female range in pre-pubertal children, and rise progressively with advancing pubertal development. Adult levels are achieved only after the completion of genital development and thereafter levels increase up to the 4th decade. The values in pre-pubertal boys are slightly higher than those reported by others (Saez and Bertrand 1968; Winter and Faiman 1972; Boon et al. 1972). The testosterone values in pubertal and young mature subjects are also different from those of Winter and Faiman, who found no further changes in these levels after the age of 16 years. The lower mean testosterone and high levels of LH in the mature teenagers compared with adults suggest that the setting of the feedback system may change during maturation, and that adult levels of these hormones may not be attained before the age of 20–25 years. Oestradiol levels are low in pre-pubertal boys and increase in the late stages of puberty.

The values we obtained for the binding capacity of SHBG are comparable to those reported by Vermeulen et al. (1969, 1972) in that the binding capacity of SHBG is high before puberty, and decreases to adult levels before the completion of pubertal development. The finding of adult male binding capacity in plasma pools from subjects at different stages of genital development, and of testosterone levels below the normal range for men in the same pools, indicates that the mechanism which controls the elaboration of SHBG is sensitive to relatively low circulating levels of testosterone.

No attempt has been made in these human studies to correlate morphological changes in the testis, or the development of spermatogenesis with clinical and hormonal features. It would appear, however, that spermatogenesis may be complete at a relatively early stage of puberty, coinciding with testicular enlargement, and preceding achievement of full development of secondary sex characteristics (Richardson and Short 1978). It would clearly be of interest to examine closely the relationships between FSH levels and developing spermatogenesis in man.

3.1.4 Pituitary Responses to LHRH

A number of investigators have described the characteristics of the pituitary gonadotrophin responses to single injections of LHRH before and during puberty (see review by Franchimont and Burger 1975). In summary, accompanying the progressive rises in basal LH levels with advancing pubertal development there is an increasing response of LH to the injection of LHRH, with a marked increase between stages I and II of puberty, and a further increase at stage III. FSH responsiveness is much less marked, and the magnitude of the response relative to basal FSH levels is less than after the onset of puberty.

Because of the biphasic secretion of LH in response to continuous LHRH infusion (Chap. 3) we studied changes in LH and FSH secretion in response to this stimulus in six pre-pubertal boys aged between 9 and 12 years, with testicular volumes of 2–3 ml and plasma testosterone concentrations which ranged from 0.5–2.0 ng/ml. We also studied another five boys between the ages of 13 and 16 years who were in pubertal stages III–V with testicular volumes of 15–20 ml, and plasma testosterone concentrations which ranged from 1.7–10.4 ng/ml. Studies started between 0800 and 1000 h, when LHRH was given by continuous intravenous infusion of a dose of 1 μg/min for 4 h. We obtained blood samples at 15 min intervals before and during the infusion, and used radioimmunoassays to measure serum LH, FSH and testosterone.

The results of these studies in the pre-pubertal boys are shown in Fig. 3.1. In contrast to the biphasic secretory responses seen in adults, the LH responses in these boys are monophasic; there is an early increase in serum LH levels and maximum values are reached after 30–60 min, after which LH levels remain stable until the end of the infusion. It may be noted that in three boys (subjects *3*, *5* and *6*, who were older than the two youngest boys, subjects *1* and *2*) there is evidence of pulsatile secretion. One boy (subject *4*) shows a biphasic pattern during the early part of the infusion but does not show the continuous increase seen in adults. Although basal levels of LH are lower in these boys than adults, the area under the LH curve (measured by planimetry) is not significantly different from adults.

The serum levels of FSH increase gradually and progressively during the infusions as they do in adults, but there is no biphasic pattern. There is one difference: the area under the FSH curve in pre-pubertal boys is significantly greater than that in adult men ($P < 0.01$). Basal levels of testosterone are lower than in adults and show no significant increases during the infusions.

The results of similar studies done in pubertal boys are shown in Fig. 3.2. The LH responses are again monophasic, and in general resemble those of the pre-pubertal boys. By contrast the FSH responses are less and are not significantly different from those of adult men. Levels of plasma testosterone do not change during the infusion.

The monophasic response of LH to continuous LHRH infusions in sexually immature boys contrasts with the biphasic response characteristic of adult men. Similar monophasic responses have been noted in other forms of sexual immaturity, e.g. in pre-pubertal girls, in patients with hypogonadotrophic hypogonadism, and thin patients with anorexia nervosa (Bremner et al. 1978). In addition, the biphasic pattern is absent in some patients with pituitary tumours.

The reasons for the absence of a biphasic LH pattern in sexual immaturity are not known. A possible explanation is that endogenous LHRH production in various forms of sexual immaturity is qualitatively less and does not occur in an episodic fashion as it does in adults. The absence of episodic LH secretion suggests the absence of episodic endogenous LHRH production. Chronic administration of LHRH has been demonstrated to induce gonadal maturation

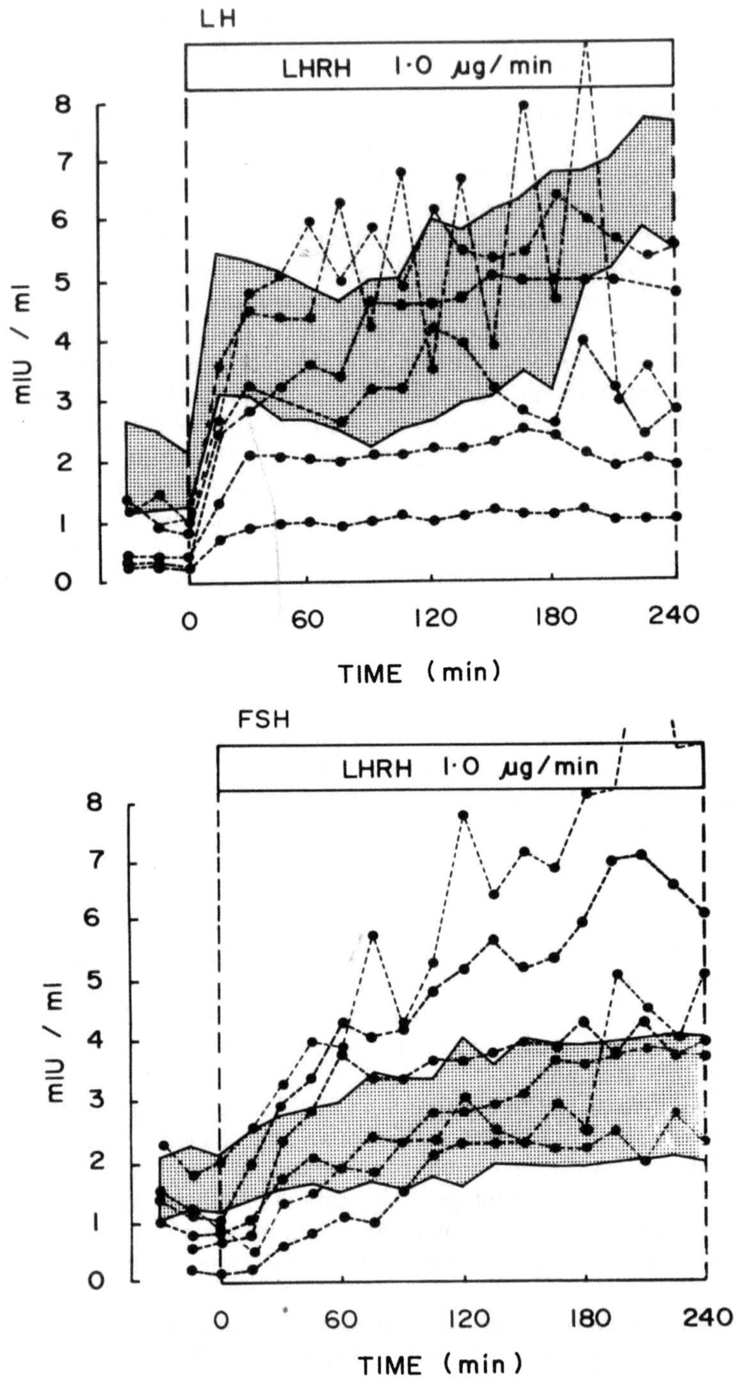

Fig. 3.1. Serum LH and FSH values before and during 4-h LH-RH infusions (1.0 µg/min) in pre-pubertal children. *Shaded areas* are ranges of gonadotrophin values for normal adults during similar infusions. Subjects plotted in ascending order, numbers 1–6, taking curve order at 60 min

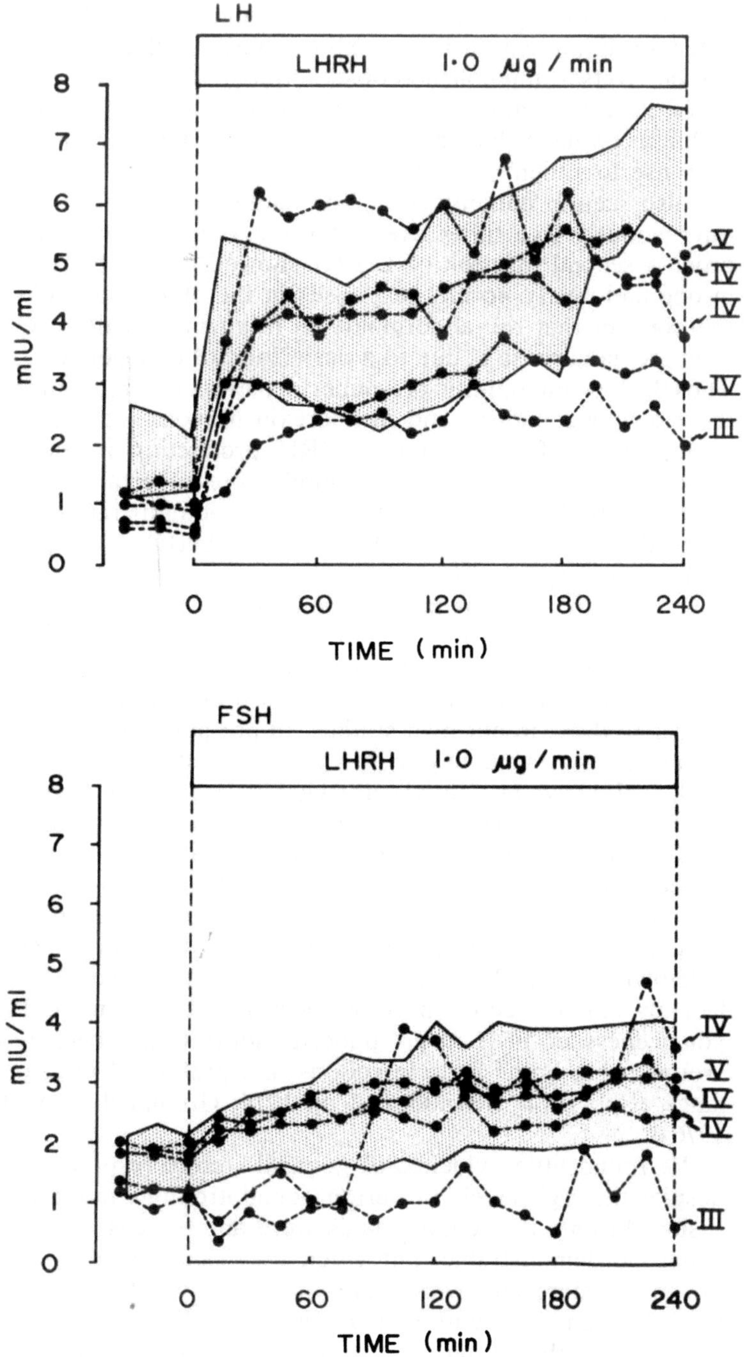

Fig. 3.2. Serum LH and FSH values before and during 4-h LH-RH infusions (1.0 μg/min) in stages III, IV and V, pre-pubertal children

in patients with hypogonadotrophic hypogonadism (Bergada et al. 1973) and ovulation in patients with anorexia nervosa (Nillius and Wide 1975; Bremner and de Kretser, unpublished observations).

The repeated administration of LHRH to hypogonadotrophic patients will within a few days change the LH response from a monophasic "pre-pubertal" response to a biphasic "adult" pattern (Bremner et al. 1978). Similar changes are also seen in patients with anorexia nervosa. When we gave 10 μg LHRH intravenously five times every day for 4 days to two patients with this disorder a second infusion of LHRH showed normal gonadotrophin responses in one and nearly normal responses in the other. Such observations support the concept that the abnormality in pituitary gonadotrophin responsiveness in anorexia nervosa is due to a deficiency of endogenous LHRH production. Thus the low monophasic pre-pubertal pattern of LH responses in hypogonadotrophic hypogonadism and in anorexia nervosa are almost certainly due to a deficiency of endogenous LHRH production in each case. Since this pattern, which is similar to that found in pre-pubertal children, can be changed to the "adult" biphasic LH response by administration of LHRH, it seems likely that an important mechanism of pubertal development is an increase in the episodic secretion of LHRH.

Several other groups have presented data from studies of constant LHRH administration to normal pre-pubertal children or boys with delayed puberty (Bermudez et al. 1974; de Lange et al. 1974; Reiter et al. 1976a). The pattern of gonadotrophin increase found by de Lange et al. and by Reiter et al. are similar to those in our own studies. In pre-pubertal children the LH response is monophasic, while in pubertal children and adults it is biphasic. Bermudez et al. (1974) have presented somewhat different results which show a relatively small increase in LH early in the infusions in pre-pubertal boys, with maximal levels being obtained at 3–4 h of a 4-h infusion.

The patterns of FSH increase during LH infusion are gradual, monophasic and greater in pre-pubertal boys than in intrapubertal boys or adults. The reasons why FSH increases are relatively large in pubertal individuals are unknown, but may be related to deficiency of endogenous LHRH or a relative lack of inhibin secretion from their immature gonads. Relative hyper-responsiveness of FSH in pre-pubertal subjects has been reported by several groups using both single injections and prolonged infusions of LHRH (Delange et al. 1974; Bermudez et al. 1974; Grumbach et al. 1974; Reiter et al. 1976a).

We found little evidence of gonadal steroid responsiveness in our studies despite the high levels of serum gonadotrophins induced by the LHRH infusion. In only a few individuals were any increases in plasma levels of testosterone demonstrable, but when they occurred they were small and late in the infusion, and were never statistically significant. These results give no indication that acute changes in gonadal steroid levels have any role in determining the patterns of pituitary gonadotrophin responses to LHRH. Other studies of prolonged LHRH infusions have found small but significant increases in plasma testosterone levels in normal men and intrapubertal children (de Lange et al. 1974; Bermudez et al. 1974; Reiter et al. 1976b). In the ram, by contrast to men, plasma testosterone levels increase markedly during LHRH infusion, but we found no evidence that the changes in plasma steroid levels were important in the acute modulation of pituitary responsiveness to LHRH (Bremner et al. 1980).

The fact that patients with hypogonadotrophic hypogonadism and anorexia nervosa resembled in many ways normal pre-pubertal children in terms of gonadotrophin responses to LHRH opens interesting possibilities for future research into the mechanisms of puberty. Both these disorders offer experimental groups that could serve as models of the pre-pubertal state; these patients can receive exogenous hormonal administration on an experimental basis that would be unacceptable in pre-pubertal children. For example, the demonstration that endogenous LHRH administration may switch the patterns of gonadotrophin responsiveness from the "pre-pubertal" to the "adult" pattern has implied that similar changes in endogenous LHRH production may be important in normal puberty. With the availability of patient groups that can serve as models of the pre-pubertal state, and of the major hormones (LHRH and steroids) that control pituitary secretion, a clearer understanding of pubertal changes in the pituitary should be possible over the next few years. For example, recent studies of the pulsatile administration of LHRH (Carmel et al. 1976) have shown that it is possible to reproduce the pattern of gonadotrophin changes occurring during puberty and to induce ovulation and spermatogenesis in patients with hypogonadotrophic hypogonadism.

3.2 Studies in Rats

The laboratory rat has been used extensively as an experimental animal for studies in reproductive endocrinology. Initial studies to evaluate pituitary-testicular relationships during post-natal development in the rat have not included the immediate perinatal period (Swerdloff et al. 1971; Goldman et al. 1971; Ojeda and Ramirez 1972). Since the process of spermatogenesis in the rat requires 48 days (Clermont 1972) and the time from birth to sexual maturity is only 50 days, it is possible that important events may occur within the first few post-natal days to initiate sperm production. There is evidence of a gonadal-hypophyseal feedback mechanism very early in the neonatal life. Yaginuma et al. (1969) showed that if male rats are hemi-castrated on the day of birth the remaining testis develops compensatory hypertrophy 3 days later. Also, the demonstration of increase in gonadotrophin secretion in neonatal male rats following castration (Goldman et al. 1971) provides further evidence for such a relationship. Because of the possibility that there may be hitherto unrecognised changes during these early stages of sexual maturation, we have undertaken a series of studies of hormonal changes from the time of birth to sexual maturity.

3.2.1 Changes in LH, FSH and Testosterone Concentrations with Age

Earlier studies have used bioassay methods to examine changes in gonadotrophin secretion during sexual maturation of male rats (Kragt and Ganong 1968; Lisk 1968; Labhsetwar 1970). They measured LH and FSH in pituitary

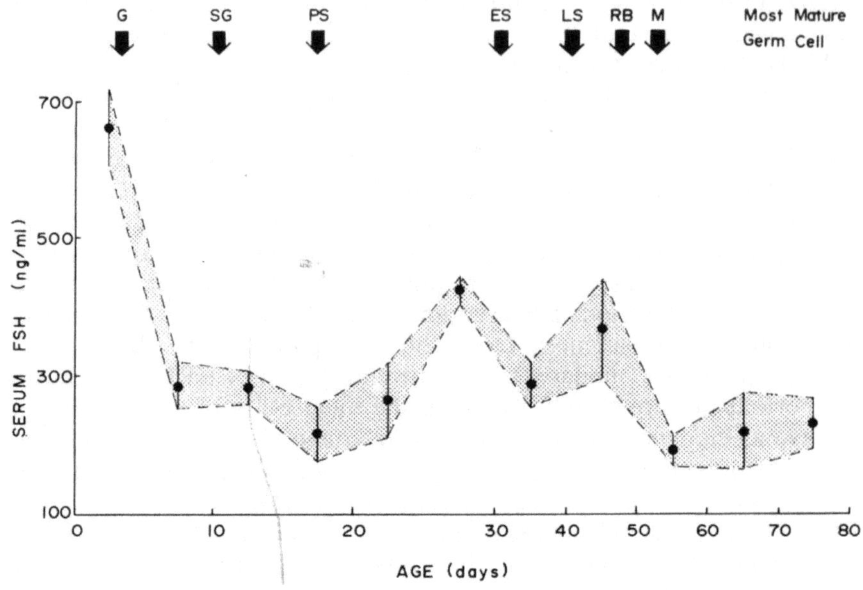

Fig. 3.3. Profile of FSH levels during the development of the male rat. The times at which different germinal cells appear in the testis are represented: *G*, gonocytes; *SG*, spermatogonia; *PS*, primary spermatocytes; *ES*, early spermatids; *LH*, late spermatids; *RB*, residual bodies. *Vertical bars* represent the mean ± SEM. For further details see Lee et al. (1975)

tissue since assay methods for gonadotrophins were not sufficiently sensitive to measure circulating levels. With the advent of sensitive radioimmunoassays for gonadotrophins, LH and FSH have been measured in blood samples and in pituitary tissue of developing rats. In our studies we have examined changes in immunoreactive FSH, LH and testosterone in the blood of male Sprague-Dawley rats from birth to sexual maturity (Figs. 3.3–3.5; Lee et al. 1975).

Serum FSH levels (Fig. 3.3) are significantly elevated during the first 5 days of post-natal life (mean: 660 ng/ml; range 366–941 ng/ml). An abrupt and significant decline in FSH concentrations occurs shortly thereafter, reaching levels of 136 ng/ml to 356 ng/ml (mean 285 ng/ml) between day 6 and 10. Thereafter a marked variability of FSH levels is found from days 20–25, with levels distributed over a range of 61–511 ng/ml. Between 26 and 50 days of age, FSH levels increase to values in excess of 250 ng/ml and subsequently, decline significantly between 51 and 60 days of age. This decrease coincides with the time when spermatozoa are first released from the seminiferous epithelium, that is during a period when residual bodies are first noted in the seminiferous tubules.

Serum LH levels range between 1 and 6 ng/ml from birth to 25 days and decline to reach a nadir between 26 and 30 days (Fig. 3.4). During the first 5 days of postnatal life the mean LH concentration is 3.37 ng/ml, and this level is not significantly different from levels observed during the next 20 days.

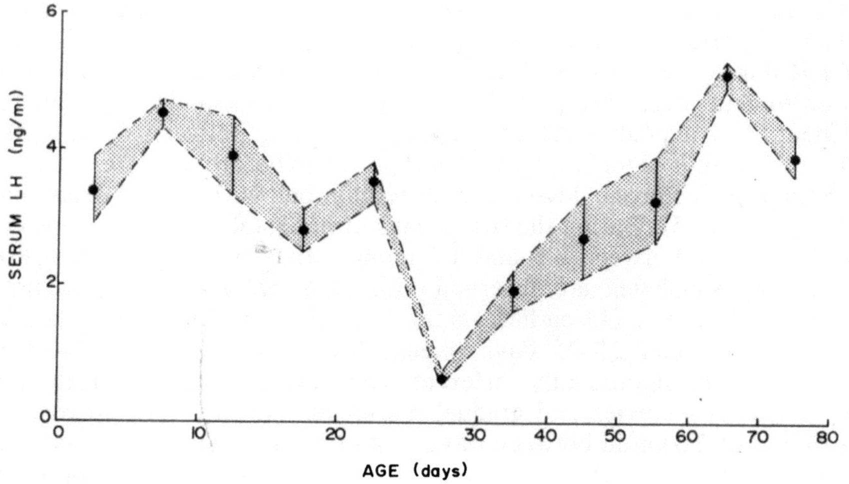

Fig. 3.4. Profile of LH levels during the development of the male rat. *Vertical bars* represent the mean ± SEM

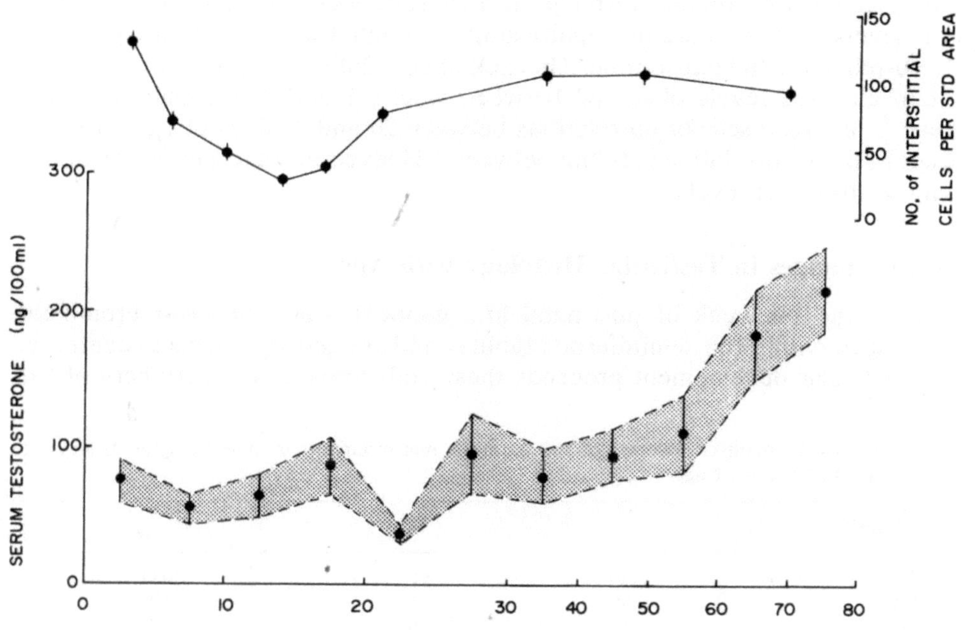

Fig. 3.5. Profile of testosterone levels during the development of the male rat. The *top panel* represents the number of mature interstitial cells per unit standard area of testicular biopsy. *Vertical bars* represent the mean ± SEM (Lording and de Kretser 1972)

Although LH concentrations between days 6 and 15 are higher than levels observed before and after this, they are not significantly different. The nadir of LH during days 26–30 is, however, significantly different from levels just prior to and after this period. Subsequent to this nadir a gradual rise is evident, and a peak level of 5 ng/ml is reached between 60 and 70 days. This LH peak is significantly higher than levels before and afterwards.

Serum testosterone levels are generally below 1.8 ng/ml from birth to 50 days (Fig. 3.5). During the first 5 days of neonatal life testosterone concentrations range between 0.5 and 1.3 ng/ml with a mean value of 0.75 ng/ml. Although lower levels are observed during the next 5 days, they are not significantly different from earlier values. A nadir of testosterone concentration is found between 21–25 days (mean: 0.4 ng/ml range: <0.25–0.45 ng/ml) but this is not significantly different from levels observed before and after this nadir. A stepwise and gradual rise occurs shortly after to reach levels in excess of 2.3 ng/ml between days 71 and 80. Testosterone levels in mature animals (days 61–80) range from 1.3 to 2.9 ng/ml and are approximately two- to threefold higher than values found during the first 3 weeks of post-natal life.

3.2.2 Relationship Between Age and Hormonal Levels

From these data we found that no significant relationships exist between FSH and LH or FSH and testosterone (Table 3.5). Whilst FSH and LH levels are negatively correlated with age, testosterone levels are positively related. LH levels, however, are not significantly correlated with age but are positively correlated with testosterone. The lack of correlation with age is due primarily to elevated levels observed between weeks 1 and 2 post-natally. When results are analysed for correlations between 20 and 30 days of age a significant positive correlation is found between LH levels and age, and between LH and testosterone levels.

3.2.3 Changes in Testicular Histology with Age

During the 1st week of post-natal life, gonocytes are the most prominent cells seen within the seminiferous tubules and are generally located centrally. As testicular development proceeds these cells move to the periphery of the

Table 3.5. Relationships between age and hormone measurements in male Sprague-Dawley rats from birth to 80 days of age

Relationship	*r*	df[a]	*P*
FSH-age	−0.46	65	<0.001
LH-age	0.08	65	NS
T-age	0.50	39	<0.001
T-LH	0.39	24	<0.05
FSH-LH	0.01	65	NS
FSH-T	−0.24	24	NS

[a] df, no. of pairs of observations−2

tubules. Sertoli cells which are located at the periphery are also present at this time and are immature in appearance, in that their nuclei lack the prominent nucleoli found in these cells in the adult testis. At about the 10th day, spermatogonia are present within the tubules. Primary spermatocytes appear within the next 2 weeks, and early spermatids by day 33. Late spermatids are present a week later and by day 47 residual bodies can be seen in some tubules, indicating that spermatozoa are being released into the lumen. Sertoli cells acquire mature characteristics at about 25 or 30 days of age, and these characteristics consist principally of a loss of nuclear chromatin, clumping and the acquisition of a prominent nucleolus.

It is well recognised that the growth of Leydig cells in the rat testis occurs in two phases (Roosen-Runge and Anderson 1959; Niemi and Ikonen 1962, 1963; Lording and de Kretser 1972). The first or fetal phase occurs from the 17th fetal day to the second post-natal week, and during this phase there is abundant lipid in the Leydig cells. The numbers of Leydig cells decrease during early post-natal life and reach a minimum between days 14 and 17. In the second phase very little lipid is present in Leydig cells and this phase commences around the 21st to the 23rd post-natal day. During this phase the Leydig cells increase in number and the cells are "mature" in appearance, possessing smooth endoplasmic reticulum and characteristic mitochondrial cristae. This phase represents the formation of the adult generation of interstitial cells, which are maximally abundant by day 40. These two phases represent separate generations of interstitial cells, since the cells of each phase exhibit differences in histochemical and ultrastructural features (see Chap. 5).

3.2.4 Significance of Hormonal Changes in the Developing Rat

FSH. Serum FSH levels are markedly elevated during the first post-natal week, and are at least 2–4 times greater than levels observed in adult rats. During this time the only prominent germ cells seen in the tubules are the gonocytes. These elevated levels of FSH may be involved in the initiation of the spermatogenic process, by promoting the division of gonocytes to form spermatogonia (Clermont and Perey 1957) since the spermatogenic process in the rat commences shortly after birth. Alternatively, these high levels may reflect a functional immaturity of the hypothalamo-hypophyseal unit. This suggestion is supported by observations that the vascular connection between the hypothalamus and pituitary develops only after the fifth post-natal day (Glydon 1957; Fink and Smith 1971), and that catecholamine fluorescence in the median eminence of the hypothalamus does not intensify until the same time (Smith and Simpson 1970). Although speculative, catecholamines in the hypothalamus may be involved in control of gonadotrophin secretion (Fuxe and Hokfelt 1969). It seems unlikely that the source of elevated FSH levels seen at birth is of maternal origin since there is good reason to believe that FSH does not cross the placenta. If this is true the fetal pituitary has quite a high capacity to secrete FSH.

There are several possible reasons why FSH secretion is increased during the neonatal period. One is that this hormone may be involved in the transformation of gonocytes to spermatogonia. Another is that FSH is almost certainly responsible for the rapid division of Sertoli cells during the first 2 weeks of life. The specific binding of FSH to Sertoli cells and the rapid increase in FSH receptor concentrations within the testis in the first 10 days is good circumstantial evidence that FSH is involved in the division of Sertoli cells. Another potential role of FSH during the early neonatal period is the formation of the blood-testis barrier which occurs during the 2nd and 3rd weeks of life (Russell 1978). The formation of this barrier can be delayed by treating neonatal rats with specific anti-FSH antisera (Adey, unpublished observation). Similarly, treatment with 25 μg oestradiol benzoate in 4-day-old male rats delays spermatogenesis in these animals as well as the pubertal rise of FSH and testosterone (Brown-Grant et al. 1975; Rich and de Kretser 1978).

The rate of testicular growth in the rat is greatest between 25 and 60 days of age, and preceding this increase in testicular growth rate is a rise in pituitary serum FSH levels, suggesting that FSH may be involved (Labhsetwar 1970; Ojeda and Ramirez 1972; McCann et al. 1974; Ketelslegers et al. 1978). Furthermore, an increase in the total number of FSH receptors per testis occurs after the 3rd week. Maximum receptor numbers are established by 60 days of age at a time when complete spermatogenesis and maximum testis size are attained.

The elevated FSH levels seen in rats between the fourth and seventh postnatal week may be involved in the process of spermatid maturation, while the subsequent decline after day 50 when spermatogenesis is complete suggests that an intact and mature seminiferous epithelium may elaborate a factor or factors capable of exerting a feedback influence on FSH secretion. This would be consistent with the concept first introduced by Mottram and Cramer (1923) that spermatogenic tissue produces a hormone which is responsible for feedback inhibition of a gonadotrophic hormone. McCullagh (1932) named this factor "inhibin" and evidence to support the existence of such a substance has been provided by several workers (see reviews by Setchell and Main 1974; Franchimont et al. 1975a,b; Baker et al. 1976a; de Jong 1979). If the decline in serum FSH in the intact rat is the result of feedback inhibition by a product of the seminiferous epithelium, then selective damage to the spermatogenic tissue at a time well before the decrease in FSH levels should prevent this fall in FSH. This has been demonstrated in elegant studies by Swerdloff et al. (1971), in which rats made cryptorchid at the age of 21 days exhibited higher FSH levels at 49 days than those intact rats at a time when mature sperm are present in the intact animal. It should be noted, however, that the fall in FSH levels coincides with the period of rising serum testosterone concentrations (Figs. 3.3, 3.5) and the possibility of a long-term negative feedback mechanism between testosterone (or one of its metabolites) and pituitary FSH secretion during development cannot be excluded. It is also of interest that the initiation of the FSH rise in rats is in concert with rising LH levels which continue to rise after FSH levels have declined. This dissociation strongly suggests independent control systems for these two hormones.

LH and Testosterone. We have referred to evidence for a relationship between the testis and pituitary in newborn rats. Our observations of elevated

LH and testosterone concentrations during the early neonatal period, and a secondary increase in these hormones after the fourth post-natal week, indicate that the testis develops in two distinct stages.

During the first phase, regression of the fetal generation of Leydig cells appears to be accompanied by a decrease in circulating testosterone levels, reaching a nadir at about the third post-natal week. Similar observations have been made by Ketelslegers et al. (1978). They noted that the decline in plasma testosterone is not due to a decrease in testicular LH receptors, but more likely to a diminishing number of fetal Leydig cells.

Previous investigations concerning the maturation of Leydig cell function in rats involved the measurement of testosterone in the testis and in peripheral venous blood (Resko et al. 1968). Using pooled plasma they found testosterone concentrations of 1 nmol/litre in the 5-day-old male rat, and only 0.1 ng/ml in the 10-day-old male rat. Between the ages of 10 and 30 days testosterone concentrations remain at levels between 0.1–0.15 ng/ml. At the age of 40 days a rise in testosterone concentrations to 0.6 ng/ml occurs; approximately twice that concentration is reached in adulthood. The concentrations of testosterone in testicular tissue follow a similar pattern, decreasing with increasing age until about 30 days when an increase is seen. The pubertal rise in testosterone is in accord with our own findings of increasing circulating testosterone levels occurring after the fourth post-natal week, coinciding with the formation of the adult generation of Leydig cells (Lee et al. 1975).

The presence of testosterone in the testis and blood at 1 and 5 days of age suggests that the testis is capable at this early post-natal age of steroid synthesis and secretion (Pahnke et al. 1975). Although androstenedione, a precursor of testosterone, is present in the testis between 1 and 5 days of age, it was not detected in blood. However, Hashimoto and Suzuki (1966) measured testosterone and androstenedione in testicular venous blood of the mature adult rat and found a difference in the type of androgen secreted between the two groups. A predominance of androstenedione is secreted in the pre-pubertal rat, a pattern which changes at about the time of puberty (40–46 days of age). Similar findings have been previously reported in the bull, in which the androstenedione/testosterone ratio in testicular venous blood becomes considerably reduced with increasing age (Lindner 1961a). A change in testicular steroidogenesis with age in rodents has also been reported by Nayfeh et al. (1966, 1975), and by Podesta and Rivarola (1974). Androstanediol is formed from cholesterol in larger amounts in the immature rather than in the mature testis. Testosterone is the major steroid formed in incubations of adult testes. Plasma androstenedione levels are found to be elevated in 20- to 35-day-old rats, at a time when plasma testosterone levels are minimal. There is also an increase in testicular 5α-reductase activity at this time. The formation of androstanediol is also found to be especially high in seminiferous tubules of rats at 26 days of age, at a time when meiotic divisions are first observed (Rivarola et al. 1972). These observations of changes in testicular metabolism of androgens may be important in the initiation and progression of spermatogenic activity.

Other studies have shown that plasma levels of LH are elevated in neonatal rats, and decline to minimum values from days 12–15, and from these low levels, LH rises gradually to reach a maximum at about 70 days (Ojeda and Ramirez 1972; McCann et al. 1974). Independently Miyachi et al. (1973) have demonstrated peaks of LH between the ages of 17 and 20 days in male Holtzman rats, and coincident with the LH peaks are peaks in the levels of serum testosterone. In most studies the increase in LH concentrations takes place from 25 days of age (Miyachi et al. 1973; Döhler and Wuttke 1974), and the parallel rises in the levels of LH and testosterone seen between days 30 and 65 correlate well with the formation of the adult generation of Leydig cells (Lording and de Kretser 1972). During this second phase of testicular development increased secretion of testosterone from the testis is associated with an increase in the weights of seminal vesicles and ventral prostate (Resko et al. 1968; Knorr et al. 1970; Grota 1971; Bloch et al. 1974). There is a rapid increase in testis weight, Leydig cell numbers and several enzymes essential for testosterone biosynthesis at about 20 days of age (Knorr et al. 1970). The numbers of testicular LH receptors also increase rapidly and reach a maximum by 50–60 days, coincident with the attainment of maximum plasma testosterone concentrations, maximum testis size and maximum Leydig cell numbers in the testis (Ketelslegers et al. 1978). Although plasma testosterone concentrations reach maximum levels at the same time as the maximum number of LH receptors are found, the increase in LH receptors in the testis precedes the pubertal rise in circulating testosterone levels. There is now ample evidence to propose that LH receptors are partially under the influence of LH action (Odell et al. 1973; Chen et al. 1977). From these findings it seems probable that the pubertal rise of FSH initiates the increase in the number of testicular LH receptors and that these receptors become responsive to circulating LH levels with a subsequent increase in testosterone secretion. It is not clear how FSH accomplishes this role since FSH receptors have not been identified on Leydig cells.

Other hormonal factors that influence testosterone secretion, particularly prolactin and growth hormone, have been evaluated. Both growth hormone and prolactin can markedly enhance the effect of LH on testosterone secretion, suggesting that the modulation of the response of Leydig cells to LH can be regulated by FSH, growth hormone and prolactin, and that these hormones may play important roles in the process of pubertal development (Swerdloff and Odell 1977).

3.3 Studies in Rams

The ram is a good animal model to study relationships between testicular development and hormonal changes from fetal to adult life, since it has a clearly defined pre-pubertal period (Dun 1955; Watson et al. 1956; Skinner et al. 1968; Courot 1974). We have used sheep to define the patterns from birth and also to investigate any changes in the sensitivity of the anterior pituitary to LHRH during sexual maturation (Lee et al. 1976a,b).

3.3.1 Changes in FSH, LH, Prolactin and Testosterone Concentrations with Age

The patterns of changes in these hormones are shown in Fig. 3.6.

FSH. Plasma levels of FSH at birth range between 11 and 22 ng/ml. During the first 5 weeks these levels increase progressively to reach a significant peak (mean: 46.7 ng/ml). Following this peak and over the course of the next 6 weeks FSH levels decrease and by 11 weeks are significantly lower than at 5 weeks (30.8 vs. 46.7 ng/ml). Between the ages of 11 and 45 weeks mean levels range between 30 and 40 ng/ml.

LH. Plasma levels of LH at birth are low (< 0.5 ng/ml) and remain at these low levels for the 1st month of life. During the 5th week there is an abrupt increase in LH levels to a peak value of 2.2 ng/ml. As with FSH, this peak

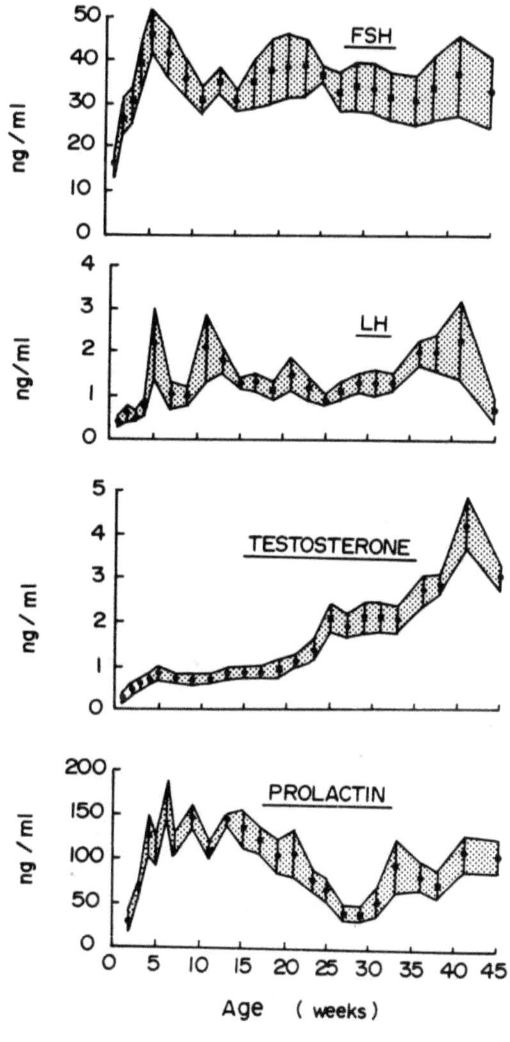

Fig. 3.6. Profiles of gonadotrophin (FSH, LH and prolactin) and testosterone levels during sexual development of the ram. *Vertical bars* represent mean ± SEM (Lee et al. 1976a). Reference preparations for gonadotrophins are NIH-FSH-S6, NIH-LH-S8 and NIH-P-S6

is followed by a sharp decline and LH levels are approximately 1 ng/ml over the next 4 or 5 weeks, after which there is a second transitory peak (Fig. 3.6). Between the ages of 15 and 33 weeks LH levels range between 0.9 and 1.3 ng/ml. From the 33rd week there is a further significant increase in LH to a mean peak value of 2.3 ng/ml at 41 weeks. Another abrupt decline in LH levels occurs at 45 weeks.

Testosterone. During the 1st week of neonatal life the mean plasma testosterone level is 0.25 ng/ml and this is followed by a gradual increase in testosterone levels during the next 4 weeks to reach 0.8 ng/ml by the fifth post-natal week. Between 7 and 19 weeks of age the mean levels range between 0.7 and 0.9 ng/ml. A progressive rise in testosterone occurs subsequently to reach a peak value of 4.3 ng/ml at 41 weeks. This peak is followed by a significant decrease to reach levels of 3 ng/ml at 45 weeks of age, comparable to levels seen in adult rams (2.95 ± 0.3 ng/ml).

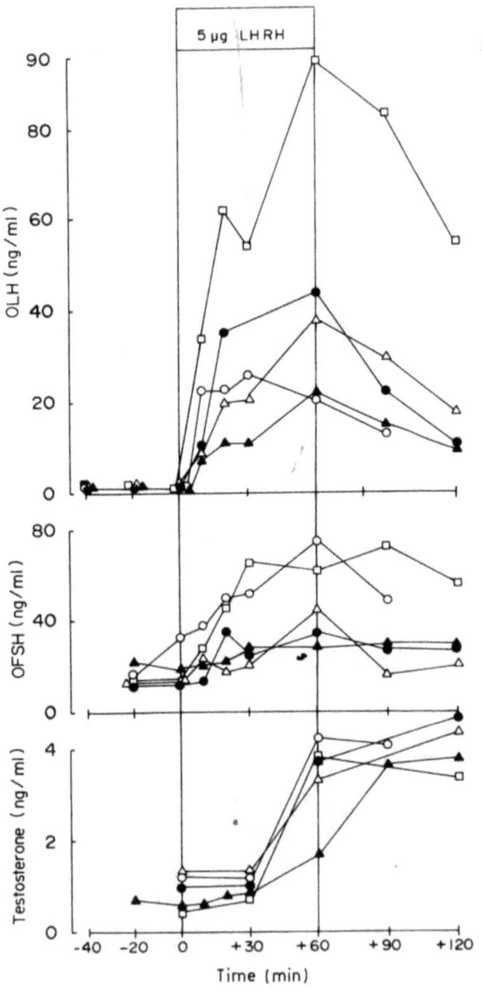

Fig. 3.7. Concentrations of FSH, LH and testosterone in the plasma of 1-day-old (nos. 78, 50, 82) and 2-day-old (nos. 260 and 56) rams after an intracarotid infusion of 5 µg LH-RH over a period of 60 min

Prolactin. The levels of plasma prolactin are 25 ng/ml during the first 2 weeks of post-natal life. These rapidly increase to reach peak levels in excess of 100 ng/ml by the fourth post-natal week. The levels remain elevated for the next 15 weeks, when a significant decline occurs, reaching a nadir between 27 and 31 weeks of age. After this nadir a further rise in prolactin levels is seen and the mean levels reached are 112 and 109 ng/ml at 41 and 45 weeks of age respectively.

3.3.2 LH, FSH and Testosterone Responses to LHRH with Age

In order to test the sensitivity of the pituitary to LHRH we gave intracarotid infusions of 5 μg LHRH over a period of 1 h to rams on the 1st and 2nd days and then at 2, 4, 6 and 8 weeks of age. The results of these studies are shown in Figs. 3.7–3.9.

LH. In all the animals studied, LH levels are significantly elevated at 10 min after the start of the LHRH infusion. The levels remain elevated during the course of the infusion, and decline once the infusion is stopped. Neonatal

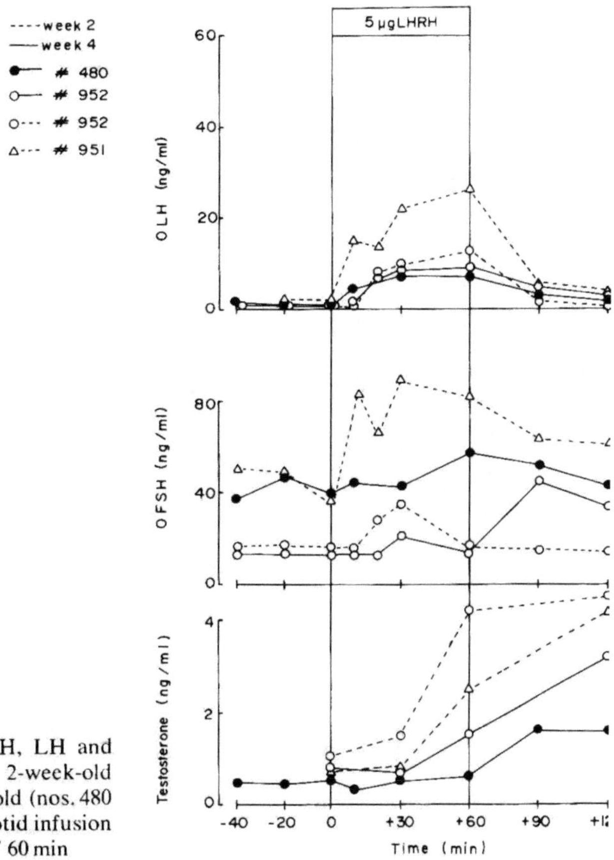

Fig. 3.8. Concentrations of FSH, LH and testosterone in the plasma of 2-week-old (nos. 951 and 952) and 4-week-old (nos. 480 and 952) rams after an intracarotid infusion of 5 μg LH-RH over a period of 60 min

animals exhibit significant LH responses to LHRH, basal values of < 1 ng/ml increasing to peak values of > 20 ng/ml by 60 min. During the next 3–4 weeks the LH responses are smaller. By the age of 2–3 months LH responses, as measured by areas under the curves, are significantly greater than responses in animals aged 2 and 4 weeks. It is pertinent to note that the body weights of the older animals (3–3 months) are almost twice as great as the 2- to 4-week-old animals (12 as compared to 7 kg) although the same doses of LHRH were used.

FSH. The response of FSH to LHRH infusions does not always follow that seen for LH. Basal FSH levels in animals aged 1 and 2 days are < 30 ng/ml, and two of five animals in this group show two- to threefold increases in FSH during the infusion. Although marginal increases are seen in most of the animals at other ages, the FSH response to LHRH in rams at 6 and 8 weeks are significantly elevated.

Testosterone. Significant increases in levels of testosterone occur within 60 min of the start of the infusion of LHRH in all animals studied. Basal

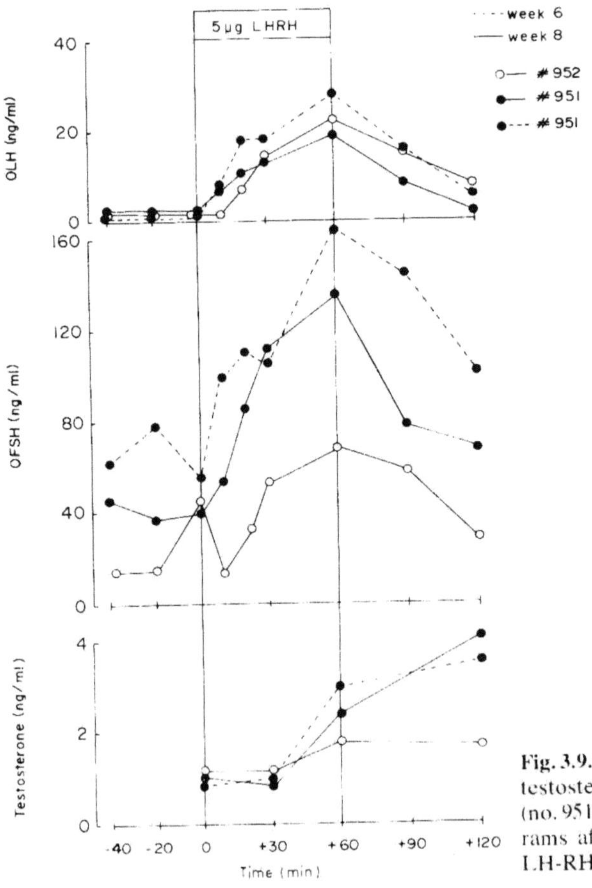

Fig. 3.9. Concentrations of FSH, LH and testosterone in the plasma of 6-week-old (no. 951) and 8-week-old (nos. 951 and 952) rams after an intracarotid infusion of 5 µg LH-RH over a period of 60 min

testosterone levels are less than 1.2 ng/ml and are increased to levels of 2.0 ng/ml or more after 60 min of infusion. These levels remain elevated for the next hour, and are usually higher than levels observed at the time of the end of the LHRH infusion.

3.3.3 Changes in Testicular Histology with Age

These are shown in Fig. 3.10. The seminiferous tubule diameter of the ram testis remains relatively uniform in size during the first 17 weeks of life,

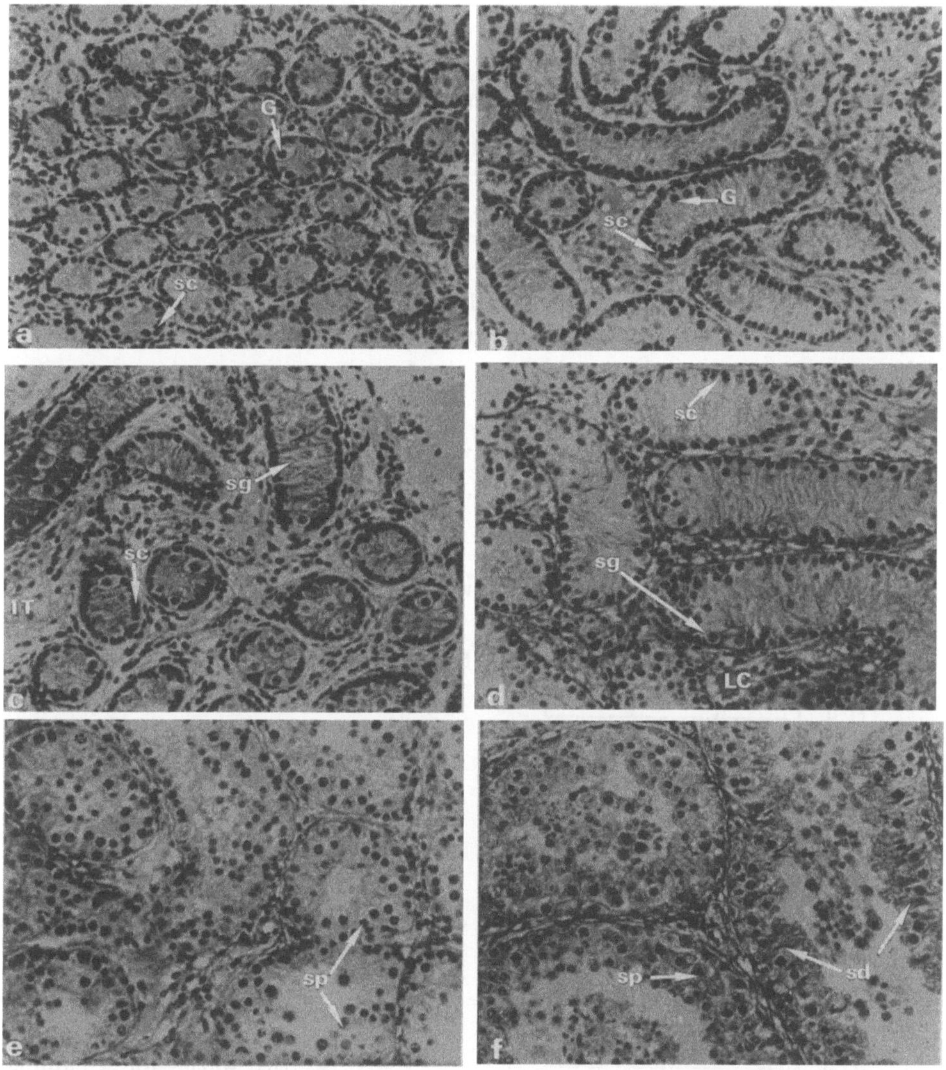

Fig. 3.10. Light micrographs of testis from rams aged 5 (**a**), 18 (**b**), 24 (**c**), 34 (**d**), 36 (**e**) and 39 (**f**) weeks old. *G*, gonocytes; *SC*, Sertoli cells; *sg*, spermatogonia; *sp*, spermatocytes; *sd*, spermatids; *LC*, Leydig cell

and throughout this phase the cords maintain a similar appearance with Sertoli cells at the periphery and gonocytes centrally located. The earliest cell change is the maturation of the Sertoli cell between 17 and 21 weeks after birth. Spermatocytes are first seen in biopsies taken between 31 and 36 weeks, and spermatogenesis is fully established by 45 weeks, when the animals become sexually mature.

Leydig cells have proved difficult to identify during the course of sexual development, and are not really recognisable until the time of sexual maturation. This time, between 36 and 45 weeks, coincides with the peak of circulating testosterone levels. The difficulty in the identification of Leydig cells has also been experienced by others (Hay and Deane 1966; Skinner et al. 1968).

3.3.4 Significance of Hormonal Changes

Our studies have shown the changes that occur in the secretion of pituitary gonadotrophins and in the morphology of the testis in the Merino/Corriedale rams during sexual development. The circulating levels of gonadotrophins and testosterone increase shortly after birth and reach peak levels between 5 and 7 weeks of age. The responsiveness of the anterior pituitary increases at the same time as the levels of gonadotrophin increase, but rapid increases in plasma testosterone levels following infusions of LHRH occur at all ages.

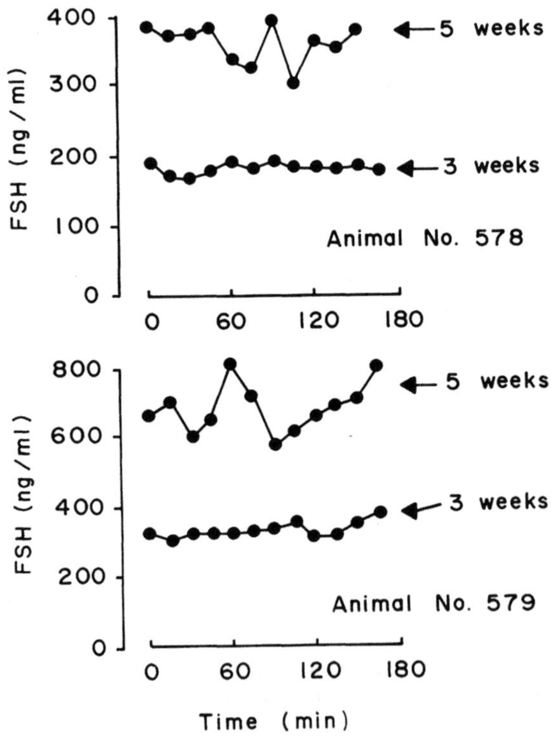

Fig. 3.11. Plasma FSH levels in two neonatally castrate lambs (nos. 578 and 579; castrated within 48 h of birth) at 15-min intervals for 3 h at the ages of 3 and 5 weeks. All samples were assayed in a single assay

We were not able to correlate changes in hormone levels with specific cytological changes in the testis. It is possible that increases in FSH and LH may reflect some alteration in the sensitivity of the hypothalamus or pituitary which facilitates the onset of puberty. The augmentation of the secretion of FSH and LH in response to infusions of LHRH at about the same time that the basal serum levels of gonadotrophin increase supports the concept of a change in the interrelationships between the hypothalamus, pituitary and gonad. If ram lambs are castrated at birth, levels of FSH are 2 or 3 times greater at 5 weeks than at 3 weeks of age (Fig. 3.11). These increases in circulating levels of FSH which occur in the absence of the testes suggest that a change in the hypothalamic control of FSH occurs in the absence of the testes and testosterone. We support the proposition that the feedback inhibition of FSH secretion is already established on the first neonatal day, and that the control of FSH secretion comes from testicular secretion other than testosterone. Since Sertoli cells or gonocytes are the only seminiferous tubule cells present in the neonatal lambs, the question of whether FSH inhibitory factors are secreted by these cells remains unknown.

The elevated levels of FSH seen during the period of sexual maturation may increase the sensitivity of Leydig cells to LH; this has previously been suggested for the rat by Odell et al. (1973). It may also explain why the rise in testosterone levels is seen at 23 weeks of age, an increase that occurs before the secondary rise in LH levels between the 33rd and 35th weeks. It is also of interest that prolactin and testosterone concentrations begin to rise during the time of the secondary LH increase. It is possible that prolactin may also enhance the sensitivity of Leydig cells to LH.

The physiological role of prolactin in the ram is not known. Prolactin-deficient mice treated with prolactin show enhanced spermatogenic activity (Bartke and Lloyd 1970), indicating a role for prolactin in testicular function. The localisation of labelled prolactin in the Leydig cell and ventral prostate of rats has led to the concept that prolactin sensitises the testis to LH and has a role in the growth of secondary sex glands during sexual development (Rajaniemi et al. 1974; Aragona et al. 1977; Bartke and Dalterio 1976; Negro-Vilar et al. 1977). In the ram dramatic changes occur in the secretion of prolactin during the course of sexual development (Fig. 3.6). Between 3 and 5 weeks of age prolactin levels are 2–3 times higher than levels seen in newborn lambs. This increase in prolactin during the neonatal period occurs concomitantly with increases in LH, FSH and testosterone. Prolactin levels remain elevated for the next 4 months, which are the summer months and periods of long daylight. Prolactin levels subsequently decline and reach a nadir between the 6th and 7th months, which are the times of shortest daylight. We believe that photoperiod influences the secretion of prolactin in sexually developing rams. In adult rams high levels of prolactin have been found during long daylight periods and low levels during periods of short daylight (Pelletier 1973).

Changes in the secretion of prolactin during the 1st year of sexual development in the ram are probably of physiological importance. In a longitudinal study of Ile de France rams, transient increases in prolactin concentrations are observed during the third post-natal week, and secondary prolactin peaks occur between the 7th and 12th weeks, which are periods of diminishing daylight. These are contrary to our findings of low prolactin levels during the winter, but the difference between the two studies is the season when the lambs were born. Our study involved lambs born during the spring, whereas the Ile de France rams were born during the autumn. In both studies increased prolactin levels are associated with the establishment of spermatogenesis, indicating that prolactin is involved with testicular development in the ram.

It is possible that seasonal factors other than photoperiod, such as fluctuations in nutritional conditions and temperature, may influence sexual development in the ram (Dyrmundsson 1973). The rate of sexual development is highly dependent on the growth rate of the animal, and consequently ram lambs experiencing faster growth rates during rearing tend to attain puberty earlier in the season (Dun 1955; Watson et al. 1956; Courot 1962; Dyrmundsson and Lees 1972). To date there is no direct evidence of any relationship between photoperiod, environmental temperature and pubertal development in the ram. However, there are some observations on the effects of day length and level of feeding on serum prolactin levels in growing rams which suggest that the increased growth rate during the summer may be associated with increased prolactin secretion, since prolactin is known to have growth-stimulating effects (Horrobin 1973; Forbes et al. 1975).

In an extensive study of testicular development in Merino rams Watson et al. (1956) found the general histological characteristics of the testes to be closely related to testicular weight and this in turn to body weight. Spermatozoa are not seen in the lumen of seminiferous tubules in any animal weighing less than 27 kg, and are present only in those which weigh more than 28 kg. Animals with this body weight are aged 5–6 months. In our study of crossbred Merino/Coriedale rams the full complement of spermatogenesis is established by 45 weeks, which is much later than in other breeds of sheep (Table 3.6). Despite differences at the time at which spermatozoa are first seen in the ram testis, the body weights of different breeds of rams at the time of sexual maturity are quite similar. As indicated earlier the rate of sexual development may be dependent on growth rate, and in our series of animals the gain in weight was relatively slow. It would therefore be interesting to determine the ratio of testicular size to body weight for these various breeds, and to determine if a constant ratio exists

Table 3.6. Body weight and age of rams at appearance of spermatozoa in testes

Breed (no. of rams)	Locality	Age when spermatozoa are present (weeks)	Approx. body wt. at puberty (kg)	Refs.
Ile-de-France (56)	France	20–22	35	Courot (1962, 1971)
Merino (110)	Australia	18–32	27	Watson et al. (1956)
Namaqua Africander (12)	South Africa	28	32	Skinner (1970)
Suffolk (54)	England	16	35	Skinner et al. (1968)
Merino-Corriedale (29)	Australia	39–45	30	Lee (1976)

between breeds at the time of sexual maturity. This ratio (if it is constant) would consequently provide a reliable index for the assessment of sexual maturation in rams.

Response to LHRH. The pituitary-testicular axis in rams is responsive to LHRH stimulation from the time of birth (Lee et al. 1976b). This is in accord with previous findings in neonatal lambs which receive injections of crude ovine hypothalamic extracts or purified porcine gonadotrophin releasing factor (Foster et al. 1972b). Our studies also show that there is an increase in pituitary sensitivity to LHRH at approximately 5–8 weeks of age. This increase in pituitary responsiveness to LHRH coincides with the peak levels of serum gonadotrophins in developing rams at about 5 weeks. It is reasonable to conclude that a change in sensitivity on the hypothalamic-pituitary-testicular axis occurs at this time, perhaps representing the time of initiation of the pubertal process. The study of Crim and Geschwind (1972b) supports this conclusion; rams castrated at the age of 60 days exhibit a greater LH elevation following the operation than those of other ages. Additional evidence is the finding of a rapid increase in pituitary gonadotrophin content in Suffolk rams from 42 days of age during post-natal development (Skinner et al. 1968).

Another interesting feature in the LHRH stimulation studies is the rapid increase in testosterone concentrations which follow the LHRH infusions. Significant rises occur within 60 min of the start of the infusion. This differs from observations made in men (Roth et al. 1973; de Kretser et al. 1975a) when the magnitude of the response is small and significant elevations in serum testosterone levels occur much later (8–12 h). The finding of rapid increases in testosterone secretion in newborn rams at a time when mature Leydig cells cannot be identified in the testis suggests that the undifferentiated elongated mesenchymal cells in the intertubular spaces are capable of steroid biosynthesis.

3.4 Overall Comments

The results presented in this chapter are longitudinal studies of profiles of hormonal changes that occur from birth to sexual maturity in male rats and rams, and before puberty to adulthood in man.

Despite differences in the times at which sexual maturity is established, the patterns of hormonal secretion are quite similar. The early post-natal increases in gonadotrophin secretion noted in man (Forest et al. 1976) may have their counterpart in the rises in FSH and LH at 5 weeks noted in rams, and in the high FSH levels in the neonatal rat. In man and in rats early pre-pubertal rises in FSH have been noted and can be correlated with growth and testicular size and spermatogenesis (de Kretser et al. 1977). The role of the pubertal rise in FSH in the rat is to induce increased sensitivity of the testis to LH (Odell et al. 1973; Odell and Swerdloff 1976). In man, levels of FSH rise more abruptly during the early stages of puberty, but as puberty advances and testicular volumes increase, the levels of FSH plateau and frequently decline before the completion of puberty (Burr et al. 1970;

Winter and Faiman 1972; Grumbach et al. 1974; Baker et al. 1976c). Changes in the levels of FSH prior to and during puberty are consistent with the view that as the testis matures it elaborates a feedback signal that controls the secretion of FSH (Swerdloff et al. 1971). In rams, however, no definite rise in FSH coincident with the onset of spermatogenesis can be demonstrated (Lee et al. 1976a; Walton et al. 1978). The clearly defined rise which occurs within 4–6 weeks after birth does not appear to coincide with any particular change in the testis.

The concomitant increases in LH and testosterone during the pubertal period in man, rats and sheep suggest that these hormones are closely related. Both LH and testosterone rise progressively during the later stages of puberty, reaching a new feedback equilibrium which persists into adulthood. The precise role of the LH-stimulated rise in testosterone on the spermatogenic process remains unclear. Steinberger (1971) has reviewed the evidence indicating that testosterone is necessary for certain key steps in the spermatogenic process, mainly the transformation of gonocytes to primitive type A spermatogonia, during diakinesis and possibly during spermatid differentiation. Rivarola et al. (1972) have suggested the need for 5α-reduced metabolites of testosterone between the 21st and 26th days is necessary for the initiation of the meiotic stages of spermatogenesis.

Episodic secretion of LH and testosterone appears to be necessary for normal reproductive activity. In man, this is absent before the onset of puberty, and initially occurs nocturnally in association with the early stages of puberty (Boyar et al. 1972). In the ram, episodic secretion of LH and testosterone is present very early during the post-natal period (Foster et al. 1978) and in the breeding season, but is diminished or absent in the non-breeding season (Bremner 1977; Lincoln 1979). The finding that body weight may be a reliable index of sexual maturity in the ram is of interest. The concept that puberty is more closely related to weight than to age is well known in other mammals (see review by Frisch 1974). Data for rats, mice, pigs and cattle indicate that sexual maturity (defined by vaginal opening or by the first oestrus) is attained at the same weight for slow-growing as for fast-growing animals. Furthermore, the mean weight of girls at menarche (47 kg) has been found to be similar for early and late maturing girls (Frisch, 1974). Whether the attainment of a critical body weight is required for the establishment of spermatogenesis in the ram (or other male species) requires further investigation.

The role of the adrenal and pineal glands in the process of sexual maturation is unknown. Delayed puberty in female rats has been shown to occur after adrenalectomy (Ramaley and Bunn 1972; Ramaley 1974) whereas pinealectomy leads to precocious puberty in the male (Thieblot and Blaise 1963; Roth 1965). Although the advancement of puberty in the male following pinealectomy is probably due to a removal of pineal factors that inhibit gonadotrophin secretion, the precise role of the pineal gland in the control of sexual maturation remains unclear and requires further investigation. Likewise the role of the adrenal, the effects of nutrition and the role of growth hormone and prolactin on pubertal development require further exploration (Ramirez 1973; MacKinnon et al. 1978; Ramaley 1979).

4 Changes in the Pituitary-Testicular Axis with Age

H.W.G. Baker and B. Hudson

4.1 Introduction

That testicular function may be deficient in old men has been recognised from antiquity. Throughout history there are examples of attempts to rejuvenate Hebrew kings, Popes and eminent physicians with various interesting treatments, including warmth from young maidens, ingestion of human milk, infusion of blood from young men and injection of testicular extracts (Dragstedt 1969). Over the last 40 years, age-related testicular degeneration has been studied scientifically in various species (Korenchevsky et al. 1953; Bishop 1970; Andrew 1971; Vassileva-Popova and Yanev 1975; Rigaudiere et al. 1976; Riegle et al. 1977; Gray 1978; Everitt 1980). In man, Kinsey et al. (1948) found sexual activity declined progressively with age and that about three of every four men in their eighties were impotent. Studies by other workers indicate that sexual performance falls faster than sexual interest. Also, maintenance of sexual activity in the elderly is related to the health of the individual, survival and health of the wife and a high sex drive in youth (Newman and Nichols 1960; Verwoerdt et al. 1969; Pfeiffer et al. 1969, 1972; Pfeiffer and Davis 1972; Martin 1975). The duration of penile erections occurring with rapid eye movement sleep also declines progressively with age (Karacan et al. 1975). Coital performance in old men and changes in the male sexual response were detailed by Masters and Johnson (1966). The loss of secondary sexual hair in the elderly was studied by Hamilton (1951) and Melick and Taft (1950). Reduced testicular size and histological evidence of impaired spermatogenesis in old men was reported by Bennett et al. (1950). Blum (1936) found a high incidence of azoospermia in senescence. Increases in pituitary content and urinary excretion of gonadotrophins with age were demonstrated by bioassay and reduced urinary and spermatic vein androgens by chemical methods (Henderson and Rowlands 1938; Pedersen-Bjergaard and Tonnesen 1948; Albert 1956; Engle and Pincus 1956; Hollander and Hollander 1958; Johnsen 1959; Morer-Fargas and Nowakowski 1965).
Development of methods for measuring the concentrations of pituitary and gonadal hormones in the general circulation has led to a large number of contemporary investigations and several reviews of changes in the pituitary-testicular relationship with age (Baker et al. 1976c, 1977; Vermeulen 1977; Harman 1978). Despite some minor differences in interpretation there is general agreement on the nature of these changes. In this chapter, the data are reviewed using the results of a study performed in Melbourne for illustrative

purposes (Baker et al. 1976c). Some consideration of methodological problems and speculations on the causes and significance of senescent testicular failure are included.

4.2 Methods

4.2.1 Testing the Pituitary-Testicular Axis

Figure 4.1 outlines procedures for testing the pituitary-testicular axis at different levels. Clinical indices of testicular size, secondary sexual hair distribution and sexual function give some guide to androgen action at the target tissue level. Luteinising hormone (LH), follicle-stimulating hormone (FSH), androgens and oestrogens are measured in serum or plasma by radioimmunoassay or competitive protein binding techniques. The binding capacity (q) of the sex hormone binding globulin (SHBG) may be measured by ammonium sulphate precipitation or equilibrium dialysis and free steroid levels may be calculated or estimated by similar methods. The intravenous

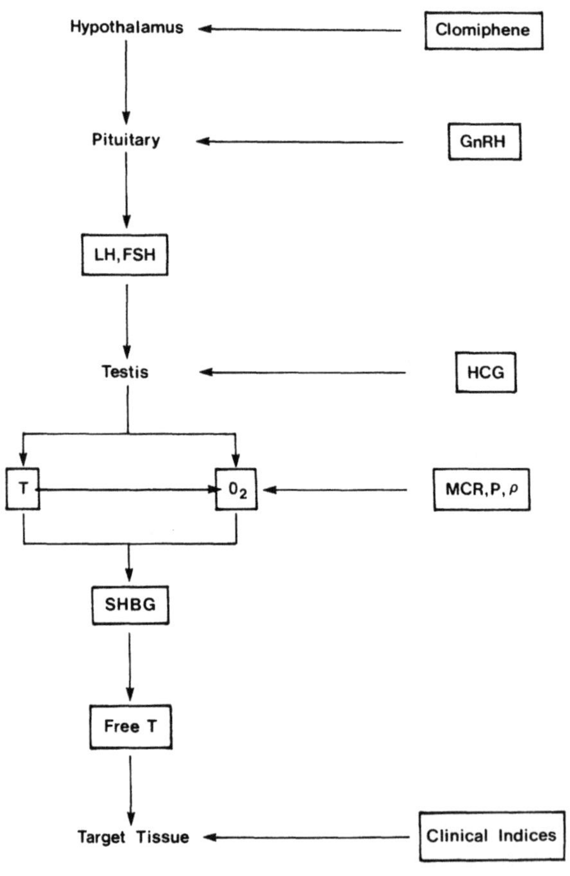

Fig. 4.1. Testing the pituitary-testicular axis

infusion or injection of radio-labelled steroid and isolation and measurement of the radioactivity of the precursor steroid itself and its products makes possible the measurement of metabolic clearance and blood production rate (MCR,P) of the precursor and the transfer constant (ϱ) for peripheral conversion of precursor to product. Pituitary and hypothalamic function may be tested by measuring serum LH and FSH after administration of synthetic gonadotrophin-releasing hormone (GnRH) and clomiphene (Chap. 2). Leydig cell reserve is examined by measuring the rise in serum testosterone levels following injection of human chorionic gonadotrophin (hCG) (Chap. 5).

4.2.2 Selection of Subjects

There are several theoretical problems with the experimental design of reported studies of hormone changes with aging. Most have been cross-sectional studies in which different men in various age groups have been investigated at one point in time. Obviously the more appropriate longitudinal design is difficult to apply to humans. Another problem is that in many studies, including our own, the elderly subjects were patients in geriatric or general hospitals. Although investigators were careful to exclude men with severe illness, defined endocrine disorders and those taking drugs likely to interfere with the study, the criticism cannot be avoided that illness rather than age may have contributed to the hormonal changes. It is possible that the observed abnormalities would be less frequent and less severe in healthy old men from the general community. Some workers have attempted to select subjects on the basis of good health and the hormonal changes were less marked in their studies. However, they had very few men over the age of 70 years (Snyder et al. 1975; Lewis et al. 1976; Harman 1978).

4.2.3 Statistical Methods

Usually single determinations of the basal hormone levels have been used. Santen and Bardin (1973) have shown that one measurement of serum LH gives a poor estimate of the mean circulating level because of the episodic secretion of this hormone. Similar considerations would apply to FSH, testosterone and oestradiol, which also exhibit circhoral fluctuations in blood levels (Baker et al. 1975). This problem is offset to some extent by the inclusion of large numbers of subjects in the studies. However, the presence of episodic secretion may cause the skewed distribution of results of single hormone determinations in a group of subjects. Several investigators have recognised that logarithmic transformation is necessary before applying statistical methods which depend on the normal distribution (Rubens et al. 1974; Stearns et al. 1974; Baker et al. 1976c).

In general, analyses have been performed to determine the significance of correlations between hormone levels and age, and between pairs of hormone results. In the Melbourne study it was found that few statistically significant correlations remained once the effect of age was removed. This indicates that care is needed in applying such statistical data to causal relationships between the changes in one hormone and another.

4.3 Summary of Results

4.3.1 Virility, Testicular Size and Histology

As shown in Fig. 4.2 reduced secondary sex hair, impotence and testicular atrophy occur with increasing frequency in older age groups (Stearns et al. 1974; Tanoa et al. 1975; Baker et al. 1976c). The effect of age on testicular histology has been studied mainly in autopsy material and there are some inconsistencies between the reports. Constant changes with age appear to be progressive thickening of the seminiferous tubule basement membrane, interstitial fibrosis, pigmentation of Leydig cells and focal tubule sclerosis (Sniffen 1950; Lynch and Scott 1950; Tillenger 1957; Sasano and Ichigo 1969; Bishop 1970; Andrew 1971; Suoranta 1971; Kaden 1975). Other changes are variable in occurrence. Even in extreme old age, spermatogenesis may appear normal. However, generalised hypospermatogenesis is common and germ cell arrest, germ cell aplasia or seminiferous tubule hyalinisation are occasionally seen (Sniffen 1950; Tillenger 1957; Sasano and Ichigo 1969; Frick 1969; Suoranta 1971; Tanoa et al. 1975; Kaden 1975). The damage is more severe at the periphery of the arterial supply of the testis and focal degenerative changes are often associated with arteriolar thickening and defective capillary beds (Sasano and Ichigo 1969; Suoranta 1971). The number of Leydig cells declines with age (Sarjent and McDonald 1948; Sniffen 1950; Tillenger et al. 1955; Tillenger 1957; Frick 1969; Harbitz 1973).

Although some studies of the effect of age on semen quality have been reported, there are no detailed studies which include large numbers of men

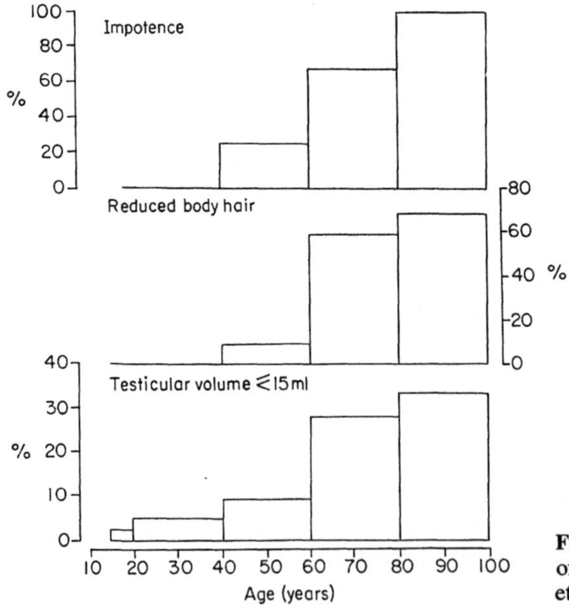

Fig. 4.2. Frequencies of clinical evidence of testicular failure in aging men (Baker et al. 1976c)

of all ages (Blum 1936; MacLeod and Gold 1953; Natoli et al. 1972; Tanoa et al. 1975). Surprisingly the larger studies show no decrease in sperm concentration with age. MacLeod and Gold found decreased motility, no change in sperm morphology and increased sperm concentration in men between 20 and 50 years of age. Natoli et al. found a fall in the proportion of sperm with normal morphology and decreased motility but no change in concentration between 45 and 91 years. From the histological studies and the hormonal data covered below it is likely that many old men are oligospermic.

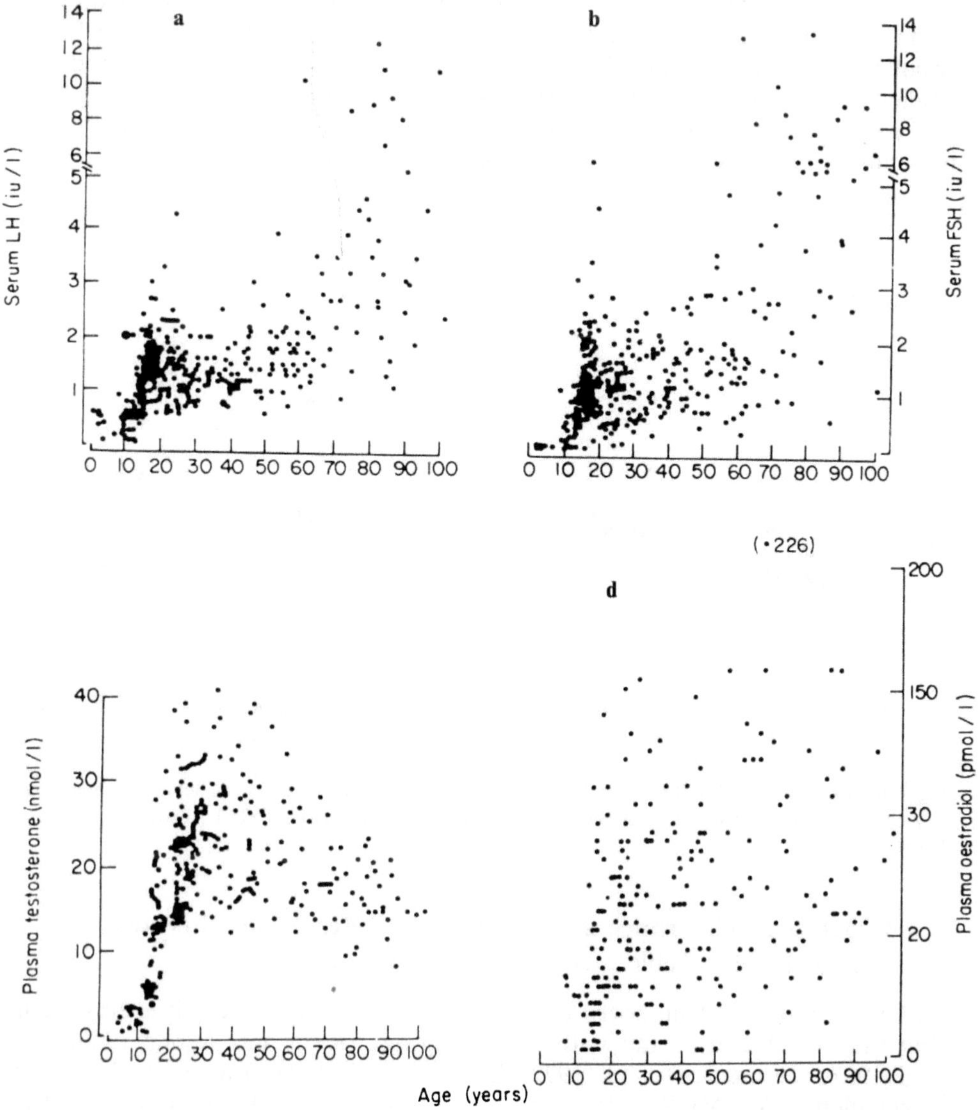

Fig. 4.3. Levels of LH, FSH, testosterone and oestradiol in males of different ages (Baker et al. 1976c)

4.3.2 Gonadotrophin and Sex Hormone Levels (Figs. 4.3–4.5)

With few exceptions there is a general agreement among the published reports for the following changes in hormone and SHBG levels with age: rising LH and FSH, falling testosterone, rising SHBG capacity, falling free testosterone and rising oestradiol (Table 4.1). There are significant positive and negative correlations between these results and age (Table 4.2). Low levels of dihydrotestosterone and other androgens and high levels of oestrone have also been reported in old men (Rubens et al. 1974; Kley et al. 1974; Giusti et al. 1975; Pazzagli et al. 1975; Pirke and Doerr 1975b; Lewis et al. 1976; Vermeulen 1977; Pirke et al. 1977). It would appear that these changes do not occur suddenly at any particular age but are gradual and progressive from about the age of 50 years. This point will only be defined by longitudinal studies of individual men. It is worth noting that the range of results is wide, and some men over the age of 70 years have values within the ranges seen in younger men between 20 and 50 years.

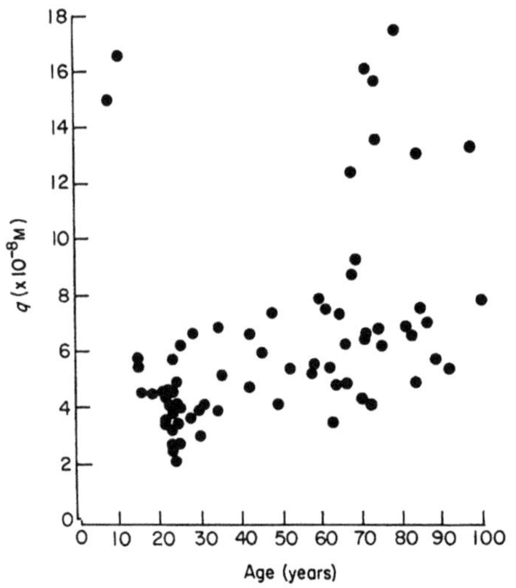

Fig. 4.4. Sex hormone binding globulin capacity (q) in males of different ages (Baker et al. 1976c)

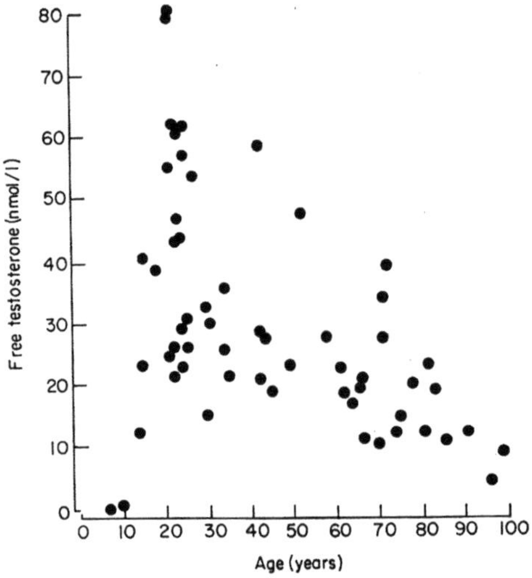

Fig. 4.5. Free testosterone levels in males of different ages (Baker et al. 1976c)

4.3.3 Metabolic Clearance and Production Rates of Sex Steroids (Figs. 4.6–4.8; Table 4.2)

Although only small numbers of subjects have been studied, it seems clear that the MCR^T and P^T fall with advancing age (Kent and Acone 1966; Isurugi 1967; Vermeulen et al. 1972; Bayard et al. 1973; Baker et al. 1976c; Vermeulen 1976). MCR^{O_2} also seems to be reduced with age, but P^{O_2} is the same in young and old men (Bayard et al. 1973; Baker et al. 1976c). The peripheral conversion of testosterone to oestradiol also probably increases

Table 4.1. References for changes in hormone levels with age in men

Increased LH and FSH		Reduced testosterone		Increased SHBG		Reduced free testosterone		Increased oestradiol	
Swerdloff and Odell	1968	Kirschner and Coffman	1968	Vermeulen et al.	1972	Vermeulen et al.	1972	Pirke and Doerr	1973
Schalch et al.	1968	Frick	1969	Pirke and Doerr	1973	Nieschlag et al.	1973	Rubens et al.	1974
Ryan and Faiman	1968	Vermeulen et al.	1972	Baker et al.	1976c	Rubens et al.	1974	Kley et al.	1974
Burger et al.	1972	Pirke and Doerr	1973	Vermeulen	1977	Kley et al.	1974	Baker et al.	1976c
Nieschlag et al.	1973	Nieschlag et al.	1973			Stearns et al.	1974	Hallberg et al.	1976
Wide et al.	1973	Rubens et al.	1974			Pirke and Doerr	1975	Vermeulen	1977
Rubens et al.	1974	Stearns et al.	1974			Snyder et al.	1975	Muta et al.	1981
Stearns et al.	1974	Mazzi et al.	1974			Baker et al.	1976c		
Isurugi et al.	1974	Giusti et al.	1975			Vermeulen	1977		
Mazzi et al.	1974	Konno et al.	1975			Muta et al.	1981		
Tanda et al.	1975	Tanda et al.	1975						
Baker et al.	1976c	Baker et al.	1976c						
Greenblatt et al.	1976	Greenblatt et al.	1976						
Hallberg et al.	1976	Hallberg et al.	1976						
Lindholm et al.	1976	Vermeulen	1977						
Vermeulen	1977	Muta et al.	1981						
Muta et al.	1981								

with age (Fig. 4.8). This may contribute to the maintenance of P^{O_2}. Mannelli et al. (1979) found the concentrations of testosterone and androstenedione in spermatic venous blood decreased with age while oestradiol levels were unchanged. Increased conversion of androstenedione to oestrone has also been demonstrated in senescence (MacDonald et al. 1971; Hemsell et al. 1974). The reason for and mechanism of the changes in steroid interconver-

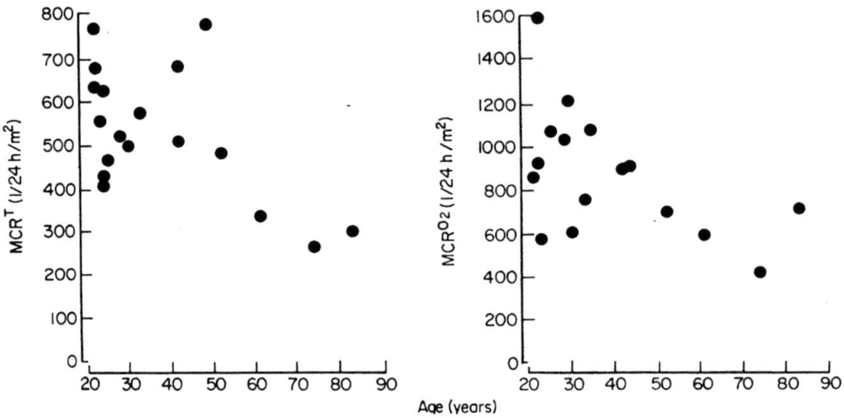

Fig. 4.6. Metabolic clearance rates of testosterone and oestradiol in men of different ages (Baker et al. 1976c)

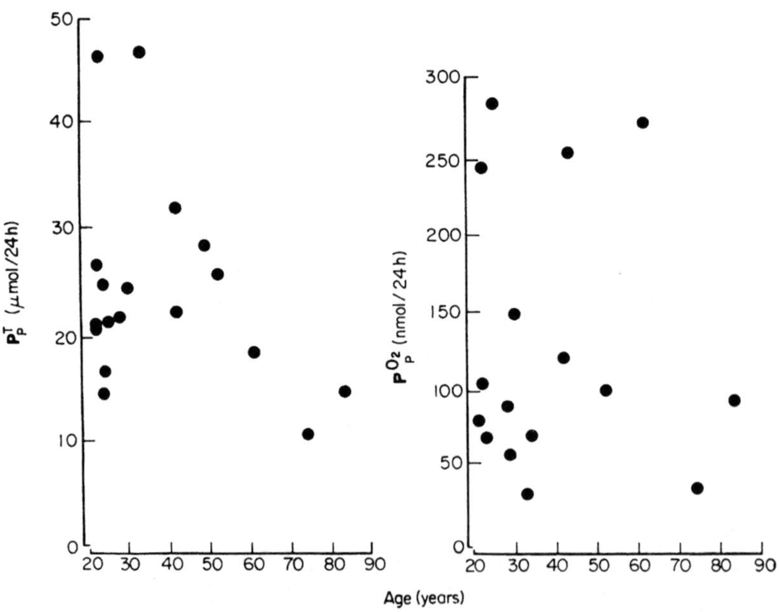

Fig. 4.7. Plasma production rates of testosterone and oestradiol in men of different ages (Baker et al. 1976c)

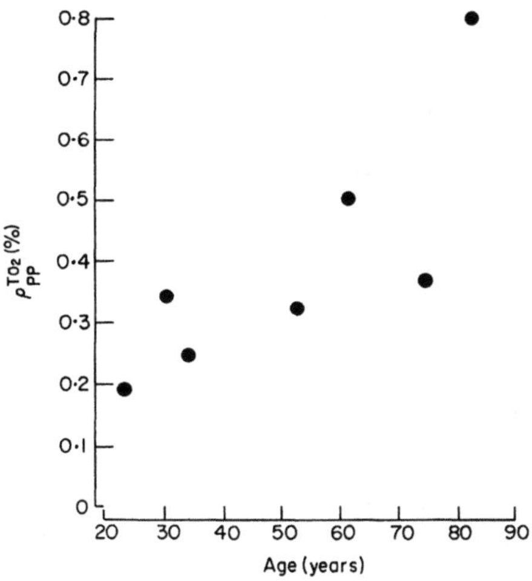

Fig. 4.8. Transfer constants for the peripheral concentration of testosterone to oestradiol in men of different ages (Baker et al. 1976c)

sion are unclear at present. Increased peripheral conversion of testosterone to oestradiol has also been demonstrated in men with cirrhosis and Klinefelter's syndrome, and thus it may be a common accompaniment of primary hypogonadism (Wang et al. 1975; Baker et al. 1976b).

4.3.4 Dynamic Tests of Gonadotrophin and Testosterone Secretion

The results of pituitary and Leydig cell stimulation tests are difficult to interpret because of the large numbers of factors involved including variations in the delivery of the stimulant to the tissue of interest, modulation of responsiveness by endogenous factors and changes in the clearance of the product of interest from the circulation. Although the results reported by other investigators are generally similar the conclusions vary. In elderly subjects injection of synthetic GnRH causes a rise in the elevated basal levels of FSH and LH, but in some reports the relative increment (stimulated/basal) is less than in young subjects (Hashimoto et al. 1973; Mazzi et al. 1974; Rubens et al. 1974; Haug et al. 1974; Snyder et al. 1975; Kumahara et al. 1975; Lindholm et al. 1976; Muta et al. 1981). This may indicate a degree of decreased function of the pituitary gonadotropes in elderly men (Snyder et al. 1975). Also, Muta et al. (1981) found a relative resistance to the gonadotrophin-suppressing effects of testosterone and oestradiol in old men. However, it is clear from the elevated basal gonadotrophin levels that senescent testicular failure is basically a primary gonadal disorder. Clomiphene tests have not been used extensively, and there are insufficient data to review (Geller et al. 1970).

Similar problems of interpretation also apply to Leydig cell stimulation tests. Both before and after hCG administration, plasma testosterone levels are lower in old men than in young men, but the relative rise is similar or reduced in the elderly (Frick 1969; Frick and Kincl 1969; Longcope 1973; Nieschlag et al. 1973; Rubens et al. 1974; Mazzi et al. 1974). This type of

Table 4.2. Relationships between age and hormone measurements in men (Baker et al. 1976c)

Measurement	*r*	df	*P*
Plasma testosterone	−0.34	210	<0.001
Plasma oestradiol	0.18	178	<0.05
Serum LH	0.59	214	<0.001
Serum FSH	0.60	215	<0.001
q	0.57	60	<0.001
% free testosterone	−0.52	48	<0.001
Free testosterone	−0.63	48	<0.001
% free oestradiol	−0.49	50	<0.001
Free oestradiol	−0.42	47	<0.01
MCR^{T} (1/24 h)	−0.61	15	<0.01
MCR^{T} (1/24 h/m^2)	−0.53	15	<0.05
MCR^{O_2} (1/24 h)	−0.56	13	<0.05
MCR^{O_2} (1/24 h/m^2)	−0.50	13	<0.1
P_P^T	−0.34	15	NS
$P_P^{O_2}$	−0.10	13	NS
$\varrho_{PP}^{TO_2}$	0.81	5	<0.05
Testicular volume	−0.19	81	<0.01
Reduced body hair score	0.83	134	<0.001
Reduced sexual function score	0.85	134	<0.001

response has been variously interpreted as evidence of either primary (Nieschlag et al. 1973; Rubens et al. 1974) or secondary hypogonadism (Longcope 1973).

4.4 Significance of Senescent Testicular Degeneration

4.4.1 Mechanism of Hormone Changes with Age

The evidence reviewed suggests an increasing frequency of primary testicular insufficiency with age. A reasonable explanation for the hormone changes is as follows. Seminiferous epithelial degeneration results in reduced testicular size and elevated FSH levels, possibly because of reduced inhibin production (Baker et al. 1976a). Leydig cell impairment leads to reduced androgen secretion and low circulating levels. The increased plasma protein binding of testosterone coupled with the low total levels results in a marked lowering of free testosterone levels with reduced MCR^{T}, high LH levels and clinical features of androgen deficiency. The reasons for the other changes are less clear. The reduced MCR^{O_2} and increased peripheral conversion of testosterone to oestradiol would contribute to the maintenance of oestradiol production rates and elevated plasma oestradiol levels. It is possible that increased testicular or adrenal secretion of oestradiol may also occur in the elderly (Murakami et al. 1976; Mannelli et al. 1979). High oestrogen levels may in turn be a stimulus for increased SHBG levels (Kley et al. 1974). The latter suggestions are rather tentative because each of the changes correlate better with age than with each other, and when the effect of age is removed in the analyses most of the correlations lose their statistical significance (Baker et al. 1976c). Further studies will be required before the mechanism of the hormone changes with age is completely understood.

4.4.2 Further Studies

Several other aspects of senescent testicular failure warrant more investigation. Target tissue responsiveness may be impaired with age. Studies of senescent laboratory animals suggest reduced responsiveness to a number of steroid hormones (Roth 1974; Roy et al. 1974). This may result from a reduced number of receptors in the target cells (Roth 1974; Roy et al. 1974; Shain et al. 1975). In man, Vermeulen et al. (1972) found decreased conversion of testosterone to 3α-androstanediol and an increased ratio of 5β to 5α metabolies in the urine of old men, which can be interpreted as evidence of underutilisation of testosterone by target cells. It is also possible that receptors for gonadotrophins may be reduced or altered with age. For example there is some evidence that the affinity of th LH receptors may decrease with age (Vassileva-Popova and Yanev 1975). Also, LH receptors are "down regulated" by high hormone levels (Purvis et al. 1977). There is evidence from perfusion studies of rat testes that testosterone secretion may be reduced in the presence of excessive stimulation (Baker et al. 1977). Furthermore, it is possible the clearance of gonadotrophin may be decreased in the elderly because the decline in LH and FSH levels following a GnRH-induced peak is slower than in young men (Rubens et al. 1974; Snyder et al. 1975). The nature and biological activity of gonadotrophins may also change with age (Dufau et al. 1977a).

4.4.3 Aetiology of Testicular Damage

While it is probable that senescent testicular failure is an entity, its cause remains as mysterious as the aging process itself. Superficially at least, it is quite distinct from the menopause and climacteric in women in that it does not occur regularly or suddenly at any particular age. Because the seminiferous epithelium and Leydig cells are both affected, theories must explain the disordered function of both testicular compartments. This consideration would seemingly exclude a change in the seminiferous tubules as the initial event. However, decreased Leydig cell activity has been demonstrated in several disorders in which the seminiferous epithelium is believed to be primarily involved (de Kretser et al. 1975c). There is a reduced testosterone response to hCG in young men with germinal cell arrest or aplasia. This finding highlights the relative lack of knowledge of the relationships between the interstitial and tubular compartments of the testes. It may be possible that a progressive deterioration in Sertoli cell function, or depletion of germinal elements might be primary causes of the age-related testicular degeneration. Of the many other possibilities, vascular insufficiency and autoimmunity might be mentioned. Although the location of histological changes in the testes can be related to alterations in the microvasculature, this does not necessarily indicate the changes are ischaemic in origin. In fact the vascular changes may themselves be secondary to other processes (Sasano and Ichijo 1969; Suoranta 1971). With regard to auto-immunity it is interesting that the incidence of circulating sperm auto-antibodies increases with age, and inflammatory cells may be seen in the senescent testis (Frick 1969; Suoranta 1971; Fjallbrant 1975). Further studies including quantitative testicular histology are indicated.

4.5 Clinical Relevance

In the past the possibility that androgen deficiency might contribute to aging in men was entertained, and some equivocal studies of the effect of androgen replacement were reported (Korenchevsky et al. 1953; Freeman et al. 1956; Reiter 1963; Wesson 1964; Rigby et al. 1964; Editorial 1975; Albeaux-Fernet et al. 1978). A re-evaluation of androgen replacement therapy in the geriatric population might be worthwhile.

Knowledge that androgen production changes with age has led to new studies in patients with prostatic disease and evidence is accumulating that dihydrotestosterone levels are elevated in men with prostatic hypertrophy (Stearns et al. 1974; Horton et al. 1975; Vermeulen 1977). The tissue levels of dihydrotestosterone are increased in benign prostatic hypertrophy (Siiteri and Wilson 1970). The condition can be produced experimentally in castrated dogs by treatment with 3α-androstanediol, a steroid converted to dihydrotestosterone in the prostate, and the prostatic hypertrophy is greatly enhanced by simultaneous administration of oestradiol (Moore et al. 1979). Such studies may lead to a better understanding of the cause of this common condition and to effective medical therapy and prevention.

Increased oestrogen levels may also be related to the occurrence of "idiopathic" gynaecomastia in old men (Hall 1959). This possibility has not been investigated by modern methods.

Finally, further clinical research on the development of senescent testicular failure may give some insight into the aetiology of idiopathic oligospermia, which is a major cause of reduced fertility in younger men. The range of histological abnormalities in the aged testis is remarkably reminiscent of the findings in biopsies from men being investigated for infertility (Chap. 4).

4.6 Summary

A large number of endocrinological studies of testicular function in men of different ages suggest that primary testicular failure becomes common and more severe with aging. There is an increasing frequency of impotence, reduced secondary sex hair and testicular atrophy. Serum LH and FSH levels rise, androgen production rates and levels fall and oestrogen levels rise. The clearance of oestradiol falls but the production rate is maintained, in part, through increased peripheral conversion of testosterone to oestradiol. The levels of SHBG rise and free testosterone levels are reduced. Leydig cell responsiveness to hCG is probably reduced but gonadotrope responsiveness to GnRH reasonably maintained in the elderly. There are histological changes in the seminiferous epithelium of old men but these are non-specific. Senescent testicular failure is mainly a primary gonadal disorder but its cause and significance are only poorly understood.

5 Spermatogenesis and the Sertoli Cell

K.A. Rich and D.M. de Kretser

The pioneering studies by Greep and co-workers (Greep et al. 1936) established that two gonadotrophic hormones FSH and LH could be extracted from mammalian pituitary glands. From these observations and the studies of Smith on hypophysectomised animals (Smith 1930) the concept was developed that FSH acted on the seminiferous tubules and LH on the interstitial cells of the testis. Advances in the techniques available to isolate proteins has enabled purification and characterisation of the amino acid sequences of the peptide subunits FSH and LH. These purified glycoprotein hormones have been used to study the site and mechanism of action within the testis and have led to a better understanding of the gonadotrophic control of the testes. More recently, numerous studies have implicated prolactin as a third gonadotrophic hormone involved in the control of testicular function (see review Risbridger et al. 1981a). In view of the demonstration of receptors for prolactin (Aragona and Friesen 1975) and LH (de Kretser et al. 1971) on Leydig cells, the action of these hormones are considered in Chap. 6.

The concept that FSH acts on the seminiferous tubules has received much support in recent years. Prior to considering the mechanism of action of this hormone, a review of the numerous developments in our understanding of the structure and function of the seminiferous epithelium is attempted, to place the role of FSH in perspective.

Over 90% of the testicular mass in the rat is made up of the seminiferous tubules, which produce spermatozoa. The seminiferous tubules are highly coiled and form a complex pattern of convolutions. Basically they form loops that empty at both ends into the rete testis, which is drained by a number of ducts forming the ductuli efferentes. These ducts leave the testis and gradually fuse into a single, highly convoluted duct that forms the head, body and tail of the mammalian epididymis. Spermatozoa and seminiferous tubule fluid are transported in these tubules and ducts to the epididymis, wherein sperm maturation occurs. Fluid resorption occurs in the head and body of the epididymis while the tail is concerned with sperm storage (Setchell 1969).

5.1 Spermatogenesis

In the sexually mature mammal, the seminiferous epithelium consists of a non-proliferating population of Sertoli cells and germ cells at various stages of the spermatogenic process. The detailed studies of Clermont (1972) have

demonstrated an orderly sequence of development for each species and have established the concept that for each species the time taken for spermatogenesis is a biological constant. The process can be subdivided into three phases:
1. Replication by mitosis of the stem cells or spermatogonia.
2. Meiosis involving the primary and secondary spermatocytes and reduction of the diploid to the haploid chromosomal status.
3. Spermiogenesis, the complex metamorphosis resulting in the transformation of a "conventional" cell, the spermatid, into the spermatozoon.

5.1.1 The Spermatogenic Cycle

In the rat testis, spermatogenesis is observed to occur about a radial axis of co-ordination within each seminiferous tubule. This allows the development of germ cells to be traced by means of analysing the specific cellular associations of many different germ cells at various stages of maturation. LeBlond and Clermont (1952a) defined the characteristic changes taking place in the acrosome of the spermatid during its development (spermiogenesis) and correlated these changes with each of the specific cellular associations. The development of spermatids in the rat was subdivided into 19 steps; however, examination of the seminiferous tubules in cross section reveals only 14 well-defined cellular associations since step 1 to 8 spermatids are always associated with more mature spermatids (step 15 to 19). Thus, when spermatid development reaches step 15, a new generation of spermatids is formed in that area of seminiferous tubules, and the cycle repeats itself. On the basis of these findings, LeBlond and Clermont (1952b) defined the cycle of the seminiferous epithelium as "that series of changes occurring in a given area of the seminiferous epithelium between two successive appearances of the same cellular association".

The formation of specific cellular associations and the sequence of their appearance in a given area of the seminiferous tubule are highly synchronised. The numerical relationships between the various cell types within a cellular association and their absolute numbers within a cross section of a seminiferous tubule are highly consistent (Clermont 1972). The definition of these quantitative relationships of the seminiferous epithelial cells led to the development of exceedingly precise techniques for quantitative evaluation of cellular changes in the seminiferous tubules after damage to the spermatogenesis (Chowdhury and Steinberger 1964; Clermont and Morgentaler 1955; Oakberg 1956).

Once the conceptual and mathematical models for the spermatogenic process were established for the rat, similar models were developed for a number of other species. However, definition of the cycle of the seminiferous epithelium in man proved difficult since histological examination of the seminiferous tubules failed to reveal well-defined cellular associations. Using a similar principle to that described for other mammalian species, Clermont (1963) proposed that in man the entire cycle consists of six stages (Fig. 5.1). However, the detailed composition of the various cellular associations, as well as the numerical relationship remains poorly defined (Steinberger and Tjioe 1968).

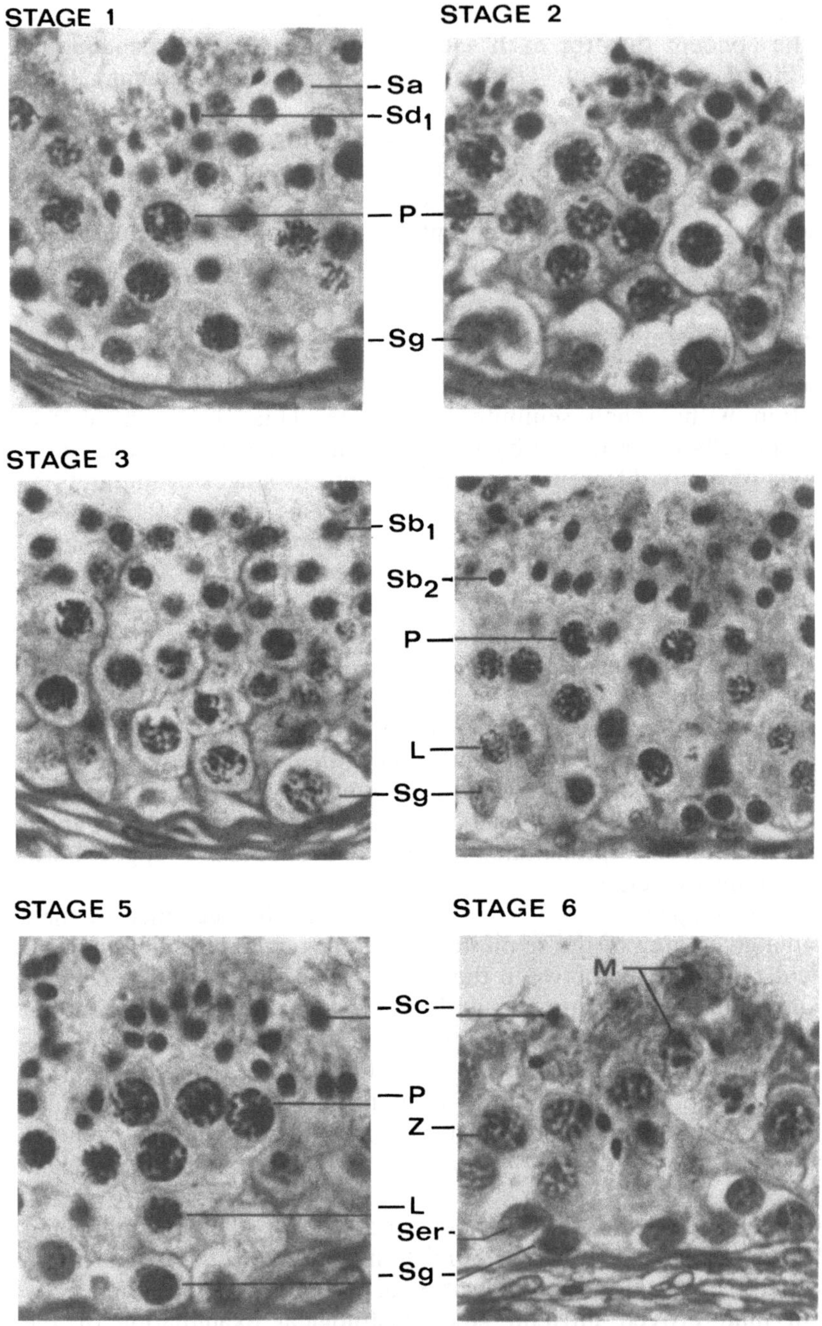

Fig. 5.1. Light micrographs illustrating the seminiferous cycle in the human testis using the staging proposed by Clermont (1963). *Sg*, spermatogonia; *L*, leptotene; *Z*, zygotene; *P*, pachytene primary spermatocytes; *Sa, Sb,* Sb_2, *Sc, Sd,* indicate spermatids; *Ser,* Sertoli cell nuclei; *M,* Meiosis (de Kretser et al. 1981)

5.1.2 Kinetics of the Spermatogenic Process

An analysis of the kinetics of spermatogenesis must consider the interaction between the temporal and spatial aspects of this process. Von Ebner (1871) formulated the concept of the wave of the seminiferous epithelium, and Regaud (1901) extended this concept and postulated that the "wave is in space what the cycle is in time".

Perey et al. (1961) confirmed the basic wave concept of von Ebner and Regaud, and by employing quantitative techniques, defined the wave in the seminiferous tubules of the rat testis with much greater precision. Extensive analysis of serial cross sections of the rat testis revealed that specific stages of the cycle are arranged in consecutive order along the tubule so that adjacent segments are either less or more advanced by a single stage; a wave of spermatogenesis therefore moves from the centre of the testis to the periphery, or in the reverse direction. The duration of each stage is not consistent, so that a length of tubule showing one particular stage of spermatogenesis might be much shorter than a length of tubule showing another stage.

In the rat each seminiferous tubule contains, on average, 12 complete spermatogenic waves, each approximately 2.6 cm in length (Perey et al. 1961). The mechanisms involved in synchronisation and the origin of the wave pattern are not clear. The pattern is probably set during fetal life or soon after

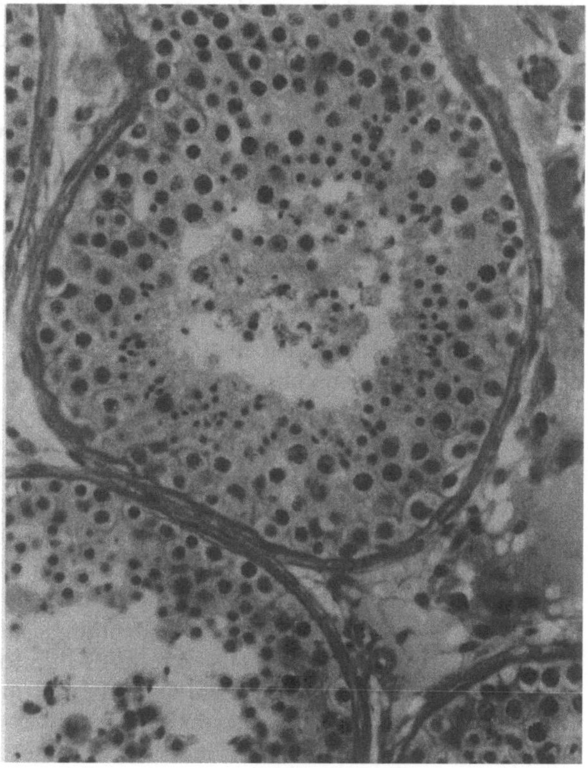

Fig. 5.2. Light micrograph of the human testis, showing that a number of stages of the seminiferous cycles can be seen in single cross sections of seminiferous tubules

birth (Clermont and Perey 1957). Although it seems possible that the Sertoli cells are in some way involved in the maintenance of this pattern, which depends on the mitotic activity of spermatogonia, details of the underlying mechanism are still unknown.

In contrast to that of other mammals, the human seminiferous epithelium in individual seminiferous tubules lacks a uniform wave of spermatogenesis. Thus, when a single tubule is examined in cross section, two or more stages may be present side by side in pie-shaped fashion (Fig 5.2). Chowdhury (1971) has suggested a clone concept for human spermatogenesis whereby each spermatogonium or a small group of spermatogonia form a clone of germ cells which proceed in their development independently of the surrounding groups of cells.

5.1.3 Duration of Spermatogenesis

The entire process of spermatogenesis or formation of spermatozoa from the least differentiating germ cell (A_1 spermatogonia) requires four cycles of the seminiferous epithelium in the rat. Using a variety of techniques the duration of spermatogenesis has been determined for a number of species. The difference in the duration of spermatogenesis is not only a species-species characteristic, but may also vary among various strains of rats: in the Long-Evans strain it was found to be 48 days (Steinberger 1962), but 51.6 days in the Sprague-Dawley strain (Clermont and Harvey 1965). In a study of the duration of the mitotic cycles of spermatogonia in the rat, Huckins (1971) observed that every 12.5 days a new sequence of spermatogonial maturation was initiated by the A_1 spermatogonia. Thus a new cycle of the seminiferous epithelium is initiated every 12.5 days.

In the human testis, Heller and Clermont (1964) used the incorporation of tritiated thymidine to demonstrate that the spermatogenic process took 70 ± 4 days.

5.1.4 Requirements for Quantitation of Spermatogenesis

The complex changes within the seminiferous epithelium, particularly in man where two to three cell associations may occupy one cross section of a seminiferous epithelium, make it necessary to provide quantitative data to support subjective impressions. Where specific cellular associations may be recognised, it is possible to quantitate the epithelium at that phase and to sample an adequate number of sections from different animals. However, in certain types of testicular damage, spermatids which simplify the recognition of specific cell associations may be absent and recourse may be necessary to using the primary spermatocyte and spermatogonial populations.

In states where cell associations are not easily recognisable or in the human testis due to overlap of these cell groupings, alternative methods have been suggested. Counting germ cells in relationship to known lengths of the seminiferous epithelium has been used (Steinberger and Tjioe 1968) whereas others have resorted to relating germ cell numbers to Sertoli cells (Skakkebaek and Heller 1973). The latter method assumes that the Sertoli cells do not alter their numbers, a proposition that does not hold during early development or during testicular damage.

5.2 The Sertoli Cell

The Sertoli cells are the only non-germ cell elements within the seminiferous tubules. They were first described by Sertoli in 1865 as columnar cells with cytoplasmic processes extending from the basement membrane to the lumen of the seminiferous tubule. The processes envelop the neighbouring germ cells to provide them with physical support and this close association has led to the concept that the Sertoli cells exert a "nurse" type of function. According to Regaud (1901) Sertoli believed that these cells formed a syncytium in the human testis, but as a result of his later studies in the rat, Sertoli (1878) reversed his opinion and maintained that they were independent of each other. This issue was settled by the electron microscopic studies of Fawcett and Burgos (1956), who demonstrated that the lateral and apical Sertoli cell surfaces were bounded by distinct cell membranes, cellular boundaries which were not readily visible with the limited resolution of the light microscope.

While the cytological differentiation of the germ cells has been exhaustively studied and described in elaborate detail, the fine structure of the Sertoli cells and their functions in the maintenance of spermatogenesis are still poorly understood. Von Ebner (1871) is credited with introducing the concept of a symbiotic relationship between the Sertoli cells and the developing germ cells. He defined the spermatoblast as the functional unit of the seminiferous epithelium and described it as consisting of a cluster of synchronously developing germ cells embedded in a club-like swelling of the apical portion of the supporting cell. Although the term spermatoblast fell into disuse, Elftman (1950) and Roosen-Runge (1962) stressed the usefulness of regarding the Sertoli cells and their associated germ cells as symbiotic units, even though evidence bearing on the nature and extent of the physiological interdependence of the two populations was still largely lacking.

In recent years, the Sertoli cells have become the subject of intensive investigations since evidence accumulated indicating that they may represent a target site for the action of FSH in the testis and secrete and androgen-binding protein (ABP), which responds to stimulation with FSH (reviewed in detail by Hansson et al. 1975a; and by Means 1975).

5.2.1 Morphological Characteristics

The cytoplasm of the Sertoli cell extends from the basal lamina to the lumen of the seminiferous tubule. Elftman (1963), using a silver-staining method, described the Sertoli cells "standing on the basement membrane in patterned array not unlike trees in an orchard". In tangential sections, the basal layer of spermatogonia is seen to be arranged in rings, or, more accurately, in a network organised around the bases of the Sertoli cells. This arrangement

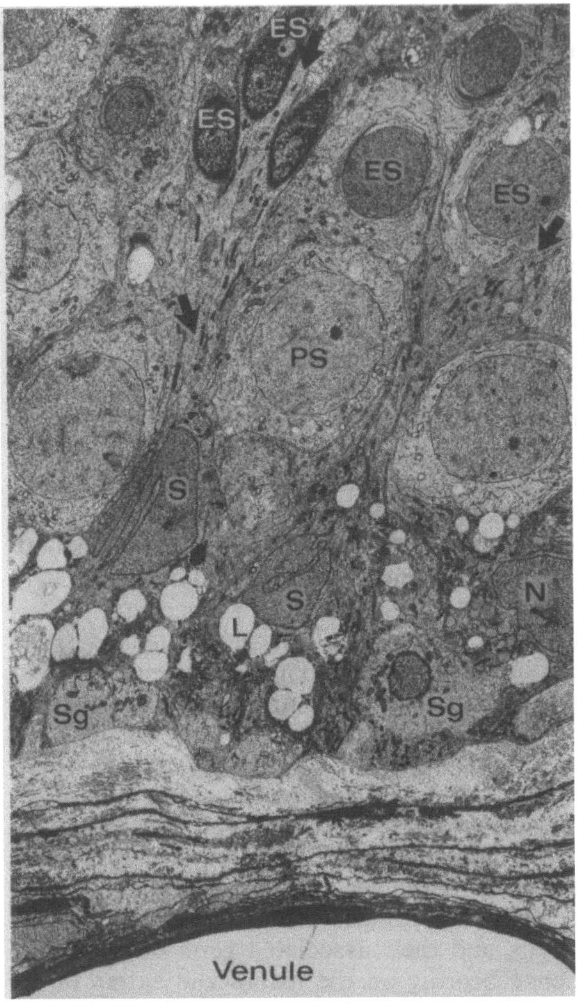

Fig. 5.3. General view illustrating the arrangement of the Sertoli cells *(S)* and germ cells. *Sg*, spermatogonia; *PS*, primary spermatocyte; *ES*, early spermatid; *LS*, late spermatid. Note processes of Sertoli cell cytoplasm *(arrows)*, lipid inclusions *(L)* and nuclei *(N)*. The lamina propria and a venule are shown. Micrograph by courtesy of Dr. J.B. Kerr. × 2500

of the spermatogonia determines the distribution of the more advanced germ cell stages derived from them, which when displaced upwards, maintain their close relationship with the sides of the supporting Sertoli cells. Thin processes of Sertoli cell cytoplasm extend laterally between the associated germ cells and partially or often completely surround them (Fig. 5.3).

5.2.2 Nucleus

The nucleus of the Sertoli cell was described by classical cytologists as irregularly oval or pyramidal with its long axis perpendicular to the lamina propria of the seminiferous tubule. The nuclei frequently form a single row lying central to the spermatogonia though some changes in the position of the nuclei occur in different phases of the spermatogenic cycle. Examination of thinner sections by electron microscopy has shown its shape to be much more complex than was appreciated with the light microscope. The nuclear features of mature Sertoli cells include an infolded nuclear membrane, a relatively homogeneous nucleoplasm, and a single tripartite nucleolus. The nucleolus proper, which incorporates RNA precursors, appears in the electron microscope as a reticular structure accompanied by two electron-dense, smaller structures composed of heterochromatin. These structures do not incorporate RNA precursors, stain positively with Feulgen reagent, and are referred to as heteropycnotic bodies, juxtanuclear bodies or satellite karyosomes. The functional significance of the tripartite nucleolar structure is not understood at present (Fawcett 1975).

5.2.3 Cytoplasm

The basal and perinuclear regions of the Sertoli cell contain a rich supply of organelles and inclusions. Mitochondria are usually randomly distributed but in the human, aggregations are often seen immediately adjacent to the basement membrane of the tubule. Granular endoplasmic reticulum is found predominantly in the basal cytoplasm as parallel stacks of cisternae. Smooth endoplasmic reticulum is scattered throughout the cytoplasm as a system of small vesicles or anastomosing tubules. Increased aggregations are observed in many species within the cytoplasm that immediately surrounds the heads of developing spermatids. This complex may serve as a specialised form of support, enabling cohesion to be maintained between the spermatid and Sertoli cell although it may be involved in metabolic exchange between these cell types (Fawcett 1975).

Concentric arrays of smooth endoplasmic reticulum, often surrounding lipid inclusions, are found in the basal aspects of the cell. Earlier ultrastructural studies referred to these structures as lamellar bodies but frequently the membranes were connected by many small annuli resembling the size and shape of nuclear pores. These features suggest that they are similar to the annulate lamellae found in other tissues. The Golgi apparatus is not a single organelle localised in a constant position as it is in the many other cell types. Instead, in electron micrographs, it appears to consist of multiple separate Golgi elements scattered through the basal cytoplasm and occasionally in the supranuclear region. Each Golgi complex of the Sertoli cell consists of a few short, parallel cisternae and associated small vesicles. There are no larger vacuoles or membrane-bound granules to suggest the segregation and concentration of secretory products (Fawcett 1975) although secretion of ABP by the Sertoli cell has now been firmly established (Fritz et al. 1976; Rommerts et al. 1978). As yet no specific function can be assigned to the Golgi apparatus in this cell type.

Various crystalline inclusions are observed in the cytoplasm of the human Sertoli cell; the reason for their presence is obscure. Such filamentous inclusions are collectively referred to as crystals of Charcot-Böttcher (Fawcett and Burgos 1956).

Lysosomal structures are scattered throughout the cytoplasm and are assumed to aid in the destruction of degenerating germ cells and residual bodies released by the spermatids during spermiation (Reddy and Svoboda 1967). A phagocytic function for the Sertoli cells was originally suggested by Maximow (1899). Subsequent studies have demonstrated that Sertoli cells ingest damaged germ cells, vital dyes and particulate matter (Clegg and McMillan 1965).

Parallel arrays of microtubules within the intermediate and particularly the apical regions of the Sertoli cell have been described in numerous studies (Fawcett 1975). The abundance of microtubules is most obvious in Sertoli cells supporting late cap-phase and more advanced spermatids. In the Sertoli cells microtubules have usually been interpreted merely as cytoskeletal elements providing internal support for the columnar portion of the cell, but they may also be actively involved in the movements of cytoplasm that are responsible for the displacements of the late spermatids upwards or downwards in the epithelium at different stages of spermiogenesis (Fawcett 1975). Means et al. (1978) have recently proposed that the cytoskeletal network comprising microtubules and microfilaments may be controlled by changes in calcium ion flux, via the intracellular receptor protein calcium dependent regulator (CDR), and that by affecting these intracellular components, FSH may regulate specific protein secretion and motility of the Sertoli cell.

The lipid content of Sertoli cells is highly variable from species to species both in respect of its total amount and in the size of the lipid droplets. In the rat, lipid droplets are most abundant in stages IX to II of the spermatogenic cycle (Kerr and de Kretser 1975). The lipid present immediately after spermiation is presumed to be derived largely from phagocytosis of residual bodies. After heat, X-irradiation or oestrogen treatment, the amount of Sertoli cell lipid is observed to increase, sometimes quite markedly (Collins and Lacy 1969).

These observations led Lacy (1962) to propose that in the normal cycle the ingestion of the residual bodies by the Sertoli cells provides material utilised by those cells in the synthesis of one or more steroids that act as local hormones, stimulating spermatocyctes to complete meiosis and thus replenish the supply of spermatids for the next cycle. On the other hand, Kerr and de Kretser (1975) obtained evidence suggestive of a transfer of these lipid inclusions from the Sertoli cells to primary spermatocyctes late in meiotic prophase. There is as yet no evidence that the lipid is utilised by the Sertoli cell for steroid biosynthesis, although the Sertoli cells have been shown to be capable of forming testosterone from exogenous progesterone (Tcholakian and Steinberger 1978) and to aromatise exogenous testosterone to oestradiol in vitro (Dorrington and Armstrong 1975).

Many investigations suggest that the Sertoli cell qualifies on morphological grounds as a cell with the potential for steroid biosynthesis. There is agreement amongst morphologists concerning the organelles which are commonly present within steroid-secreting cells (Christensen 1975). These characteristics include an extensive smooth endoplasmic reticulum, a prominent Golgi apparatus, mitochondria of variable shape and internal structure, often with tubular cristae, numerous lysosomes and lipid inclusions which vary in number depending on the species. The foregoing discussion has indicated that these structures are indeed characteristics of the Sertoli cell.

5.2.4 Inter-Sertoli Cell Junctions

Many substances in the blood plasma are retarded or excluded from the lumen of the seminiferous tubule. This barrier to the penetration of substances has been termed the blood-testis barrier and has been documented from both a physiological (Setchell and Waites 1975) and a structural standpoint (Dym and Fawcett 1970; Fawcett et al. 1970). The morphological basis for this barrier is attributed to the presence of parallel rows of occluding junctions between adjacent Sertoli cells. The effectiveness of the junctions in functioning as a permeability barrier was demonstrated by Dym and Fawcett (1970), and by Dym (1973). They found that if electron-opaque extracellular tracers such as lanthanum or peroxidase were injected interstitially or during perfusion fixation, their continued passage into the seminiferous epithelium was always prevented by the occluding Sertoli cell junction.

The occluding junctions are one component of what has been termed the "junctional complex" or "junctional specialisation". These junctional complexes are found near the base of the epithelium, and are characterised by sub-surface cisternae and bundles of filaments on the inner surfaces of the apposed cell membranes of adjacent Sertoli cells (Flickinger and Fawcett 1967). The filaments have been shown to contain actin (Toyama 1976) and thus may have a contractile function. In these extensive junctional complexes the outer leaflets of the membranes in some areas of the junction are 150–200 Å apart, but in other areas they approach to within 20 Å of one another as in the gap junctions or nexuses of other cell types (Fig. 5.4). In addition, there are often multiple focal tight junctions along the length of the junctional complex where the outer leaflets of the apposing membranes appear to be fused (Dym and Fawcett 1970).

These unique junctional specialisations between Sertoli cells probably have multiple functions. In addition to the obvious general function of helping to maintain the structural integrity of the epithelium, the areas of very close approximation of the membranes (20 Å) probably constitute low-resistance pathways providing for cell-to-cell communications, whereas the linear tight junctions effectively seal the intracellular cleft and consistute the intra-epithelial component of the blood-testis barrier (Fawcett 1975).

The Sertoli cell junctional complexes divide the seminiferous epithelium into basal (spermatogonia and pre-leptotene primary spermatocytes) and adluminal (later stages of germ cells) compartments. The complexes may provide a structural basis for the maintenance of a different milieu in each of these compartments, which may be crucial during specific stages of germ cell development. Such a function of the junctional complexes seems to be suggested by their development in the rat between the 15th and 18th post-natal day, at the time when spermatocytes appear in the seminiferous tubules. Formation of the specialised junctions coincides with the cessation of Sertoli cell proliferation (Steinberger and Steinberger 1971) and occurs in the absence of germ cells (Means et al. 1976). Furthermore, de Kretser and

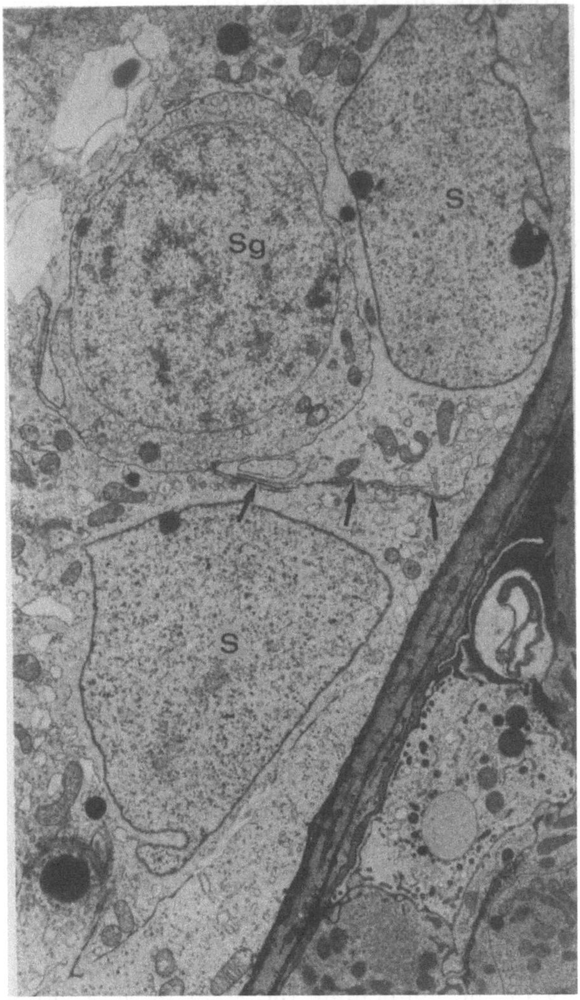

Fig. 5.4. Occurrence of specialised cell junctions *(arrows)* between adjacent Sertoli cells *(S)*. Note the presence of lanthanum in the intertubular tissue and in the intercellular space between spermatogonia *(Sg)* and Sertoli cell *(S)*. Micrograph by courtesy of Dr. J.B. Kerr. × 6600

Burger (1972) have shown that Sertoli cell tight junctions are not present between the immature Sertoli cells of adult men with hypogonadotrophic hypogonadism, but were formed in response to administration of exogenous gonadotrophins.

The existence of the inter-Sertoli cell junctions means that the Sertoli cells form a continuous epithelial layer, which thus prevents diffusion of substances into the intercellular spaces. Therefore every substance of nutritional or regulatory character has to pass through the cytoplasm of the Sertoli cell in order to reach the germ cells residing in the adluminal compartment.

It is clear that the junctional complexes must periodically allow movement of the germ cells from the basal to the adluminal compartment. Several investigators have considered the mechanism by which this might occur. Nicander (1967) observed Sertoli-Sertoli junctional specialisations to be present both below and above young spermatocytes. Both Nicander (1967) and Dym and Fawcett (1970) postulated breakdown and formation of tight junctions as the mechanism by which cells are transferred from the basal to the adluminal compartment. Ross and Dobler (1975) agreed that tight junctions above the Sertoli cell break down, but believed that the sub-surface specialisations remained intact. They proposed that as the spermatocyctes move between two Sertoli cells, they attach to the freed junctional surface and remain attached until their release into the tubule lumen.

However, Russell (1977) was unable to find any junctional specialisations facing leptotene spermatocytes, and demonstrated that the occluding junctions between adjacent Sertoli cells remained intact during the upward movement of the leptotene cells and did not dissociate until the new junctional complex below was well established. The Sertoli cells thus play an active role in the transfer of spermatocytes to the adluminal compartment. Russell (1977) has described that the leptotene spermatocytes may exist in a transitional compartment formed by cytoplasmic extensions and tight junctions of Sertoli cells both basal and adluminal to the spermatocyte. While Dym and Cavicchia (1977) also observed that a number of early spermatocytes were enclosed by Sertoli-Sertoli cell tight junctions both above and below in their study of the monkey testis, they refuted the idea of an intermediate compartment.

These results indicate that the inititiation of meiosis occurs while the early spermatocytes (pre-leptotene and leptotene) are still in the basal compartment of the epithelium and may not require the special micro-evironment provided by the Sertoli cells in the adluminal compartment. The ultimate fate of the Sertoli-Sertoli tight junctions above the zygotene spermatocytes remains a subject of controversy. However, it has recently been suggested that specific proteases, such as plasminogen activator, may play a role in the breakdown of these junctions. Cultured Sertoli cells secrete a plasminogen activator into the medium, the production of which is stimulated by FSH (Lacroix et al. 1977).

5.2.5 Sertoli Cell Maturation

Classically, only fully mature Sertoli cells are referred to by this name, while their precursors are usually termed supporting or sustentacular cells. In the pre-pubertal testis, the immature Sertoli cells exhibit a characteristic ovoid nucleus with the chromatin scattered throughout the nucleoplasm and usually clumped at the nuclear membrane. Maturation of the testis transforms the immature Sertoli cells into tall elaborately shaped cells with a characteristic prominent nucleolus (Sniffen 1952; Flickinger 1967).

In all species proliferation of the Sertoli cells ceases shortly after birth. In the rat and the ram, the Sertoli cells cease dividing and remain in constant interphase concurrent with the initiation of the meiotic prophase of the primary spermatocytes (Clermont and Perey 1957). Cessation of Sertoli cell division may be linked to a functional change within the seminiferous epithelium necessary for the continued meiotic maturation of the germ cells in close association with the Sertoli cell. Additionally, the nuclear and nucleolar characteristics, the specialised inter-Sertoli cell junctions and the development of smooth endoplasmic reticulum appear to be dependent on gonadotrophic stimulation (Flickinger 1967; de Kretser and Burger 1972). Many studies have noted that all phases of germ cell differentiation occur in intimate contact with the Sertoli cell, which exhibits extensive cytoplasmic ramifications throughout the depth of the seminiferous epithelium. Many of the modifications to the Sertoli cell noted during studies on the maturation of the mammalian testis are consistent with the proposal of Roosen-Runge (1962) that the Sertoli cell plays an important if not central role in the initiation of the spermatogenic cycle.

5.2.6 Secretory Products

5.2.6.1 Seminiferous Tubule Fluid

It has been recognised for some time that the seminiferous tubules secrete a fluid which carries the spermatozoa out of the testis and into the epididymis. Secretion of seminiferous tubule fluid in the rat testis begins at around 25 days of age, corresponding to the time at which early spermatids are first evident and a few days after the formation of the blood-testis barrier. The rate of formation of free-flow tubule fluid is approximately 21 μl/h/testis in adult rats (Setchell 1970). It is thought that most of the fluid collected from the efferent ducts after ligation is derived from the seminiferous tubule. Although the contribution of the rete testis to tubule fluid formation is relatively small, the equilibration between components in tubule fluid and interstitial lymph may occur in the rete area (see Fritz and Dorrington 1977).

Studies using micropuncture techniques have shown that seminiferous tubule fluid contains very high concentrations of potassium and bicarbonate, and low levels of sodium and chloride, in comparison to that of blood plasma (Tuck et al. 1970; Levine and Marsh 1975). It has also been shown that the tubule fluid collected from both human and rat testes contains very much less protein but proportionately more specific proteins than that of blood plasma (Kormano et al. 1971; Koskimies and Kormano 1973; Koskimies et al. 1973).

The Sertoli cell is believed to be responsible for the production of seminiferous tubule fluid, although direct evidence for this is still lacking (Waites 1977). The evidence for the Sertoli cell origin of this secretion is based on the finding that testes which had been depleted of germ cells by pre-natal treatment with the drug busulphan continued to produce tubule fluid (Setchell 1969). It has been suggested that fluid secretion in the tubules may be dependent on the development of the tight junctions between adjacent Sertoli cells for creation of a standing gradient in the adluminal compartment. If solute was pumped by the Sertoli cells from the interstitial extracellular fluid into the intercellular spaces above the occluding junctions, making the fluid there hypertonic, water would then be drawn in to make the intercellular fluid isosmotic. Fluid would then flow along the intercellular spaces into the lumen of the seminiferous tubules. This mechanism has been proposed by Setchell (1969), but remains unproven.

The fact that the seminiferous tubules do not have a lumen, and fluid secretion by the epithelium does not begin until about the time of first appearance of occluding junctions between Sertoli cells (Flickinger 1967; Vitale et al. 1973) strongly suggests that fluid secretion in the tubules may be dependent on development of the necessary morphological relations in the epithelium for creation of a standing gradient in the adluminal compartment.

The hormonal regulation of seminiferous fluid production is ill defined. Local heating of the testes, surgically induced cryptorchidism and hypophysectomy all lead to a decrease in total fluid secretion (Setchell 1970; Setchell and Waites 1972; Hagenas et al. 1978). Evidence for impaired secretion of fluid in states of testicular damage comes from the study by Levine and Marsh (1975) showing altered ionic composition of primary tubule fluid in sterile tubules of busulphan-treated animals, in comparison to adjacent tubules with active spermatogenesis. The sterile tubules were found to have decreased potassium and increased sodium levels. The disruption of the lymph-tubule fluid potassium gradient may result from damage to the Sertoli cells, or from impaired Sertoli cell–germ cell interactions. Furthermore, as discussed in Chap. 7, numerous agents which disrupt spermatogenesis, interfere with the capabilities of the Sertoli cells to secrete fluid.

5.2.6.2 Androgen-Binding Protein

The first secretory protein to be characterised and shown to derive from the Sertoli cell was the testicular androgen binding protein, ABP. Paradoxically, ABP was first identified in the epididymis and only later found to derive from the testis (French and Ritzen 1973), more specifically from the Sertoli cell (Fritz et al. 1974; Tindall et al. 1974; Hagenas et al. 1975). With the discovery of ABP and methods for its quantitation (Ritzen et al. 1981), a biochemical marker of Sertoli cell secretory function was available for study of the hormonal regulation of Sertoli cell function.

Direct evidence for production of ABP by the Sertoli cell was derived from experiments conducted in vitro with cultures of isolated Sertoli cells (Steinberger et al. 1975; Fritz et al. 1976). Cultured Sertoli cells were shown to secrete ABP into the medium and to respond to FSH stimulation with increased ABP production (Steinberger et al. 1975; Fritz et al. 1976; Rommerts et al. 1978). Testosterone has also been shown to be effective in stimulating ABP secretion in vitro (Louis and Fritz 1977).

ABP has been well characterised in the rat (Ritzen et al. 1973; Musto et al. 1978) and in the rabbit (Weddington et al. 1975b). In the rat, ABP was shown to be a protein with a molecular weight of about 90000. It shows a high affinity for 5α-dihydrotestosterone, with a K_D of approximately 10^{-9} *M*, while other steroids show little binding. ABP is secreted with the fluid from the seminiferous tubules through the rete testis and the efferent ducts into the epididymis, where it is degraded or taken up by the epithelial cells lining the epididymal duct.

ABP has been found to be closely similar to the testosterone-oestradiol binding globulin (TeBG), which circulates in the blood of most species, including man. In fact the presence of TeBG in the human has complicated the clear demonstration of the existence of ABP in this species. This controversial issue has not yet been settled, and there are proponents both for (Hsu et al. 1977) and against (Vigersky et al. 1976) the existence of ABP in the human. More recently Purvis et al. (1978) have claimed that from the proportion of transcortin found within testicular cytosols made from human testes, the ABP activity measured is the result of contamination by TeBG. However, the recent demonstration that Sertoli cells in culture can maintain other plasma proteins, e.g. transferrin, must now raise doubts about the above explanation (Skinner and Griswold 1980). Measurement of ABP in the rat is, however, simplified by the absence of TeBG in the blood of this species (Corvol and Bardin 1973).

Comparison of partially purified preparations of ABP and TeBG in the rabbit has shown that they cross-react immunologically (Weddington et al. 1975b). After purification, the only difference in their physical characteristics was a slightly different charge (Hansson et al. 1975c). Thus very similar, if not identical, glycoproteins seem to be produced by two different organs (testis and liver) under completely different regulatory control.

The purification (Musto et al. 1978) and the subsequent development of a radioimmunoassay (Gunsalus et al. 1978a) for rat ABP has made possible the measurement of vastly smaller levels of ABP than was possible using the polyacrylamide gel system developed by Ritzen et al. (1974). Antibodies against purified ABP were utilised to detect an immunoreactive material in the peripheral blood of male rats. It was shown that this material binds steroid and is the same size as native ABP (Musto et al. 1978). It was hoped that antibodies raised against the purified rat ABP could have been used to study human ABP. Unfortunately, it has been found that the antisera show no cross-reactivity with testicular and epididymal extracts from a wide variety of mammalian species, including man.

Since the polyacrylamide assay system could not detect ABP in plasma it was thought that it was secreted only in a luminal direction. However, Gunsalus et al. (1978b) were able to detect immunoreactive ABP in the serum of male, but not female rats. Surprisingly, ABP was also detected in the amniotic fluid of both male and female rat fetuses but the significance of this finding is unknown at present (Musto et al. 1978).

Further studies by this group indicating that ABP is released into the blood from the testis, most probably from the basal aspect of the Sertoli cells, raises the possibility that seminiferous tubule function could be studied by monitoring ABP levels in plasma. Preliminary results of plasma ABP levels in rats with seminiferous tubule damage failed to show any major changes, despite markedly decreased levels of immunoreactive ABP in the epididymis (Gunsalus et al. 1978b). However, more detailed longitudinal studies of gonadal disorders need to be carried out to determine whether the release of ABP into the blood is controlled by factors which are independent of transport to the epididymis.

It is almost a decade since the detection of ABP, and yet its physiological role is still obscure (Rommerts et al. 1976). Possible functions for ABP include a role as an intracellular carrier of testosterone or dihydrotestosterone in the Sertoli cell itself, or as a carrier of testosterone from the testis into the epididymis.

5.2.6.3 Inhibin

The existence of a testicular substance, capable of selectively suppressing the secretion of FSH from the pituitary, was postulated by McCullagh (1932). In the past 15 years, considerable evidence has accumulated in support of the original hypothesis. The proof that Sertoli cells were capable of secreting this factor was provided by the work of Steinberger and Steinberger (1976), who demonstrated that media collected from cultures of isolated Sertoli cells were capable of selectively inhibiting the release of FSH by cultured anterior pituitary cells. This finding has since been confirmed by a number of other laboratories (de Jong et al. 1978, 1978; Labrie et al. 1978) and is considered in more detail in Chap. 2.

5.2.6.4 Plasminogen Activator

Lacroix et al. (1977) have provided evidence that cultured Sertoli cells from immature rats secrete a specific protease, plasminogen activator. Like ABP, the activity of this protein was shown to be increased by addition of FSH or dibutyryl cyclic AMP to the medium during culture. The authors speculate that the protease may play a role in the opening of the occluding inter-Sertoli cell junctions to allow passage of germ cells from the basal to the adluminal compartment of the epithelium.

5.2.6.5 Other Secretory Products

The above-mentioned proteins have been identified as specific for Sertoli cells. However, Sertoli cells in culture secrete a large number of other proteins, which have not yet been characterised. Among these, albumin-like proteins are in a majority (Rommerts et al. 1978, 1979). It is possible that most of the proteins found in primary seminiferous tubule fluid are actually derived from the Sertoli cells (Kormano et al. 1971; Koskimies and Kormano 1973). Furthermore, some of the most potent regulators of gonadal differentiation in the embryo appear to derive from the Sertoli cells or their precursors; these are the meiosis-preventing substance (MPS) (Byskov and Saxen 1976; Byskov 1978) and Mullerian-inhibiting hormone (Josso et al. 1977).

The glutamate, inositol, and other small molecular weight substances characteristic of the tubule fluid are also probably the products of Sertoli cells. The recent report that Sertoli cells in culture can convert glucose to inositol (see Fritz and Dorrington 1977) lends support to this proposal; however, the capacity of other testicular cell types to do so has not yet been determined.

It has been pointed out elsewhere that the Sertoli cells have a number of cytological characteristics of steroid-secreting cells and are said to have the capacity to synthesise testosterone from steroid precursors in vitro (Tcholakian and Steinberger 1978; Welsh and Wiebe 1978). It is not possible, however, to establish whether the testosterone found in the rete testis fluid is secreted by the Sertoli cells or whether it traverses the epithelium from the interstitium (Setchell et al. 1978). Whether this capacity is physiologically important in vivo remains to be demonstrated. Androgen is essential for spermatogenesis, but certainly most of it is produced by the Leydig cells in the interstitial tissue.

5.2.7 Steroidogenic Activity

The Leydig cells have generally been accepted as the major site of steroid biosynthetic activity in the testis. The possibility that the seminiferous tubule might also possess the capacity to produce steroids was suggested by the occurrence of tumours in the dog, believed to originate from the Sertoli cells, which secrete oestrogens (Huggins and Moulder 1945). The abundance of smooth endoplasmic reticulum in the Sertoli cell has been interpreted as morphological evidence of steroidogenic capacity (Christensen 1975).

Several investigators have reported the ability of isolated seminiferous tubules to form various androgens, including testosterone, from endogenous precursors or from exogenous C_{21} compounds (Christensen and Mason 1965). However, Sertoli cells are deficient in both 3β-hydroxysteroid dehydrogenase and in cholesterol side-chain cleavage activity, which are only present within the Leydig cells of the testis (Hall et al. 1969).

Preparations of Sertoli cells from immature rats have been shown to possess 3β-hydroxysteroid dehydrogenase and 5α-reductase activity (Dorrington and Fritz 1975). More recently, these investigators have also reported aromatisation of exogenous testosterone to oestradiol by cultured Sertoli cells from immature rats, and the stimulation of its production by FSH (Dorrington et al. 1975). However, the question as to whether Sertoli cells in the adult rat testis produce oestradiol is a controversial issue at the present time, since Valladares and Payne (1979) have shown that aromatase activity in the adult rat testis is located within the interstitial cell fraction. The ability of FSH to stimulate oestrogen synthesis in Sertoli cells is lost by 30 days of age (Dorrington et al. 1978). Nonetheless, it is generally accepted that Sertoli cells from the immature or adult rat testis are capable of forming testosterone from exogenous progesterone precursors in vitro (Tcholakian and Steinberger 1978; Welsh and Wiebe 1978) and more recently from more distant precursors.

The physiological significance of the capacity for testosterone synthesis and metabolism by the Sertoli cell is not clear at the present time. It would seem feasible that either testosterone or its metabolites may affect some biological activity within the Sertoli cell, be made available to the developing germ cells, or alternatively have some effect outside of the seminiferous tubule. The presence of oestrogen receptors in interstitial cells (Mulder et al. 1974) and a direct effect of oestradiol on testosterone synthesis in the testis has been demonstrated (Samuels et al. 1964; Chowdhury et al. 1977). It has been proposed that oestrogens formed by the Sertoli cells may affect testosterone biosynthesis in the Leydig cells, and that interaction between products formed by the interstitial and tubule compartments may be of importance in the overall expression of steroidogenic activity in the testis (discussed in Chap. 6). Furthermore, Cigorraga et al. (1980) have demonstrated that the induction of desensitisation of the testis following large doses of hCG can be blocked by tamoxifen and have therefore implicated oestradiol in this process (discussed further in Chap. 6).

5.2.8 Hormonal Regulation of Sertoli Cell Function

The formation of the concept that many, if not all, of the hormonal effects on spermatogenesis are executed through the Sertoli cells is one of the most important developments in the understanding of the control of testicular function in recent years. Studies on the function of the Sertoli cells, and its response to hormones, became possible with the discovery of a specific Sertoli cell marker, ABP. A schematic drawing of the current concept of the sites of hormone action on the testis is shown in Fig. 5.5.

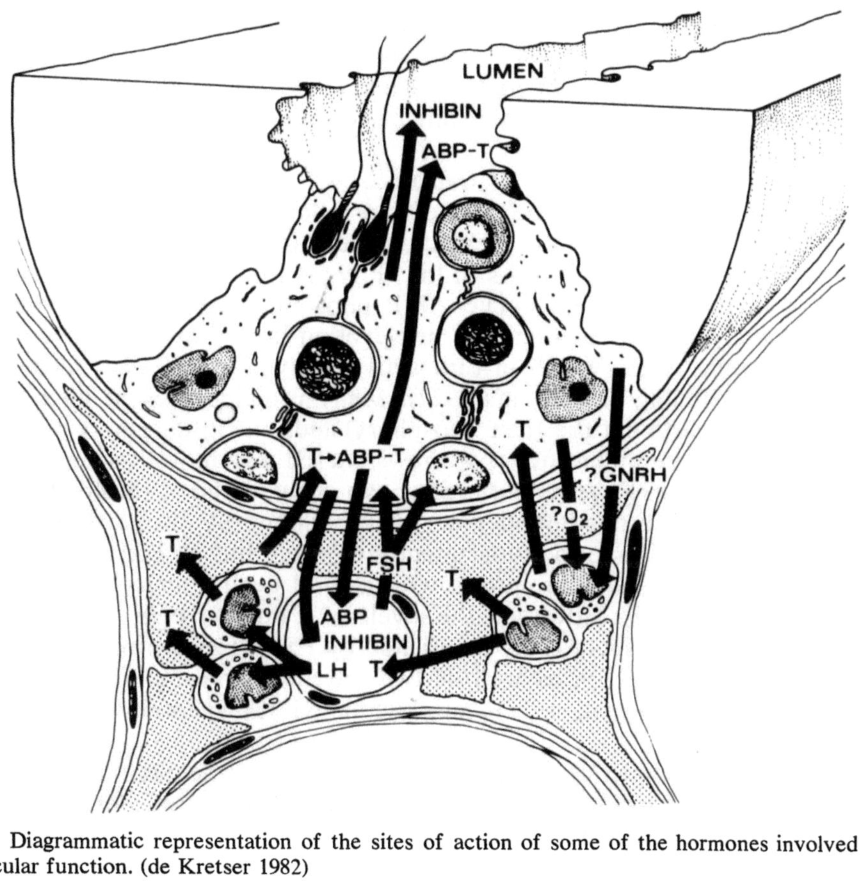

Fig. 5.5. Diagrammatic representation of the sites of action of some of the hormones involved in testicular function. (de Kretser 1982)

5.2.9 Actions of FSH on the Sertoli Cell

One of the first reports of the effects of hormones on the Sertoli cell was the study by Murphy (1965) showing morphological changes in the Sertoli cells following injection of FSH into hypophysectomised rats. Later electron microscopic studies by Castro et al. (1970, 1972) showed that ferritin-labelled FSH bound preferentially to the Sertoli cell, rather than to germ cells. Recent studies by Orth and Christensen (1977), using radio-iodinated FSH, have confirmed and extended the earlier observations. They demonstrated that the receptor sites for FSH were localised in the basal region of the seminiferous epithelium, a finding which may have important functional implications. More recent findings by these investigators have suggested that, in addition to Sertoli cells, spermatogonia have binding sites for FSH (Orth and Christensen 1978).

The sequence of biochemical events in the rat testis which are initiated by the action of FSH has been extensively studied in recent years by Means and co-workers (reviewed by Means et al. 1976). In order to demonstrate specific effects on the Sertoli cells after in vivo administration of hormones, these workers have routinely used animals with "Sertoli cell-enriched" (SCE) testes, in which the majority of germ cells have been destroyed as a result of pre-natal irradiation. Studies to be described later in this book suggest that testicular function in these pathological testes may not be entirely normal, since the Sertoli cells are also damaged by the irradiation treatment. However, the dysfunction of the Sertoli cells in fetal irradiated testes has a gradual onset, and is not severe in the immature animals used by Means and co-workers in their studies.

Studies on the responses of immature SCE rats to in vivo administration of FSH have allowed elucidation of the following sequence of events. The binding of FSH to receptors located on the plasma membrane of Sertoli cells (Fakunding et al. 1976) results in the activation of adenyl cyclase and a decrease in the activity of cyclic AMP phosophodiesterase. Together these altered enzyme activities lead to an elevation in the intracellular concentration of cyclic AMP, which in turn activates cyclic AMP-dependent protein kinase (Fakunding and Means 1977). Many proteins present in every subcellular compartment are then phosphorylated, but to date no single protein substrate has been identified that shows altered activity following phosphorylation. All of these events outlined above occur within 1–3 min of exposure to FSH and reach maximal degrees of stimulation by 30 min. Rates of RNA and protein synthesis are subsequently elevated but no convincing data are available to link these processes with altered cyclic nucleotide metabolism (Means et al. 1976). However, the levels of a number of proteins have now been shown to be specifically stimulated by FSH. These proteins include the secretory protein ABP, as well as two intracellular proteins, protein kinase inhibitor (Beale et al. 1977) and γ-glutamyl transpeptidase (Hodgen and Sherins 1973).

More direct evidence for the action of FSH on the Sertoli cell has come from studies of isolated Sertoli cells in culture. Cultured Sertoli cells from immature rats respond to FSH by increasing mitotic activity (Griswold et al.

1977) and by increasing the secretion not only of ABP, but also of cyclic AMP (Dorrington et al. 1975), plasminogen activator (Lacroix et al. 1977), oestradiol (Dorrington and Armstrong 1975), and metabolites of androstenedione (Welsh and Wiebe 1976, 1978).

FSH is known to be necessary for the initiation of spermatogenesis in the immature rat, but once spermatogenesis is established, it can be maintained in the hypophysectomised rat by testosterone or dihydrotestosterone (Ahmad et al. 1973). The maintenance of spermatogenesis by gonadotrophin or androgen supplementation is paralleled by the stimulatory effects of these hormones on ABP production (Hansson et al. 1976). Thus the two hormones which are known to be crucial for spermatogenesis have been shown to exert at least part of their effects through the Sertoli cells. Hansson et al. (1975b) claim that the effect of FSH administration on ABP synthesis in the hypophysectomised rat is dramatically enhanced in rats maintained on high doses of androgens, and thus the two hormones act synergistically on the Sertoli cell. However, Tindall et al. (1978a) were unable to demonstrate such a synergistic effect using a similar experimental design.

5.2.10 Effects of Androgen on the Sertoli Cell

Androgenic hormones alone can stimulate ABP production and maintain spermatogenesis. In accordance with these findings, cytoplasmic androgen receptors have been identified both in seminiferous tubules (Mulder et al. 1975) and in isolated Sertoli cells (Grootegoed et al. 1977; Sanborn et al. 1977). Furthermore, testosterone enhances ABP production in vitro (Louis and Fritz 1977). The fact that ABP is present in testes of *tfm* rats which lack androgen receptors (Hansson et al. 1978) suggests that androgen is not obligatory for the production of ABP by the Sertoli cell.

Thus it is clear that Sertoli cells are target cells for androgens; however, although it appears unlikely that androgens can directly affect the germ cell population of the testis, conclusive evidence is lacking. While some investigators have claimed to show the presence of androgen receptors in germ cells (Galena et al. 1974) more recent studies have produced negative findings (Grootegoed et al. 1977).

The elegant experiments performed by Lyon et al. (1975) may also be interpreted as evidence that the Sertoli cells, but not the germ cells, are target cells for androgens. These workers showed that male chimaeras of normal mice and mice carrying the *tfm* gene produced sperm bearing the *tfm* mutation on the x chromosome. It was postulated that the germ cells bearing the *tfm* mutation may have developed normally in these animals because adjacent XY Sertoli cells contributed to a localised environment conducive to germ cell development. In addition, the X chromosome bearing the *tfm* locus is normally activated no later than the early prophase of meiosis during spermatogenesis in mammals (Monesi 1974), suggesting that specific androgen receptors are not synthesised after this stage of differentiation.

The acute intravenous administration of FSH to 14- to 16-day-old rats causes a rapid (within 2 h) increase in the testicular content of ABP (Tindall and Means 1976; Kotite et al. 1978). However, since this was also found to be the case after injection of LH or testosterone, it was suggested by Tindall et al. (1978b) that all the rapid effects were caused by testosterone (in the case of FSH by contamination of the hormone preparation with LH). Furthermore, the same authors noted that addition of testosterone, and other buffer constituents such as calcium and glycerol to the homogenisation buffer stabilised ABP. Thus experimental manipulations which increase the intratesticular concentrations of testosterone could increase the recovery of ABP, thereby appearing to stimulate ABP production.

However, others have been unable to reproduce these effects (Kotite et al. 1978; Ritzen et al. 1981). Indeed Kotite et al. (1978) demonstrated stimulation of ABP activity after FSH administration even when ABP was stabilised by the addition of testosterone to the homogenisation buffer. Furthermore, Louis and Fritz (1979) have clearly shown that FSH and testosterone can stimulate the secretion of ABP from Sertoli cells in culture in an independent manner.

To date, no hormones other than FSH and androgens have been shown to enhance any Sertoli cell function. However, the addition of serum to both testicular minces in vitro or to cultured Sertoli cells has been found to increase the secretion of ABP, indicating that as yet unidentified factors may also be active (Ritzen et al. 1981; Rommerts et al. 1979). It is reasonably well accepted, however, that FSH is the primary hormone responsible for the secretion of ABP into the epididymis, although androgen appears to be also involved in its production within the Sertoli cell (Kotite et al. 1978; Tindall et al. 1978a).

5.2.11 Biochemical Changes Associated with Sertoli Cell Maturation

It has been repeatedly demonstrated that the response of the testis to FSH diminishes during pubertal maturation. FSH administration will only stimulate cyclic AMP levels, protein synthesis and ABP production in immature rats younger than about 30 days (Means et al. 1976; Steinberger et al. 1978). Isolated Sertoli cells display a diminished response to FSH in oestradiol production from testosterone (Dorrington et al. 1978) and DNA synthesis (Griswold et al. 1977) during development. The mechanisms involved in the lack of responsiveness of the adult rat testis has not been adequately explained. It does not seem to be due to increased phosphodiesterase activity, or to a decreased number of FSH receptors, since methylisobutylxanthine (MIX) will not alter the diminished FSH response, and the number of testicular FSH receptors reaches a maximum at around 60 days of age (Ketelslegers et al. 1978).

Recent studies by Parvinen et al. (1979) suggest that cyclic alterations in the functional activity of Sertoli cells associated with different stages of spermatogenesis may mean that the testis of the adult rat appears unresponsive to hormonal stimulation. These investigators have developed a method whereby individual stages of the spermatogenic cycle can be identified and isolated by dissection of the living tubule under the microscope (Parvinen and Parvinen 1978). They have recently shown that when tubule segments containing stages II–VI, VII–VIII, IX–XII, and XIII–XIV–I were incubated in vitro, stages VII–VIII were found to secrete 70% more ABP than the segments containing stages II–VI. It is of interest that the concentration of FSH receptors and the cyclic AMP response to FSH were inversely correlated to the secretion of ABP, suggesting that the Sertoli cells most active in protein synthesis and secretion are the least sensitive to FSH stimulation. The fact that the length of time spent in each stage during the spermatogenic cycle is predominantly represented by stages VII and VIII (Clermont 1972) could mean that the testis as a whole will appear unresponsive to FSH since the length of tubules which do respond are so poorly represented at any one time. Furthermore, the observed variations in Sertoli cell activity during the different stages of spermatogenesis may be interpreted as supportive evidence for the concept that Sertoli cells may be involved in the regulation of spermatogenesis.

6 Leydig Cell Function

Yvonne Hodgson and B. Hudson

6.1 Introduction

The role of the testis in the development of masculine features has been known for literally thousands of years. It is, however, only within the past 150 years that we have begun to understand how the testes have these effects. The location and appearances of the cells that now bear his name were first described by Von Leydig in 1857. It was only much later, in the 1930s, that the chemical nature of the hormone secreted by Leydig cells was discovered.

Considerable attention was drawn to the potential importance of the testes and their secretions by the experiments of Brown-Sequard (1889), who claimed that treatment with testicular extracts gave renewed vigour and vitality. Although Brown-Sequard's claims were never substantiated, they promoted enough interest for chemists to seek out this elixir of life. The microscopic findings of lipid inclusions in the Leydig cells led to the examination of lipid extracts of testes. Such an extract from bovine testes was ultimately shown to stimulate masculine development (McGee 1927). Testosterone was subsequently isolated from these extracts (David et al. 1935) and thereafter synthesised from cholesterol (Butenandt and Hanish 1935 Ruzicka and Wettstein 1935).

At the same time as the chemical nature of Leydig cell secretion was being investigated, the control of Leydig cell function was also commanding attention. Injuries and damage to the hypothalamus and pituitary were known to be followed by gonadal atrophy (Crowe et al. 1910; Cushing 1909, 1910), and for this reason the pituitary gland was implicated in the control of the Leydig cells. Indeed, Evans and Long (1922) used aqueous pituitary extracts to show that treatment with these could maintain gonadal function. The now classic experiments done by Smith in which he ablated the pituitary and used pituitary extracts to maintain Leydig cell (and other endocrine) function clearly revealed the relationship between the pituitary and the testes (Smith 1930). The subsequent demonstration of the existence of two gonadotrophic hormones in the female—and hence their inappropriate nomenclature for the male—led to the concept that Leydig cell function was regulated by LH and spermatogenesis by follicle-stimulating hormone (Greep et al. 1936). This concept has stood the test of time, and while we now have much clearer notions of the actions of the gonadotrophins, many questions remain unanswered.

6.2 Morphology of the Leydig Cell

Leydig cells of the mammalian testis, which are responsible for the biosynthesis of androgens, are derived from mesenchymal cells in the testicular interstitium. Most mammals exhibit fetal and adult stages of Leydig cell differentiation. Electron microscopic observations in the rat have shown that fetal Leydig cells differentiate at 16 days of development, shortly after testicular differentiation (Roosen-Runge and Anderson 1959; Lording and de Kretser 1972). The corresponding period for the human is the 4th month of gestation, where this process is associated with cellular enlargement, extensive proliferation of smooth endoplasmic reticulum, appearance of large, round mitochondria with tubular cristae and development of a prominent Golgi apparatus (Pelliniemi and Niemi 1969). Fetal differentiation of Leydig cells correlates closely with aquisition of the capacity to synthesise testosterone (Noumura et al. 1966). However, the pattern and significance of Leydig cell differentiation in the post-natal period is not as clearly defined as it is in the fetus. The rat, in which spermatogenesis begins shortly after birth (Clermont and Perey 1957), exhibits some overlap of the fetal and adult generations (Lording and de Kretser 1972). In contrast, the human exhibits a distinct biphasic pattern of differentiation, the fetal generation undergoing extensive regression at the end of the second trimester (Pelliniemi and Niemi 1969) and the adult generation reappearing only around the time of puberty. There is, however, evidence of Leydig cell activity in the neonate. Plasma levels of testosterone decline rapidly after birth only to increase again at the end of the first neonatal week. A peak concentration of about 3 ng/ml is reached by the end of the 3rd month, after which testosterone levels slowly decrease to pre-pubertal levels by the 6th month. There are no morphological data which correlate with these changes (Forest et al. 1976). It appears that the timing of adult Leydig cell differentiation is related to the duration of the post-natal pre-spermatogenic period, and the restimulation caused by the pubertal secretion of LH.

The abundance and topographical relationship of Leydig cells in the interstitial tissue of the testis varies considerably between species. From a comparative study involving 14 species Fawcett et al. (1973) concluded that there are three patterns of organisation of the intertubular tissue: (1) a small volume of Leydig cells associated with sparse connective tissue but with extensive peritubular lymphatic sinusoids, (2) clusters of Leydig cells found in abundant loose connective tissue drained by a lymphatic vessel, and (3) abundant Leydig cells that occupy nearly all the intertubular space, but have little connective tissue and few interstitial lymphatics. The rat and man, whose testicular histology has been most studied, fall into the first and second categories, respectively (Figs. 6.1, 6.2).

Rat Leydig cells are of special interest because of the extensive use of this species in studies of testicular function. Rat Leydig cells are comparatively small, averaging about 10 μm in diameter, are polyhedral or spindleshaped, and are not especially abundant. They are found in clusters which are intimately associated with the blood vessels (Fig. 6.1). The blood vessels and Leydig cells are invested by an extremely thin endothelium. Electron micro-

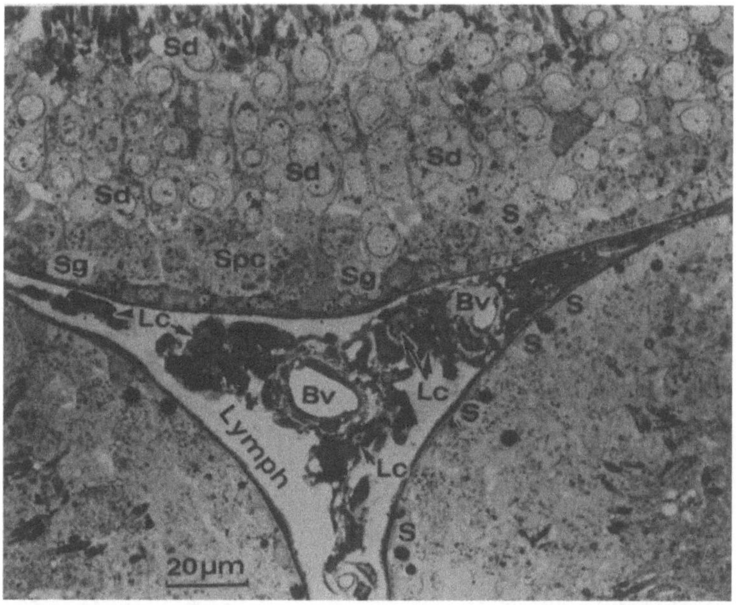

Fig. 6.1. Light micrograph of rat testis fixed by vascular perfusion, illustrating the intertubular tissue between three seminiferous tubules. Clusters of Leydig cells *(Lc)* are associated with the blood vessels *(Bv)* and are surrounded by lamphatic sinusoids. The seminiferous epithelium contains Sertoli cell nuclei *(S)* in addition to germ cells in various stages of development. *Sg*, spermatogonia; *Spc*, spermatocytes; *Sd*, early spermatids

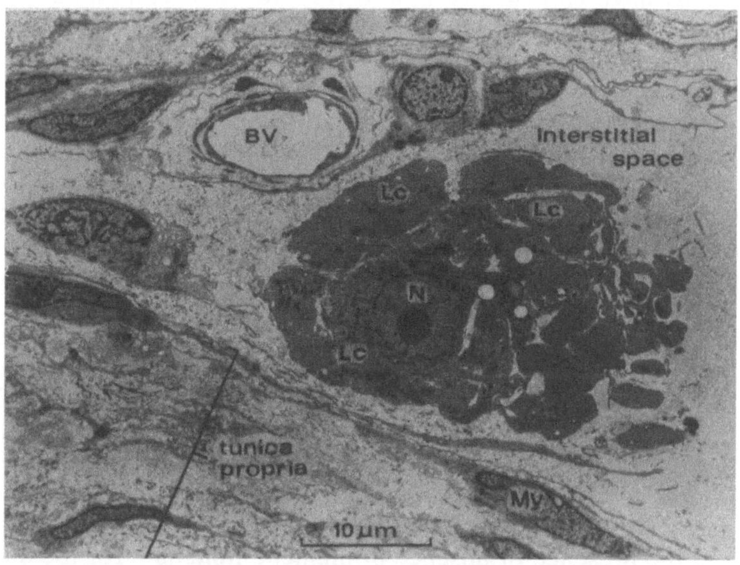

Fig. 6.2. Electron micrograph of a human testis showing a cluster of Leydig cells *(Lc)* surrounded by interstitial space. In the *lower part* of the micrograph is the tunica propria containing myoid cells *(My)* of an adjoining seminiferous tubule. *N*, nucleus of Leydig cell; *Bv*, blood vessel

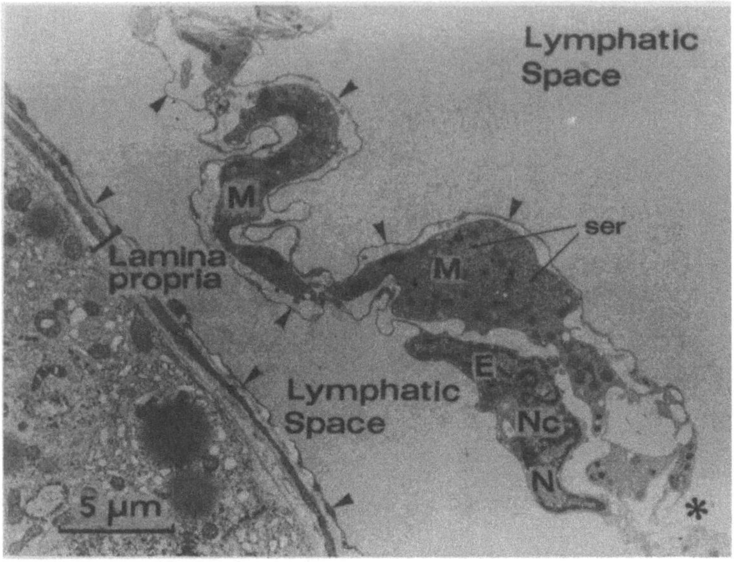

Fig. 6.3. Electron micrograph of rat testis showing Leydig cell cytoplasm containing mitochondria *(M)* and smooth endoplasmic reticulum *(ser)*. The Leydig cells are surrounded by a thin layer of lymphatic endothelial cell cytoplasm *(arrow heads)*. In some parts the endothelium is discontinuous *(asterisk)*. The main body of an endothelial cell is shown *(E)* containing the nucleus *(N)* and nucleolus *(Nc)*. The lymphatic endothelium also abuts to the lamina propria of the seminiferous tubules. Lipid droplets can be seen in the Sertoli cell cytoplasm

graphs have shown this endothelium to be discontinuous and absent over a large part of the surface of the Leydig cell clusters. Hence the Leydig cell is in direct communication with the vascular system on one side and on the other with the lymphatic sinusoids (Fig. 6.3).

Association of Leydig cells with blood vessels is not obvious in man. The interstitial space is filled with very loose connective tissue containing abundant fibroblasts (Fig. 6.2). The Leydig cells average 15 µm in diameter (Christensen and Gillim 1969) and usually are in rows or clumps, but may occur singly. Peritubular lymphatic sinusoids are not present in the human; instead, large centrally placed lymphatic vessels drain the intertubular area.

Staining of plastic-embedded tissue with toluidine blue has emphasised the heterogeneity of the population of human Leydig cells (de Kretser 1967a). Some stain darkly while others show poor staining. It is not known whether this difference is a fixation artefact or reflects a functional difference between Leydig cells. Fluorescent and autoradiographic studies of LH/hCG receptors on Leydig cells in the rat tend to confirm the latter (de Kretser et al. 1969; Hseuh et al. 1976b; Brandtzaeg et al. 1978). In addition there is a variable appearance of Leydig cells with respect to the granularity of the cytoplasm and the presence or absence of pigment, lipid and, for the human, the crystals of Reinke (Sniffen, 1950).

The Leydig cell is polygonal in form and is surrounded by a typical plasma membrane, which is frequently thrown into folds or microvilli. Its nucleus

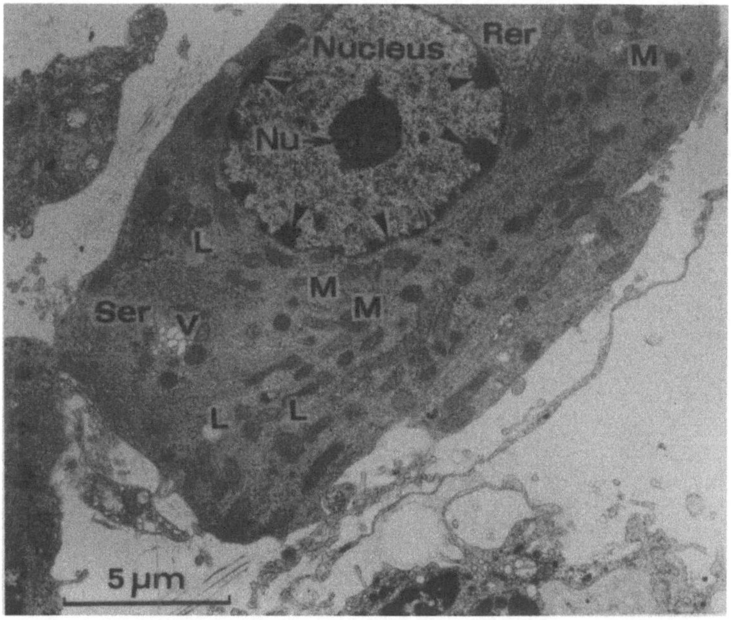

Fig. 6.4. Electron micrograph of a rat Leydig cell demonstrating an oval nucleus, surrounded by a thin rim of heterochromatin *(arrow heads)*, containing a prominent nucleolus *(Nu)*. The cytoplasmic features include abundant smooth endoplasmic reticulum *(Ser)* and mitochondria *(M)*, several lipid droplets *(L)*, rough endoplasmic reticulum *(Rer)* and vesicles *(V)*

is large and ovoid with a thin rim of heterochromatin (Fig. 6.4). The nucleus exhibits one or two prominent nucleoli. The most prominent ultrastructural feature, in common with many other steroid-secreting cells, is the abundance of smooth endoplasmic reticulum. This is believed to reflect the extent to which Leydig cells rely upon synthesis of cholesterol for androgen biosynthesis (Christensen 1965). Comparative studies show a direct correlation between the amount of smooth endoplasmic reticulum in Leydig cells and the maximum steroid output of the testis (Ewing et al. 1979; Zirkin et al. 1980). In humans the smooth endoplasmic reticulum is well developed and appears as an extremely compact network of vesicles ranging in diameter from 550 to 4 500 Å with tubules ranging in diameter from 250 to 1 000 Å (Fig. 6.5; de Kretser 1967a). In the rat the smooth endoplasmic reticulum is moderately developed and composed entirely of interconnecting tubules, forming a network throughout the cytoplasm. These tubules of smooth endoplasmic reticulum are more irregular in diameter and arrangement in the rat than in man. In both species tubules of smooth endoplasmic reticulum enclose a cavity that is separate and distinct from the background cytoplasm and extends as a continuous channel throughout the cell. From detailed morphometric studies in the rat, Mori and Christensen (1980) have calculated the smooth endoplasmic reticulum occupies 23.7% of cytoplasmic volume and has a total surface area 11 times that of the plasma membrane. This vast area of smooth endoplasmic reticulum contains many of the enzymes necessary for

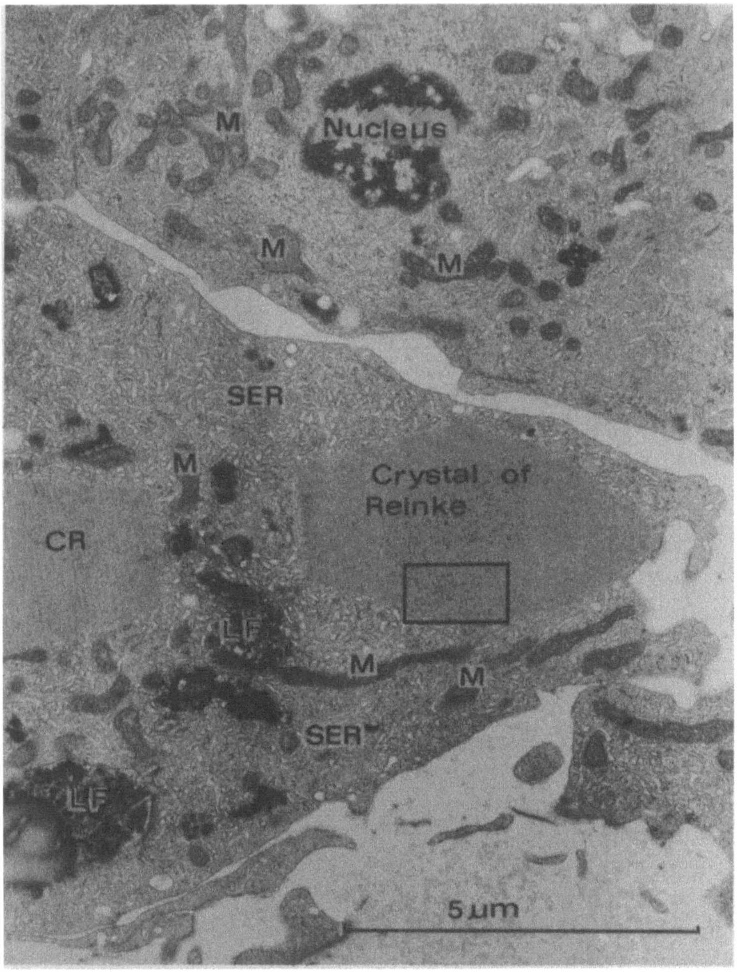

Fig. 6.5. Electron micrograph of human Leydig cells fixed by vascular perfusion. Vesicles and tubules of smooth endoplasmic reticulum *(SER)* are evident in both cells. Mitochondria *(M)* and lipofuscin *(LF)* are also present. The cytoplasm of the lower cell contains two crystals of Reinke *(CR)*, one of which has been magnified further in Fig. 6.7

steroid biosynthesis, allowing the Leydig cell to secrete a calculated 10800 molecules of testosterone per second.

Patches of rough endoplasmic reticulum are found scattered throughout the cytoplasm and frequently interconnect with the smooth endoplasmic reticulum. The mitochondria of human and rat Leydig cells which are similar in structure, are of moderate size and number and contain the common lamellar cristae in addition to tubular cristae characteristic of mitochondria of steroid-secreting cells (Figs. 6.5, 6.6). Some mitochondria contain what appear to be lipid inclusions in their matrix. Granules may also be found within the mitochondria. The significance of these intramitochondrial complexes is unknown. The Golgi apparatus is well developed and is commonly at one

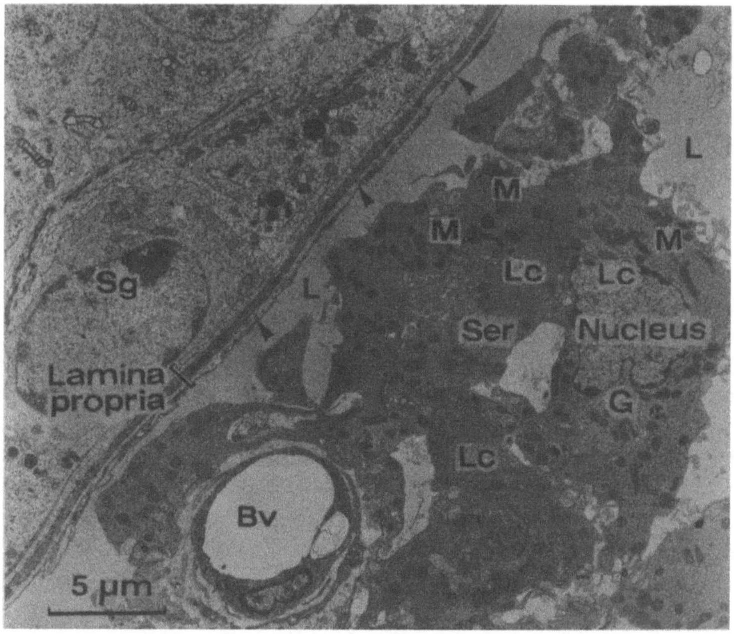

Fig. 6.6. A group of Leydig cells associated with a blood vessel *(Bv)* taken from rat. The cytoplasm of the Leydig cell *(Lc)* shows mitochondria *(M)*, smooth endoplasmic reticulum *(Ser)*, and Golgi apparatus *(G)*. Lymph *(L)* surrounds the Leydig cells and the endothelial lining *(arrow heads)* is seen adjacent to the lamina propria. A spermatogonia *(Sg)* can be seen in the seminiferous tubule

pole of the nucleus, and typically consists of between four and six flattened sacs closely pressed together (Christensen 1975).

The occurrence of lipid droplets within Leydig cells varies with the species. Human Leydig cells often contain lipid inclusions, which are unusual in the rat. In electron micrographs the lipid droplets have a homogeneous appearance, or if lipid has been extracted during the fixation or processing procedure, the droplets may appear as empty vesicles. The droplets appear to have a membrane at their surface, the thickness of which is approximately 50 Å (Christensen 1975). It is generally believed that these droplets contain cholesterol esters which are hydrolysed by soluble esterases in the cytoplasm around the lipid inclusion, thereby providing free cholesterol for steroid biosynthesis.

Also found in the cytoplasm of Leydig cells are the crystals of Reinke, lysosomes, peroxisomes, lipofuscin granules, microtubules and microfilaments. The peroxisomes, or microbodies, are usually small in diameter and irregular in shape, with an oval profile in section. They have been identified cytochemically by Reddy and Svoboda (1972) and in the rat occupy 1.2% of the cell volume (Mori and Christensen 1980). Lysosomes are usually spherical with an average diameter of 0.48 µm. Generally, they contain acid phosphatases and presumably digest material taken up by the cell or focal regions of cytoplasm that become expendable (de Duve and Wattiaux 1966) and have been implicated in the process of receptor internalisation and regulation. They stain more densely with osmium tetroxide and ferrocyanide than peroxisomes and occupy 0.6% of Leydig cell volume. The pigment granules, which are prominent in the interstitial cells, are presumably lipofuscin (Christensen 1965). The lipofuscins constitute a heterogeneous group of lipid pigments that occur in many tissues and are generally thought to be polymerisation products of oxidised unsaturated lipids.

Among the diverse organelles and inclusions in the human Leydig cell, the crystals of Reinke have probably aroused most speculation (Fig. 6.5). They do not occur in all cells, but when present, there may be several in the same cell. They are believed to be proteinaceous and are highly variable in form. They may be seen frequently as slender rods several microns long while rectangular and irregular, hexagonal forms are also common. In electron micrographs at high magnification extremely regular patterns are visible in the crystals (Fig. 6.7). Tubular structures which may represent precursors or subunits of Reinke crystals are also frequently seen within the Leydig cell, and de Kretser (1967a) has proposed a method by which these precursors may unite to form the definitive structure. Crystals with a similar periodicity have been observed in th Leydig cells of a seasonally breeding rodent, ***Rattus fuscipes***. In this species crystals are more common during the non-breeding season, a time associated with Leydig cell atrophy, and are virtually absent during the breeding season (Kerr et al. 1980). The function of these crystalline structures is unknown but their selective appearance in only some species makes it unlikely that they represent a storage form of a specific cell product. The significance of these crystals must await consideration of their biochemical characteristics together with further studies of their distribution in the normal and abnormal testis.

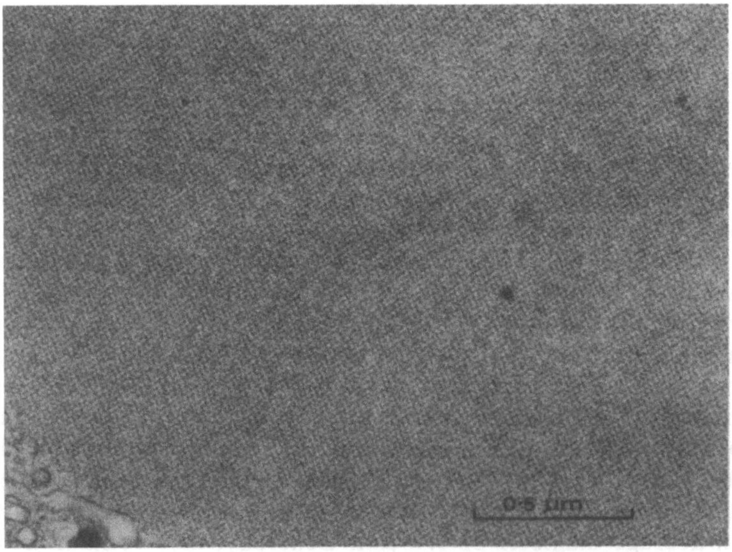

Fig. 6.7. Taken from the insert of Fig. 6.5. This electron micrograph illustrates the regular lattice array of the crystals of Reinke

In Leydig cells there are no discernible patterns in the arrangement of microtubules, although some appear to radiate from the vicinity of the centrioles within the Golgi zone. The diameter of the microtubules is about 250 Å and contrasts with that of the microfilaments, which is approximately 60 Å. The latter may be seen scattered in the cytoplasm and are particularly numerous in immature Leydig cells (Fawcett and Burgos 1960; de Kretser 1967b). It has been suggested that microtubules and microfilaments are generally supportive structures, collectively constituting a "cytoskeleton".

The view is widely held that steroid hormones are secreted by a process of passive diffusion, but we really know very little about how Leydig cells secrete testosterone or other steroids. Conventional autoradiographic studies with radioactive intermediates of steroid biosynthesis are difficult to perform because they are lipoid in nature. Secretory granules have been observed in ovine luteal cells and are protein in nature with a special affinity to bind progesterone (Gemmell et al. 1974). These authors have suggested that the luteal cells secrete progesterone in the form of granular organelles that originate in the Golgi region and are dependent on microtubules in much the same way that peptide hormones are secreted (Gemmell and Stacey 1977). An interaction between newly synthesised steroid and cytosol proteins has also been suggested by Vinson et al. (1979) for 18-hydroxydeoxycorticosterone in adrenocortical glomerulosa cells. There is no evidence of any such interaction between steroids secreted by Leydig cells and cytosol proteins of these cells, and it is tacitly assumed that newly synthesised steroids diffuse passively through the cell and cell membrane.

6.3 Steroid Biosynthesis and Secretion

Nearly 80 years ago Bouin and Ancel (1903) proposed that the major testicular hormone was secreted by the Leydig cells. In 1935 testosterone was isolated and identified as the principal androgen of the testis (David et al. 1935). The other androgens, androstenedione, DHEA and dihydrotestosterone, make little overall contribution to the effective androgen content of blood, since the former two steroids are weak androgens and the secretion rate of the latter is low. Oestradiol is also secreted by the testis, but accounts for only 10%–20% of the overall oestradiol production rate of this hormone in men. Progesterone, 17α-hydroxyprogesterone and sulphated conjugates of pregnenolone and DHEA are also secreted, but probably have no specific biological function. The Leydig cells are the site of steroid biosynthesis in the testis and testosterone is biologically the most important steroid formed. In normal men 95% of the daily production rate of testosterone, between 4 and 7 mg, comes from the Leydig cells. The pathways of steroid biosynthesis in these cells are qualitatively similar to those in other steroid-secreting tissues. Most experiments to determine these pathways have been done in vitro using rat testes and have used radioactive substrates to trace steroid synthesis and metabolism. Because the conditions that are used to study in vitro biosynthesis may be significantly different from those which exist in vivo, for instance, with respect to substrate and co-factor concentrations, some caution must be exercised in drawing conclusions about quantitative aspects of steroid synthesis and metabolism.

As with other steroid-secreting tissues cholesterol seems to be an obligatory intermediate in the biosynthesis of steroids from acetate by Leydig cells. Some intermediates which have been identified in the synthesis of cholesterol from acetate are mevalonate, squalene and lanosterol (Eik-Nes 1975). Most of the cholesterol in Leydig cells is probably derived from acetate and not from the circulating cholesterol pool. In the Leydig cell, cholesterol occurs in both free and esterified forms and the hydrolysis of cholesterol esters, mainly cholesterol sulfate, is thought to be under the influence of LH. Steroid sulfates are also present in and secreted by the testis. There is, however, little evidence that these are of much biological significance.

The enzymes required for steroid biosynthesis have been reasonably well characterised. Those required for the conversion of cholesterol to pregnenolone are within the mitochondria while those associated with the conversion of pregnenolone to testosterone are found in the endoplasmic reticulum.

The initial step in the conversion of cholesterol to androgens is the removal of the six carbon side chain with the formation of pregnenolone and isocaproic aldehyde (Fig. 6.8). This step takes place within mitochondria and requires NADPH, molecular oxygen, and an enzyme system comprising a non-haeme iron protein, a flavoprotein and cytochrome P-450 for hydroxylation and C_{17-20} lyase activity to remove the side chain. Some of the intermediate steps involved in this reaction have not been precisely defined. This reaction is controlled by LH and is the rate limiting step in testicular steroid synthesis (Hall 1966).

The conversion of pregnenolone, a Δ^5-3β-hydroxysteroid, involves two enzymes: a Δ^5-3β-hydroxysteroid dehydrogenase (pregnenolone to Δ^5-pregnene-3,20-dione) and the Δ^5-Δ^4 isomerase (Δ^5-pregnene-3,20,dione to progesterone). This enzyme complex is microsomal, and NAD is the hydrogen acceptor for the enzyme. The activity of the system is increased after gonadotrophin treatment and reduced following hypophysectomy (Purvis et al. 1973; van de Vusse et al. 1975).

Progesterone is thereafter converted by the testicular 17α-hydroxylase to 17α-hydroxyprogesterone (Fig. 6.9). This is a rapid reaction so that very little progesterone accumulates in the testis. This enzyme is also microsomal, and requires molecular oxygen and NADPH for the introduction of the

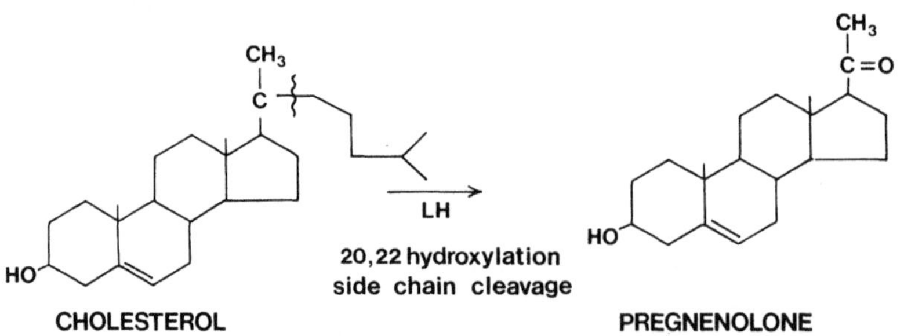

Fig. 6.8. Formulae and biochemical changes in the conversion of cholesterol to pregnenolone

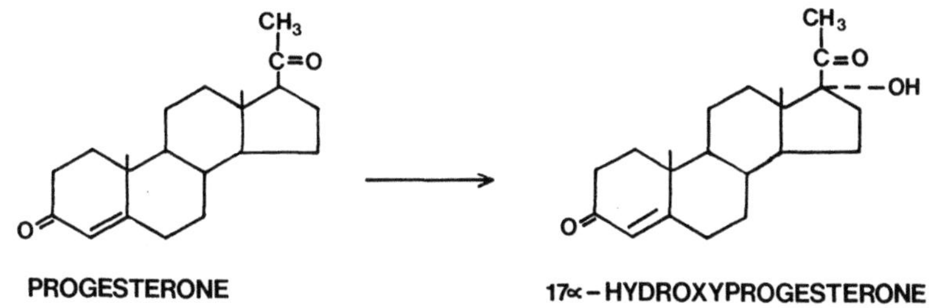

Fig. 6.9. Formulae of progesterone and 17α-hydroxyprogesterone, the conversion being catalysed by the enzyme 17α-hydroxylase

17α-hydroxyl group. It is not known whether Leydig cells contain two 17α-hydroxylase enzymes, that is a Δ^4-3-oxo-17α-hydroxylase and a Δ^5-3β-hydroxy-17α-hydroxylase. The activity of this enzyme is inhibited by the accumulation of 17α-hydroxyprogesterone in vitro but it is not known whether this occurs in vivo.

This steroid, 17α-hydroxyprogesterone, which is a secretory product of the testis, is a substrate for the C_{17-20} lyase which removes the two carbon side chain to form Δ^4 androstene-3,17-dione, a relatively weak androgen which is converted to testosterone by 17β-hydroxysteroid dehydrogenase (Fig. 6.10). This chain of steroid biotransformations: pregnenolone → progesterone → 17 α-hydroxyprogesterone → Δ^4-androstenedione → testosterone, is known as the Δ^4 pathway, and is probably the preferred route for the biosynthesis of testosterone.

The alternative pathway is the Δ^5 pathway. In this route pregnenolone, or pregnenolone sulphate, passes from the mitochondria to the smooth endoplasmic reticulum to undergo 17α-hydroxylation and form 17α-hydroxypregnenolone or 17α-hydroxypregnenolone sulphate. The two carbon side chain is cleaved by a C_{17-20} lyase to form DHEA or its sulphate. Alternatively DHEA can be converted to Δ^5-androstene-3,17-diol, which is then converted to testosterone. Through the action of the Δ^5-3β-hydroxysteroid dehydrogenase and the Δ^5-Δ^4-isomerase DHEA can be converted to Δ^4-androstenedione, and then to testosterone (Figs. 6.11, 6.12). All these intermediates have been isolated from testicular tissue, sometimes in high amounts.

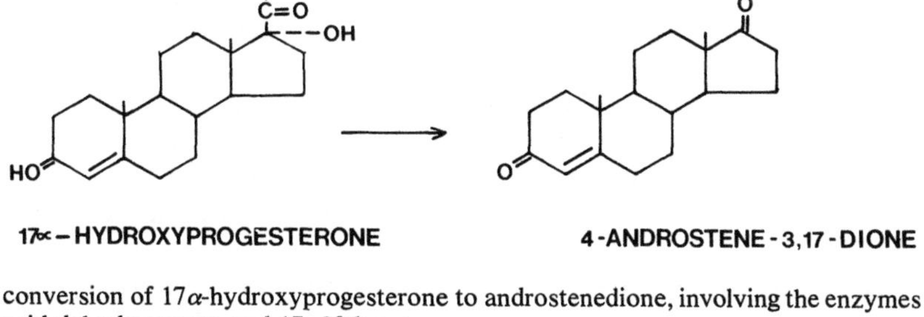

Fig. 6.10. The conversion of 17α-hydroxyprogesterone to androstenedione, involving the enzymes 3β-hydroxysteroid dehydrogenase and 17–20 lyase

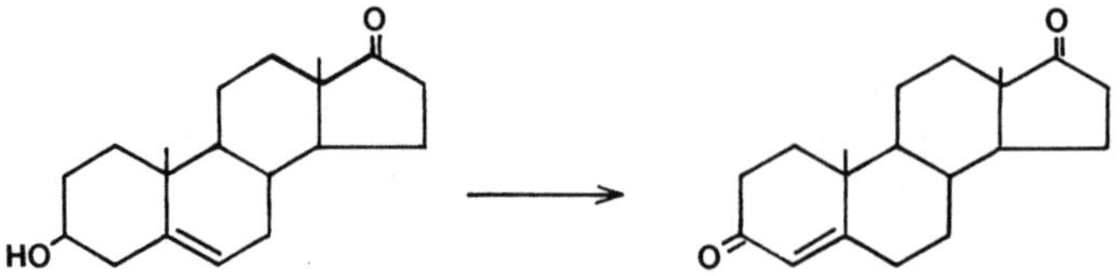

DEHYDROEPIANDROSTERONE 4-ANDROSTENE-3,17-DIONE

Fig. 6.11. Conversion of dehydroepiandrosterone to androstenedione, involving the enzymes 3β-hydroxysteroid dehydrogenase and Δ_5–Δ_4 isomerase

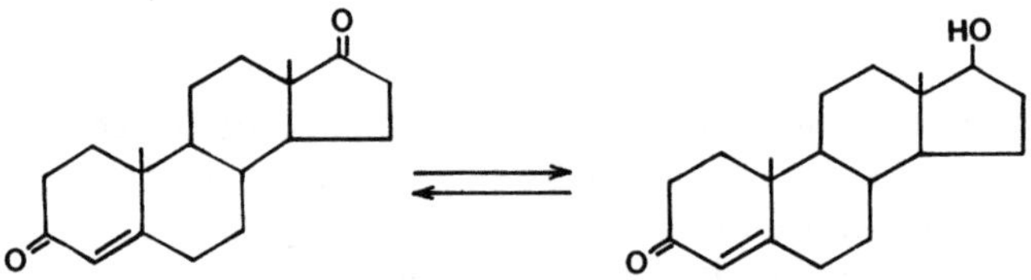

4-ANDROSTENE-3,17-DIONE TESTOSTERONE

Fig. 6.12. Conversion of androstenedione to testosterone, involving the enzyme 17β-hydroxysteroid dehydrogenase

Of the two pathways the Δ^4 pathway is probably the preferred pathway in the rat (Samuels et al. 1975) while the Δ^5 pathway is preferred in man (Yanaihara and Tracy 1972). Oestrogens are also secreted by the testes in many animals. Oestradiol is the principal oestrogen secreted by man and rat whereas the stallion produces equilins, equilinins and oestriol. In man the testicular contribution to oestradiol production is small compared to that formed by peripheral aromatisation of C-19 steroids.

Finally there is the question of whether other cells in the testis produce steroids. It is controversial whether Sertoli cells can synthesise steroids from acetate or even cholesterol. There seems to be reasonable evidence that these cells have the capacity to metabolise steroids produced by Leydig cells, for example the conversion of testosterone to dihydrotestosterone and oestradiol. (This is considered more extensively in Chap. 5.)

6.4 Regulation of Leydig Cell Function

The pituitary hormone LH plays the major role in the regulation of steroid secretion by Leydig cells. LH stimulates testosterone secretion both in vivo and in vitro. Prolactin and FSH may also be implicated in the control of Leydig cell secretion. The acute response of Leydig cells to LH involves the activation of enzymes which control cholesterol side chain cleavage, while the long-term effects involve synthesis of new proteins and an increase in the activities of several enzyme systems involved in testosterone biosynthesis.

Both LH and hCG bind with high affinity and specificity to Leydig cells, whereas closely related glycoprotein hormones do not. The binding is to receptors whose location on Leydig cell membranes has been confirmed by autoradiography and immunofluorescence and at the light microscopic level (de Kretser et al. 1969, 1971; Mendelson et al. 1975; Hsueh et al. 1976a; Conn et al. 1977; Blantzaeg et al. 1978).

Although the binding of LH or hCG to Leydig cells takes place initially on the plasma membrane, these gonadotrophins ultimately become located intracellularly (Castro et al. 1972; Ascoli and Puett 1977). We do not know whether this process of internalisation is an essential component for the trophic action of LH, or whether it merely serves to terminate hormone action and regulate receptor numbers. Because of the close structural and biological similarities between LH and hCG and the ready availability of highly purified hCG, most binding studies have been done with ^{125}I-hCG. Early studies were mainly concerned with the location of receptors for LH while subsequent studies have examined binding kinetics. Thus in the rat testis the LH receptor has a high association constant ($Ka = 4 \times 10^{10} M^{-1}$), but a low capacity – 1 pMol/g (Catt and Dufau 1978) for hCG.

The mechanism of action of LH is similar to that of many other peptide hormones: that is, by way of the adenylate cyclase, cAMP and protein kinase systems. Thus both LH and cAMP stimulate testosterone secretion by decapsulated rat testes (Dufau et al. 1971) while incubation of isolated Leydig cells with hCG or LH is followed by the synthesis and release of cAMP and testosterone (Mendelson et al. 1975). An increase in protein kinase activity accompanies this response. Reddi et al. (1971) located this enzyme in testis cytosols and showed phosphoryllation of certain histones. Although the functional importance of cAMP-dependent histone phosphorylation has not been determined, nuclear histones have been widely employed as an exogenous substrate for the study of cAMP-dependent protein kinases. Detailed studies of rat Leydig cell protein kinase have demonstrated that there is an inactive form of this enzyme which contains catalytic and regulatory subunits. The interaction between cAMP and protein kinase leads to a coupling of cAMP and the regulatory subunit, and the generation of free, active, catalytic subunits which result in the phosphorylation of nuclear histones (Reddi et al. 1971; Cooke et al. 1976; Podesta et al. 1976a,b; Dufau et al. 1977). One overall result of gonadotrophin stimulation of Leydig cells is an increase in the number of free catalytic subunits of protein kinase.

Although LH/hCG are the main trophic hormones for Leydig cells it is probable that FSH and prolactin also play a role in the regulation of Leydig cell function. When rabbit testes are perfused with supramaximal doses of LH, the addition of FSH to the perfusion results in a significant increase in testosterone secretion (Johnson and Ewing 1971). Testicular responsiveness to LH is markedly diminished in immature, hypophysectomised animals. Odell et al. (1973) have shown that this can be prevented if the animals are treated with FSH, and have suggested that increased testicular responsiveness to LH seen during sexual maturation is an effect of FSH which acts on the seminiferous tubules to regulate Sertoli cell and spermatogenic function (see Chap. 3). Thus, the number of LH receptors in the testis is increased following treatment of immature hypophysectomised rats with FSH, an effect which is related to the duration of treatment (Chen et al. 1977).

This phenomenon is also observed in vitro: thus when Leydig cells from immature hypophysectomised rats are stimulated with LH a greater response is seen in the cells from those animals which have been pre-treated with FSH (Chen et al. 1977; Purvis and Hansson 1978). LH and FSH have a synergistic effect on the activity of 3β-hydroxysteroid dehydrogenase-isomerase activity in isolated Leydig cells (Shaw et al. 1979). All these observations strongly suggest that FSH has a direct effect on and modulates Leydig cell function. Since FSH has never been shown to bind to Leydig cells, and since binding is an important premise in establishing that a hormone acts on a particular target tissue, it would seem that the effects of FSH on Leydig cells are indirect. An alternative explanation is that FSH acts by way of the alterations it induces in the tubule compartment in the testis, where FSH has been shown to bind specifically to Sertoli cells (Orth and Christensen 1978).

Prolactin, also, may augment the effects of LH on the Leydig cell. Hereditary dwarf mice which have a congenital prolactin deficiency are sterile, but the sterility can be reversed by treatment with prolactin (Bartke 1966). Prolactin has been shown also to potentiate the effect of LH, but not testosterone, in restoring spermatogenesis in hypophysectomised adult mice (Bartke 1971a). Leydig cell function can be stimulated or suppressed by manipulating prolactin secretion: thus, if adult rats or mice are treated with bromoergocryptine, which inhibits prolactin release, plasma levels of testosterone fall. Conversely testosterone levels in hypophysectomised rats are higher in those animals treated with prolactin and LH than in those treated with LH alone (Hafiez et al. 1972b). There is a greater biosynthesis of testosterone from acetate in vitro by testes from rats treated with prolactin and LH than from animals treated only with LH (Hafiez et al. 1972a).

Prolactin probably exerts its effects on Leydig cell function by modulating LH receptors. In hereditary dwarf mice LH receptors are decreased but can be increased by giving prolactin (Bohnet and Friesen 1976). A similar situation is found in hypophysectomised rats: that is, testicular binding of LH is increased by prolactin treatment (Payne and Zipf 1977) and when immature rats are treated with bromoergocryptine, LH binding in the testis is reduced (Aragona et al. 1977). Seasonal sexual regression of the testis in the golden hamster is associated with a fall in plasma testosterone levels and a reduction of testicular LH receptors, changes which can be prevented by treatment with prolactin (Bartke et al. 1975; Bex and Bartke 1977). In addition to its effects on LH receptors, prolactin may have direct effects on steroid biosynthesis; thus, levels of esterified cholesterol in the testes of dwarf mice are increased by prolactin treatment, a finding which is consistent with increased testosterone secretion in these animals after such treatment. The activities of the 3β- and 17β-hydroxysteroid dehydrogenases are also increased following prolactin treatment (Hafiez et al. 1971; Musto et al. 1972). In contrast to FSH, prolactin has been shown to bind specifically to Leydig cell membranes.

The role of oestradiol in the regulation of Leydig cell function has been a point of controversy. The existence of oestradiol receptors in Leydig cells supports the view that oestradiol has an effect on the function of these cells (Brinkmann et al. 1972; Mulder et al. 1973). Further evidence is that when oestradiol is administered simultaneously with LH and FSH to hypophysectomised rats, testis weights and plasma levels of testosterone are lower in the animals which received oestradiol than in those which did not (Kalla et al. 1980). The finding that the maximum amount of testosterone produced by decapsulated testes in vitro in response to hCG is less in the presence of oestradiol reconciles with the fact that LH evokes a lesser in vivo response in rats treated with oestradiol than in untreated controls.

Despite earlier controversies the direct evidence that the testes secrete oestrogens is substantial. Oestradiol has been measured in a higher concentration in spermatic venous than in peripheral blood (Kelch et al. 1972; Baird et al. 1973). The secretion of oestradiol is increased following the administration of hCG in men (Weinstein et al. 1974) and rats (de Jong et al. 1973). Canick et al. (1979) have shown that there is a highly significant increase in microsomal aromatase activity in Leydig cells of rats treated with hCG but there is no increase following FSH treatment. One question that has not been completely resolved is the contribution of the Sertoli cell to testicular oestradiol secretion. This question arises in view of the fact that Dorrington and Armstrong (1975) have shown Sertoli cells from young rats can aromatise testosterone to oestradiol under the stimulus of FSH. This reaction has not been demonstrated in adult rats. The Sertoli cell is unlikely to be an important source of oestradiol from the testis, since men with complete tubule destruction and presumably decreased Sertoli cell function such as in Klinefelter's syndrome may secrete more oestradiol than normal men (Wang et al. 1975).

The testis also secretes DHT, but the overall contribution to DHT production is probably less than 20%, and this probably arises from 5α-reductase activity in Sertoli cells (Wilson 1975). The testicular contribution to the daily blood production of DHT is thus not significant since most DHT arises as a result of peripheral metabolism from testosterone.

6.5 Hormonal Regulation of LH Receptors

The phenomenon of "down regulation", which has been shown for other peptide hormones and their receptors also applies to hCG/LH and Leydig cell receptors. The loss of receptors which follows a single, high dose of LH, hCG or LHRH persists for up to 6 days and is found to be dose dependent (Sharpe 1976; Haour and Saez 1977; Hsueh et al. 1976b; Catt et al. 1979). In the rat a low dose of hCG (10 IU) causes no changes in receptor content within the first 24 h but is followed by a significant fall in hCG binding at 24 h, which persists for several days. After a large dose (200 IU) there is a rapid loss of hCG binding which persists for 5 days and is restored to normal after about 7 days (Hsueh et al. 1976b). The same phenomenon is found in immature rats in which a dose of 10 IU causes a marked reduction in LH receptors within 24 h. Several hypotheses have been proposed to account for this receptor loss, but none explain the phenomenon completely. One hypothesis is that the receptors become occupied by the initially high concentrations of hCG, so that subsequent binding is inhibited, but this is unlikely since increased receptor occupancy persists for only about 12 h. Another envisages that the receptor population becomes inactivated after binding and is only slowly reactivated. Yet another hypothesis is that the receptors are completely degraded after binding so that synthesis of new receptors is necessary. Finally, the interaction between LH and its receptors may initiate a further regulatory process which leads to a loss of unoccupied receptors either through degradation or inhibition of new receptors (for review, see Catt and Dufau 1978).

The gonadotrophin-induced loss of LH receptors is accompanied by significant changes in post-receptor events, the extent and nature of which vary with the dose of hCG and the time after injection. There is a marked fall in cAMP production in vitro during the first 12 h after treatment with 200 IU hCG. The gradual return of receptor sites is accompanied by a recovery of the cAMP responses, and is believed to reflect a return of hormone-sensitive adenylate cyclase activity. During gonadotrophin-induced desensitisation there is a close correlation between LH receptor content and the cAMP response to hCG. This is consistent with the belief that most receptor sites in the testis are functionally coupled to a process which generates cAMP (Hsueh et al. 1977).

It is of interest that despite the desensitisation of the cAMP response to hCG, choleragen treatment results in normal levels of cAMP throughout the period of receptor loss and recovery. The failure of hCG during this period is interpreted as a defect in coupling between LH receptors and adenylate cyclase. The corresponding changes in testosterone responses of Leydig cells after hCG-induced receptor loss are more complex. Thus the maximum in vitro testosterone responses of desensitised cells at 2 and 4 days do not reach control values following the addition of high doses of hCG. This suppression of steroid biosynthesis does not simply result from diminished cAMP production, since it persists if endogenous cAMP is generated by treatment with choleragen or if db cAMP is added to the incubation medium. It would seem that the block in steroid biosynthesis is located beyond the level of cAMP (Tsuruhara et al. 1977). Further work by these authors has shown that there is no difference in either the number or binding capacity of intracellular cAMP receptors in the desensitised state, which suggests that the lesion is located beyond the protein kinase level. Studies by Cigorraga et al. (1978) indicate that the major steroidogenic block in desensitised cells is at the 17α-hydroxylase and C_{17-20} lyase steps. The lesions in steroid biosynthesis in gonadotrophin-desensitised Leydig cells recover before the receptors and cAMP responses return to control levels. This suggests that the decrease in LH receptors is not directly responsible for the transient abnormalities of steroid biosynthesis. This view is further supported by the finding that when rats are treated with cycloheximide there is no receptor loss after hCG but the abnormalities in steroid biosynthesis still occur despite this treatment (Haour and Saez 1977).

This period of refractoriness following hCG treatment when steroid synthesis is blocked may well be responsible for the biphasic pattern of serum testosterone levels seen after a single injection of hCG in rats (Haour and Saez 1977; Hodgson and de Kretser 1982). There is an early increase in levels of testosterone within 2h of a single hCG injection, which is followed by a return to control levels between 1 and 2 days. After 3 days there is a second increase in serum testosterone with a return to control levels at 4 days (Fig. 6.13). Similar testosterone responses have been reported for men, bulls and rams (Saez and Forest 1979; Padron et al. 1980; Sundby and Farahat 1978, Garnier and Saez 1980). The timing of the two peaks is similar in all these species but the magnitude of the two phases differs. In rats the magnitude of the second response is comparable to the first, but in men, bulls and rams the magnitude of the second phase is greater than the first. A further difference between the serum testosterone response of the rat and these species is the higher testosterone values found between the two peaks. In the rat serum testosterone levels fall to control values while they remain higher than controls in the human, bull and ram. The late response in testosterone probably results from restimulation by circulating hCG after the recovery of the Leydig cells from the refractory period induced by hCG. Thus hCG levels in serum remain elevated for several days in men, rats and sheep. This proposal is further supported by the fact that the elevation of endogenous LH induced by LHRH does not elicit a late response and further implicates persistently high circulating levels of hCG in the stimulation of the testis after recovery from the refractory period (Hodgson and de Kretser 1982; see Fig. 6.13).

Although this postulate seems reasonable there are some factors that require further evaluation. One is that the late response occurs at a time when the binding capacity of the testis for LH is reduced. Another is that at these doses of hCG, testicular steroid biosynthetic capacity is compromised as a result of reduced conversion of cholesterol to pregnenolone, which persists for at least 4 days after the administration of hCG (Tsuruhara et al. 1977). Notwithstanding the findings by several independent groups in three species the increased secretion of testosterone between 3 and 4 days is inconsistent with the known effects of hCG on desensitisation and inhibition of steroid biosynthesis (Garnier and Saez 1980; Haour and Saez 1977; Hodgson and de Kretser 1982; Padron et al. 1980; Saez and Forest 1979; Sundby and Farahat 1978).

The cause of the nadir between the early acute and late testosterone responses is unknown. One possibility is increased secretion of oestradiol following hCG treatment. It is known that testicular aromatase is stimulated and conversely the activities of 17α-hydroxylase and C_{17-20} lyase are decreased by 90% and 60% respectively after hCG (Cigorraga et al. 1980). These enzymatic inhibitions may result from the increased local production of oestradiol, a hypothesis which presumes local product inhibition by oestradiol in the Leydig cell. Blood levels of oestradiol rise after a single injection of hCG and reach a maximum at 24h and remain elevated for up to 6 days (Fig. 6.14) (Forest et al. 1979; Jones et al. 1978; Padron et al. 1980). The hypothesis that oestradiol is responsible for the refractory period has been further investigated by administration of oestradiol and anti-oestrogens following treatment with hCG. When adult male rats are given 50 μg oestradiol 48h after hCG there is no modification of the late testosterone response nor of the in vitro steroid biosynthetic activity. Nozu et al. (1981) have shown changes in oestradiol receptors within Leydig cells and an increased testicular content of oestradiol following hCG. These changes are prevented by tamoxifen. We have found that treatment with the anti-oestrogen tamoxifen either prior to or at the time of hCG administration fails to prevent the decrease in serum testosterone or the in vitro refractory period (Hodgson and de Kretser, unpublished). For these reasons we would dispute the hypothesis of Forest et al. (1979) that the refractory period is the result of oestradiol action within the Leydig cell. We are also unable to confirm the findings of Cigorraga et al. (1980) that tamoxifen prevents the block in steroid biosynthesis 3 days after hCG. Although we used a larger dose (2 mg vs. 1.5 μg), which should completely block the effect of oestradiol this should not have given conflicting results. Clearly there is a need for further study to determine the effects of oestradiol on Leydig cell function.

Although the physiological significance of the acute effects of LH in the testis is not completely clear, the practical significance is. The down regulation of LH receptors, the decrease in cAMP responses and the refractoriness to further gonadotrophin stimulation means that hCG need not be administered any more frequently than at 6- or 7-day intervals instead of the alternate day schedule which is the current custom.

The best characterised effect of chronic treatment with hCG is the change in Leydig cell ultrastructure. After 5 weeks treatment with hCG, rat Leydig cells show hyperplasia and hypertrophy (Christensen and Peacock 1980). In man there is a proliferation of smooth endoplasmic reticulum and an increase in the numbers of mitochondria and Golgi complexes (de Kretser 1967b). Furthermore there is a modification of receptor numbers and of the steroidogenic capacity of decapsulated testes following chronic treat-

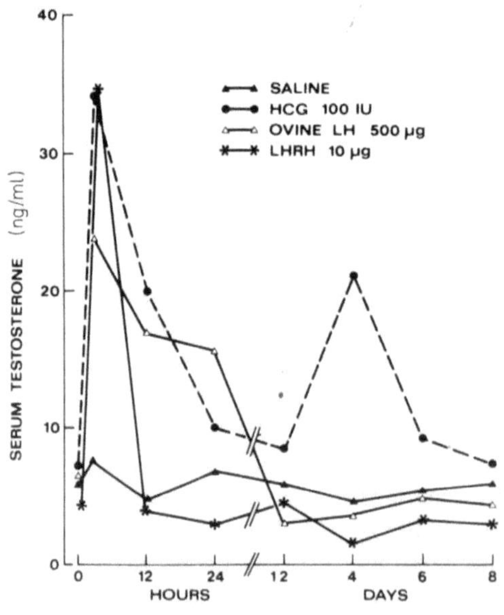

Fig. 6.13. The response of serum testosterone in rats to injections of hCG, ovine LH and LHRH is shown

ment with hCG. Although there is a loss of LH receptors in adult rats given 100 IU hCG daily for 7 days the testes can be stimulated in vitro; indeed the responses are greater than those from controls (Risbridger et al. 1981e). The finding that the testis is still responsive despite the continued presence of hCG receptor loss raises questions as to why no abnormalities of steroid biosynthesis, similar to those seen after a single injection, persist following chronic stimulation with hCG. Indeed little attention has been paid to the effects of chronic treatment with hCG on Leydig cell function; for instance, are suppression of 7α-hydroxylation and an increased formation of 5α-reduced metabolites important and, if so, how are they related to the morphological changes that are found after long-term treatment with hCG? These are issues that require further clarification.

Despite the gaps in our knowledge, hCG is useful in the diagnosis and treatment of men with testicular disorders. Over the past decade there has been a considerable increase in our understanding of the control of Leydig cell function, in particular, and how this function is most amenable to therapeutic manipulation.

6.5.1 LHRH and Leydig Cell Function

With the discovery of LHRH it was hoped that this hormone or its more potent analogues would be useful in the treatment of men with gonadal disorders and infertility. Somewhat unexpectedly it was found that chronic treatment of male rats with LHRH or more potent LHRH agonist analogues leads to a marked loss of LH/hCG receptors in the testis, decreased testosterone secretion, a reduction in the weights of the testes, prostate and seminal vesicles, and inhibition of spermatogenesis (Auclair et al. 1977; Labrie et al. 1978). This was initially interpreted as being secondary to stimulation of endogenous gonadotrophin secretion (Auclair et al. 1977). It was subsequently shown that treatment with LHRH analogues reduced the binding of hCG to Leydig cells in both FSH-treated and untreated hypophysectomised rats (Hseuh and Erikson 1979; Arimura et al. 1979). This was the first evidence for direct effect of LHRH on the testis. Thus LHRH agonists, in addition to their action on the pituitary gonadotropes, directly inhibit testicular function. More recently high-affinity binding sites for LHRH and several of its more potent analogues have been found in Leydig cell preparations. Thus, Lefebvre et al. (1980) have shown the LHRH agonist [D-Ser (TBU)^6, des-Gly-$NH_2{}^{10}$]-LHRH ethylamide binds to a single class of high-affinity sites at a K_D value of $0.12 \times 10^{-9}\,M$ and the number of sites is approximately 2500 per Leydig cell. They have also shown a correlation between the potencies of several LHRH agonists, as judged by their capacity to stimulate LH release, and their affinity for testicular binding sites.

Chronic administration of an LHRH agonist reduces the number of Leydig cell LHRH receptors to 10%–25% within 1 week but without a change in binding affinity (Sharpe and Fraser 1980). Concomitant with this is a decrease in serum testosterone levels and a transient increase in serum progesterone levels (Rivier et al. 1979). Measurement of the testicular content of these steroids after chronic treatment with high doses of an LHRH agonist has also shown reduced concentrations of testosterone but with higher than normal progesterone levels. These data suggest a defect of androgen biosynthesis at the level of the 17α-hydroxylase and 17,20-desmolase activities. In addition to its inhibitory effect on steroidogenesis and autoregulation of its testicular receptors, administration of LHRH has been reported to cause a loss of LH/hCG receptors and prolactin receptors in the testis (Catt et al. 1979). The inhibitory effects of LHRH on Leydig cell function are important for the proposed local control mechanism in the testis. Sharpe et al. (1981) have discovered an LHRH-like compound in the interstitial fluid of the testis. This substance has similar biological activities to LHRH and binds to LHRH receptors, but it is immunologically distinct from the native LHRH molecule. These authors have shown that this factor is secreted in vitro, by cultured Sertoli cells and that its production and/or secretion is enhanced by hCG. Similar peptides have been found in rat follicular fluid and in the medium from cultured granulosa cells. These have been termed gonadocrinins by Ying et al. (1981) and have been shown to be chemically distinct from LH-RH. Further clarification of the action of LHRH on the Leydig cell would aid in the assessment of the regulatory role of this new LHRH-like Sertoli cell hormone in the maintenance of normal testicular function. Treatment of men with this LHRH analogue administered daily intranasally for periods of up to 14 days results in decreased levels of testicular steroids in the blood, which may have important therapeutic implications, such as the treatment of prostatic cancer or to inhibit spermatogenesis.

6.6 Leydig Cells and Spermatogenesis

By far the largest volume of the testis is filled with an intricately coiled system of seminiferous tubules in which primitive spermatogonia differentiate into spermatozoa by the process of spermatogenesis. Endocrine control of spermatogenesis is a complex process requiring the presence of FSH and high intratesticular testosterone concentrations. Hypophysectomy causes a failure of spermatogenesis with a block at the primary spermatocyte stage (Nelson 1952). Interpretations of experiments designed to maintain or repair post-hypophysectomy spermatogenic arrest have been complicated by the fact that different investigators have waited variable lengths of time after hypophysectomy before beginning hormone treatment and many have used partially purified preparations of LH and FSH containing substantial amounts of both hormones. The ability of high doses of testosterone to maintain spermatogenesis in hypophysectomised animals is, however, well recognised (Nelson 1952; Simpson et al. 1942; see: Steinberger 1971 for review). Ludwig (1950) has shown that administration of low doses of testosterone to intact rats causes testicular damage by an indirect mechanism that involves suppression of pituitary gonadotrophins. By contrast high doses of testosterone, while exerting a suppressive action on pituitary gonadotrophins, are capable of allowing spermatogenesis to proceed in spite of markedly diminished gonadotrophin levels. Studies in boys with precocious puberty, due to interstitial cell tumors, support the concept that a high intratesticular testosterone concentration is required for spermatogenesis, as tubules adjacent to the testosterone-producing tumor undergo germinal maturation while the controlateral testis remains unstimulated despite elevated peripheral serum concentrations of testosterone (Steinberger et al. 1973). There have been many studies in both the rat and man to suggest that FSH as well as testosterone is required for the induction of spermatogenesis (Steinberger and Duckett 1967). Steinberger et al. (1973) have postulated that FSH is essential for the later stages of spermatogenesis because in the absence of FSH maturation of the seminiferous epithelium does not progress beyond the spermatid stage. They made these observations in men with complete hypogonadism in whom administration of FSH after hCG priming resulted in the completion of spermatogenesis and production of sufficient spermatozoa for fertility (Sherins et al. 1977). The presence of FSH receptors on the Sertoli cell membrane (Orth and Christensen 1977) and the ability of FSH and testosterone to stimulate androgen-binding protein (ABP) production by Sertoli cells substantiate earlier observations of the involvement of both FSH and testosterone in the regulation of spermatogenesis. While FSH is most certainly an important influence during pubertal maturation and initiation of spermatogenesis, ongoing maintenance of spermatogenesis by androgens is also very important. The close proximity of the Leydig cells to the seminiferous tubules and the ready accessibility of testosterone across the lymphatic space to the tubules aid in the maintenance of the high testosterone concentrations required in the environment of the developing germ cells.

6.7 Androgens in Blood

Testosterone is the principal androgen in blood. In the normal young adult the secretion rate of testosterone is between 4 and 7 mg/day, more than 95% of which is secreted by Leydig cells. The secretion rate of testosterone falls slowly with age (Chap. 4). The normal plasma concentration of testosterone is between 2.8 and 11.5 ng/ml, most of which is bound to plasma proteins. Binding to albumin is weak and non-specific, with an association constant of $3.6 \times 10^4 M^{-1}$. The important binding protein is a β-globulin called sex hormone binding globulin (SHBG). This protein has a high affinity (K_A $8 \times 10^8 M^{-1}$) but low capacity, $3–5 \times 10^{-8} M$, for testosterone (Vermeulen and Verdonck 1968; Rosner 1972). Testosterone is also bound to transcortin and the α1-acid glycoprotein, but this binding appears to be of minor significance.

Because of protein binding only a small amount of testosterone in plasma is free. In normal young adult men this is about 2% and represents the biologically active fraction of testosterone in plasma. The binding of testosterone to SHBG limits its entry into cells from plasma and the metabolic clearance rate of testosterone is directly related to the free or unbound fraction of testosterone in plasma. The metabolic clearance rate in men is about 500 litres/day/m², which is significantly higher than in women (about 300 litres/day/m²), who have higher levels of SHBG and a lower fraction of free testosterone—usually about 1%.

Other androgens present in blood include Δ^4-androstenedione, DHEA, DHEA sulphate, dihydrotestosterone and 5α-androstane-$3\alpha,17\beta$-diol. The former three are secreted by the testis but the testicular contribution to their overall production rates is small; moreover they are weak androgens and since Δ^4-androstenedione and DHEA are bound to albumin they are cleared much more rapidly than testosterone, with metabolic clearance rates of about 1100 litres/day/m^2. DHEA sulphate is present in blood at much higher concentrations than the other androgens and is cleared very slowly—about 8–14 litres/day/m^2. Dihydrotestosterone and 5α-androstane-$3\alpha,17\beta$-diol are more potent androgens, but are present in low concentrations, about 0.5 ng/ml and both are bound to SHBG. The production rate of DHT is about 0.25 mg, more than 70% of which arises by conversion from other androgens, principally testosterone. There is a small testicular contribution to the secretion of dihydrotestosterone but it is not certain how much is derived from Leydig cells and how much from the tubular compartment. Notwithstanding the substantial differences in blood concentrations and production rates between testosterone and dihydrotestosterone there is good evidence that dihydrotestosterone is the major active androgen and that testosterone should be regarded mainly as a prohormone.

6.8 Abnormalities of Leydig Cell Function

These may be congenital or acquired.

6.8.1 Congenital Disorders

Congenital defects of Leydig cell function are commonly associated with abnormalities of sexual differentiation. These individuals—male pseudohermaphrodites—have gonads that are exclusively testes and genital ducts and genitalia which are incompletely masculinised. They display varying degrees of genital ambiguity and phenotypic features that are female. The secretion of testosterone by fetal Leydig cells is essential for the development of male sexual structures. Testosterone itself is probably the hormone which stimulates the development of the Wolffian duct system, which becomes the vasa deferentia, seminal vesicles and epididymides, whereas dihydrotestosterone directly derived from testicular testosterone promotes the masculinisation of the external genitalia and development of the prostate.

Defects in testosterone secretion may result from a congenital absence of Leydig cells (Bethezene et al. 1976) to deficiency of enzymatic reactions involved in the biosynthesis of testosterone from cholesterol. These deficiencies are with one exception in both the Leydig cells and adrenals and at birth the degree of genital ambiguity and the amount of virilisation at puberty reflect the severity of the enzymic defect. The inheritance is autosomal recessive and clinical expression is found in homozygous individuals.

The first defect is in the conversion of cholesterol to pregnenolone (Fig. 6.8). These infants who have female external genitalia frequently die at an early age from adrenocortical insufficiency and at autopsy are found to have adrenals that are filled with lipid—hence the term congenital lipoid adrenal hyperplasia. Two patients have been described who have survived into early childhood; they are male pseudohermaphrodites with severe adrenocortical deficiency (Kirkland et al. 1973).

A deficiency in the 3β-ol dehydrogenase-Δ^5-isomerase system also leads to severe adrenocortical insufficiency and ambiguous genitalia in males (Bongiovanni 1962). Although these infants secrete increased amounts of DHEA which is weakly androgenic, this is not sufficient for masculinisation of the external genitalia and male duct structures.

A deficiency in 17α-hydroxylase was first described in a genetic female by Biglieri et al. (1966), but since then males with this condition have been described (New 1970; Mantero et al. 1971; Bricaire et al. 1972). In addition to genital ambiguities and absence of pubertal development these patients present with moderate to severe hypertension, hypokalaemia and alkalosis.

The last step in the biosynthesis of testosterone is the conversion of androstenedione to testosterone. The enzyme required for this step is 17β-hydroxysteroid dehydrogenase, and several patients have been described with this deficiency (Saez et al. 1971; Goebelsmann et al. 1973; Givens et al. 1974). These patients are genetic and gonadal males with severe abnormalities of the genitalia—labia majora and minora, clitoral enlargement and a blind vaginal pouch. Virilisation and gynaecomastia may develop at puberty, depending on the levels of androstenedione and on its conversion to oestrone and oestradiol.

At least two patients have been described with Leydig cell agenesis. These patients have a female phenotype, very low levels of testosterone and high levels of LH but normal levels of FSH. In both patients the testes were infantile in size and contained undeveloped tubules; epididymides and vasa were present in both patients. This suggests the action of testosterone at one stage during fetal development.

The commonest congenital abnormality of Leydig cells is seen in patients with Klinefelter's syndrome. In these patients there is severe damage to the seminiferous tubules leading not infrequently to complete hyalinisation of tubules. The Leydig cells appear to be increased in size and number, but often the secretion of testosterone is lower than normal despite the appearance of the Leydig cells and high levels of LH. Additional stimulation with hCG produces some increase in testosterone secretion but less than is seen in normal men. The Leydig cells are able to produce oestradiol, which may sometimes be produced in increased amounts (Wang et al. 1975; Forti et al. 1978). The reasons for the appearance of the Leydig cells in this disorder are unknown. It is of interest that Aoki and Fawcett (1978) have described changes in Leydig cells in rats in which localised damage to tubules has been induced by anti-fertility agents; these changes consist of hypertrophy of smooth endoplasmic reticulum and evidence of Leydig cell stimulation. These changes are found only in those Leydig cells in association with damaged or atrophic tubules. They raise the interesting question as to whether there may be some local feedback mechanism within the testis that is an additional controlling factor of Leydig cell function.

Cryptorchidism. Infertility in men and animals with cryptochidism is an old observation. The spermatogenic injury results from increased intratesticular temperature caused by the intra-abdominal location of the testes. Exposure of scrotal testes to heat can reproduce these changes (Rock and Robinson 1965). Initially Collins and Lacy (1969) proposed that Leydig cells were unaffected by heat, but more sophisticated studies indicate that androgen secretion may certainly be impaired in the cryptorchid testis. There are several lines of evidence: reduction of weights in the accessory organs (Clegg 1960; Tamaoki 1968; Walsh and Swerdloff 1973); decreased activity of enzymes required for testosterone biosynthesis (Llaurado and Dominguez 1963); ultrastructural changes which showed cellular hypertrophy (Kerr et al. 1979b) and impaired testosterone secretory responses to hCG. These changes in Leydig cell structure and function may yet be a further example of a local feedback system between the seminiferous epithelium and neighbouring Leydig cells (Aoki and Fawcett 1978). This concept is expanded in Chap. 7.

6.8.2 Acquired Disorders

Leydig cell function can be compromised in a number of acquired systemic disorders.

Stress. There are several observations which indicate that Leydig cell function may be affected by stress. Moderate to major abdominal surgery lasting from $^1/_2$–3 h results in a highly significant reduction in plasma testosterone levels on the day following surgery. The nadir occurs between 24 and 48 h and the levels remain low for up to 6 or 7 days (Matsumoto et al. 1970; Aono et al. 1976; Wang et al. 1978a,b). In one study plasma levels of testosterone decreased from a mean of 8 to 3.7 ng/ml and remained at this level for a further 5 days and had not returned to normal by the seventh post-operative day (Wang et al. 1978b). Plasma levels of LH showed a twofold increase during the intra-operative period and either returned to normal or remained slightly elevated during the first few post-operative days.

Wang et al. (1978a) have also shown that plasma levels of testosterone fall transiently following acute myocardial infarction. In these patients there is an increase in plasma LH which persists for a week after the infarction. Bardin and Petersen (1967) have shown in rats that there is a highly significant fall in the spermatic venous levels of testosterone following ether anaesthesia – from a mean level of 42 to 14 ng/ml. Although Bardin and Petersen interpreted this fall as being the consequence of gonadotrophin suppression, the interpretation from human studies is that stress has a direct effect on Leydig cell function. This is supported by the finding that LH levels tend to be increased rather than reduced when testosterone levels remain low post-operatively.

Psychosocial stress in men and monkeys has been shown to be associated with a decline in plasma testosterone levels. Thus Kreuz et al. (1972) found that when healthy young men are recruited into officer training programmes, two periods of stress could be identified during the training. During the first stressful period, which the recruits identified as "bad", there are significant falls in the levels of plasma testosterone but by contrast during the second stressful period, which they "enjoyed", there was no such fall. Rose et al. (1972) have shown that social stresses in rhesus monkeys are associated with fall in the levels of testosterone in plasma. When less dominant males are alone with females they have plasma levels of testosterone at 20 ng/ml or more, but when more dominant males are introduced there is a highly significant reduction in the levels of testosterone to 5.5 ng/ml or less. Unfortunately gonadotrophin measurements were not made in either of these studies involving psychosocial stress, so it is not possible to say unequivocally whether the changes result from a direct effect of stress on Leydig cells or from a suppression of gonadotrophin secretion.

6.8.2.1 Cirrhosis of the Liver

The best recognised and probably the most common of the acquired disorders is cirrhosis of the liver, in which a tendency to feminise with hypogonadism and gynaecomastia are the usual endocrine changes.

Patients with cirrhosis have low levels of free and bound testosterone, despite increases in sex steroid binding globulin and normal or increased levels of LH. Levels of oestradiol are normal or higher than normal mainly as the result of increased peripheral conversion from androgens. There is thus a reduction in the androgen/oestrogen ratio in blood (Baker et al. 1976b). It is possible that the decrease in Leydig cell function, which can be demonstrated by a reduced response to hCG, may result partly from the effects of oestrogens. It is, however, also quite possible that impaired Leydig cell function is a direct effect of alcohol since it has been shown that, plasma levels of testosterone can be reduced while LH levels remain unchanged in normal subjects with actue or chronic alcoholic excess. Not only does alcohol directly affect the Leydig cell, as shown in the rat by in vitro studies (Ellingboe and Varanelli 1979) but there is an increase in hepatic metabolism of testosterone and of the hepatic conversion of androgens to oestrogens (Gordon et al. 1979).

6.8.2.2 Chronic Renal Failure

Patients with end stage renal failure have low secretion rates of testosterone and high levels of LH. There is an impaired response to hCG (Holdsworth et al. 1977). These are indices of Leydig cell failure and are similar to the changes that may be seen in men with severe protein-calorie malnutrition (Smith et al. 1975) so that it is possible that the nutritional status in renal failure may be a contributing factor to reduced Leydig cell function in these patients.

6.8.2.3 Age

There have been several reports of declining Leydig cell function with age. This has been shown both in animals and men (Ewing et al. 1972; Prike and Doerr 1973; Stearns et al. 1974; Baker et al. 1976; Steger et al. 1979). The studies which have reported lower levels of testosterone, both free and bound, were mainly transverse studies of men in a hospital or institutional population; they also showed increasing levels of LH and FSH with age, which indicate that the changes are the result of a decline in overall testicular function. More recent longitudinal studies on men from a healthy, middle class population fail to confirm some of the earlier studies on age-related changes in testicular function (Harman and Tsitouras 1980). The discrepancy between the two sets of observations may be accounted for by the fact that many of the subjects in the earlier studies were patients in hospital, and therefore not entirely healthy, or in institutions for the aged.

6.8.3 Testicular Disorders

Infertile men with mild to moderate oligospermia have normal Leydig cell function. However, some men with more severe disorders of spermatogenesis, such as germinal cell aplasia may have low normal levels of testosterone, some elevation in LH levels and diminished responses to hCG (Baker et al. 1976a; Ishida et al. 1976). The germinal epithelium is frequently destroyed in men who have received combined chemotherapy for cancer. In many of these patients Leydig cell function is apparently normal, that is, basal levels of testosterone and LH are within the normal range (Schilsky et al. 1980). However, some patients when stimulated with LHRH show an exaggerated response in LH secretion, which suggests a mild but compensated failure of Leydig cells.

Leprosy and Myotonic Dystrophy. These are two adult onset disorders in which spermatogenic and Leydig cell failure occur.

Neoplasia and Hyperplasia. These are unusual acquired disorders of Leydig cells. When they occur in children they commonly lead to precocious sexual development as a result of an excessive secretion of testosterone. Leydig cell tumours are rare and usually benign. Very occasionally they may occur in adults and cause oestrogen excess manifest as gynaecomastia and impotence.

Leydig cell hyperplasia can result from abnormal secretion of luteinising hormone. Boys with sexual precocity due to an abnormal secretion of gonadotrophins may have a lesion of the central nervous system, such as a tumour of the pineal or hypothalamus. More often, however, no localised lesion is found but some of these children may show diffuse electroencephalographic abnormalities.

7 The Effect of Testicular Damage on Sertoli and Leydig Cell Function

D.M. de Kretser and J.B. Kerr

7.1 Introduction

Heat, irradiation, several groups of drugs and vitamin A deficiency may all disrupt sperm production. Despite the damage caused by these agents, Sertoli and Leydig cells appear normal to examination by light microscopy, and for this reason it has been assumed that these cells are resistant to damage, and are thus more robust than germ cells. However, the availability of relatively simple techniques for the measurement of testosterone, and the discovery that androgen-binding protein (ABP) is a product of the Sertoli cell, has made it possible to study the function of Leydig and Sertoli cells during the actions of agents known to disrupt spermatogenesis. These studies have shown substantial modifications to Leydig and Sertoli cell function in association with damage to the seminiferous epithelium.

7.2 Spermatogenic Damage and the Control of FSH Secretion

The rise in FSH levels that frequently follows interference to spermatogenic function has been extensively used as an argument in favour of the inhibin hypothesis (Chap. 2). In rodents it is generally agreed that elevation of FSH levels in serum almost always accompanies spermatogenic damage. The induction of cryptorchidism in the rat and in the ram leads to spermatogenic damage, and an increase in the levels of FSH (Amatayakul et al. 1971; Walsh and Swerdloff 1973; Blanc et al. 1978; Kerr et al. 1979a; Lee et al. 1981).

Similar changes also follow spermatogenic damage induced by drugs, with a reduction in FSH levels occurring with recovery (Gomes et al. 1973; Debeljuk et al. 1973a; Rich and de Kretser 1977a; Morris and Jackson 1978). Irradiation of the fetal or adult rat testis causes gross destruction of germ cells and an increase in serum levels of FSH (Bain and Keene 1975; Cunningham et al. 1975; Verjans and Eik-Nes 1976; Rich and de Kretser, 1977a; Hopkinson et al. 1978). In general, increases in FSH levels broadly correlate with the severity of the spermatogenic damage (Rich and de Kretser 1977a). However, it has been claimed that FSH levels do not increase when spermatogenic damage is induced by vitamin A deficiency or hydroxyurea treatment, despite the loss of all cell types except Sertoli cells and spermatogonia (Kreuger et al. 1974; Mecklenberg et al. 1975). More recent studies, however, have shown that increased levels of FSH (Fig. 7.1) accompany the spermatogenic damage induced by almost identical regimes of treatment (Rich and de Kretser 1977a; Huang et al. 1979).

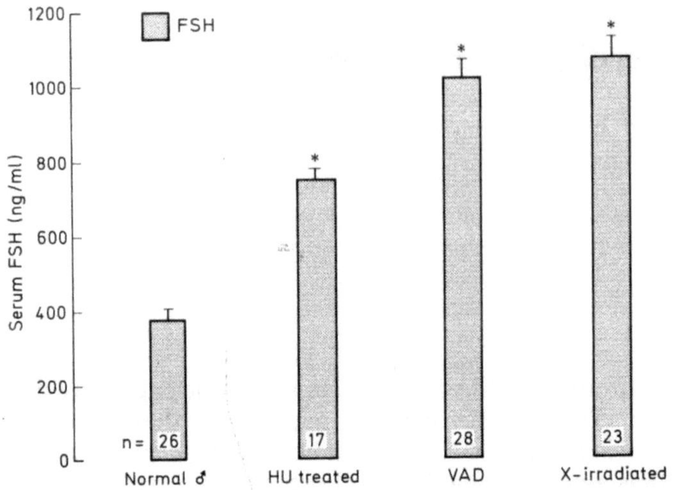

Fig. 7.1. Serum FSH levels in rats with differing testicular disorders. *HU*, hydroxyurea treated; *VAD*, vitamin A deficiency; *x-irradiated*, rats irradiated in utero at day 20 of gestation

Several studies in man suggest that there is a relationship between damage to the seminiferous epithelium and levels of FSH. This was first shown by the use of relatively imprecise bioassays for urinary FSH in men with infertility (Howard et al. 1950; Johnsen 1970). Increased levels of serum FSH have been found in men with infertility and severe germ cell damage using more sensitive and specific radioimmunoassay methods (see Fig. 3.11) (Wide and Kjessler 1969; Rosen and Weintraub 1971; Leonard et al. 1972; de Kretser

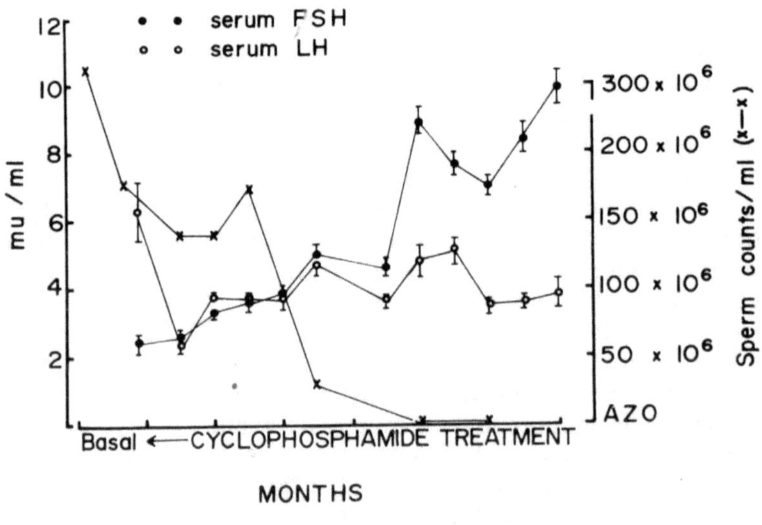

Fig. 7.2. Serum FSH, LH levels and the sperm counts of a patient before and during treatment with cyclophosphamide for renal disease

et al. 1972; Franchimont et al. 1972). These changes have also been found in men treated with cytotoxic drugs (van Thiel et al. 1972). In some men it has been possible to follow these changes prospectively. The rise in FSH that occurs following testicular damage induced by cyclophosphamide used for the treatment of renal disease is shown in Fig. 7.2.

The specificity of the relationship between the degree of spermatogenic disruption and elevation of FSH levels has proved controversial. Johnsen (1970) and Franchimont et al. (1972) claimed that spermatids are closely associated with the elaboration of the feedback signal for FSH, and if absent from the testis, FSH levels are elevated. However, Leonard and co-workers (1972), using quantitative cytology on a limited number of subjects, were not able to show any relationship between specific germ cell types and bioassayable urinary FSH levels. They postulated that an "independent testicular station" is responsible for the control of FSH.

In detailed quantitative histological studies, de Kretser et al. (1974) showed that FSH levels remained normal in some men with no spermatids in their testicular biopsy (see Fig. 3.21). However, it was possible to show an inverse relationship between the number of each germ cell type and FSH levels. In particular, if the numbers of spermatogonia were severely reduced (see Fig. 3.22), FSH levels were invariably elevated, although in some men with a normal spermatogonial complement, FSH levels were still elevated. The failure to link any one specific germ cell type with the control of FSH raised the possibility that the Sertoli cell may be involved. This prospect had largely been ignored, since in states of spermatogenic damage the number and morphology of the Sertoli cells by light microscopy appears normal. More recently, de Jong and Sharpe (1977) have shown that irradiation of the fetus can decrease the Sertoli cell complement. Although levels of FSH are almost invariably increased in men with Sertoli cell only syndrome, a fact which could be construed as evidence against the Sertoli cell as being the source of the feedback signal for FSH, the levels of FSH are considerably lower than in men with seminiferous tubule hyalinisation (see Fig. 3.11), or who have been castrated. Thus, it seems that Sertoli cells in men with the Sertoli cell only syndrome control the secretion of FSH, but the feedback signal is less than normal. It is important, therefore, to review the evidence that the secretion of FSH is regulated by Sertoli cells.

7.3 Sertoli Cell Function and Testicular Damage

It is only relatively recently that it has been possible to assess Sertoli cells other than by microscopic techniques and in isolation from germ cells. Recent developments in the understanding of Sertoli cell function have been considered previously (Chap. 5). The development of tests for Sertoli cell function has depended on the demonstration that Sertoli cells have receptors for FSH, and are the site of production of seminiferous tubule fluid and ABP.

In one of the earliest investigations of Sertoli cell function, Hagenas and Ritzen (1976) showed that following surgical induction of cryptorchidism

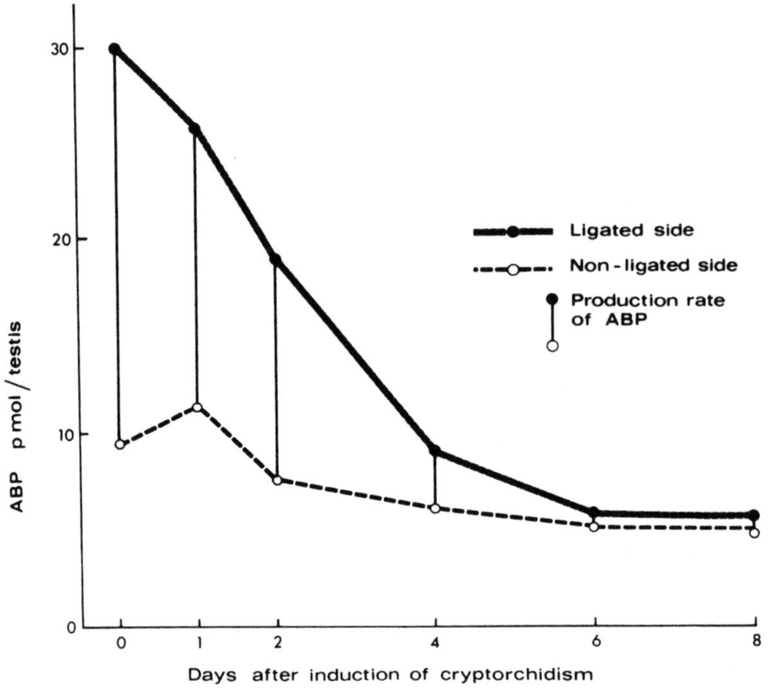

Fig. 7.3. Changes in ABP levels and production following cryptorchidism in rats. The non-ligated side represents the basal concentration in ABP whereas the ligated side represents the accumulation (production) of ABP following efferent duct ligation 16 h earlier

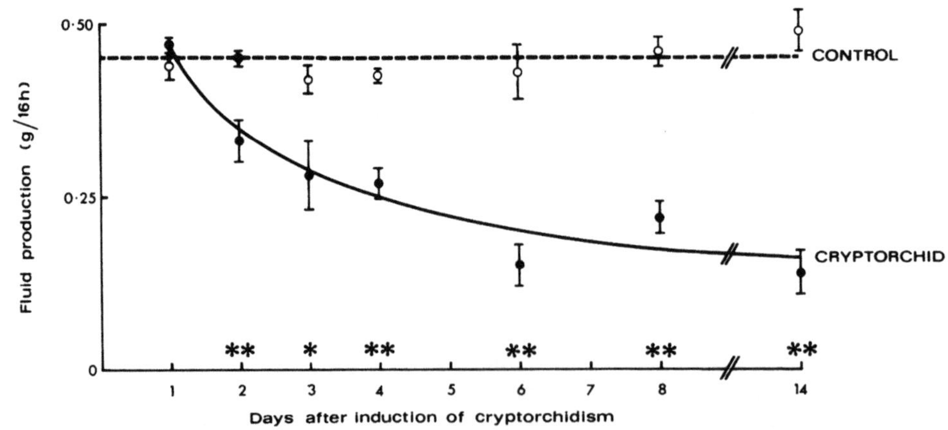

Fig. 7.4. Changes in seminiferous tubule fluid production following the induction of cryptorchidism in rats. Fluid production is measured by the difference in testis weight between one side following efferent duct ligation 16 h before and the contralateral unligated testes ** $P<0.01$; * $P<0.05$

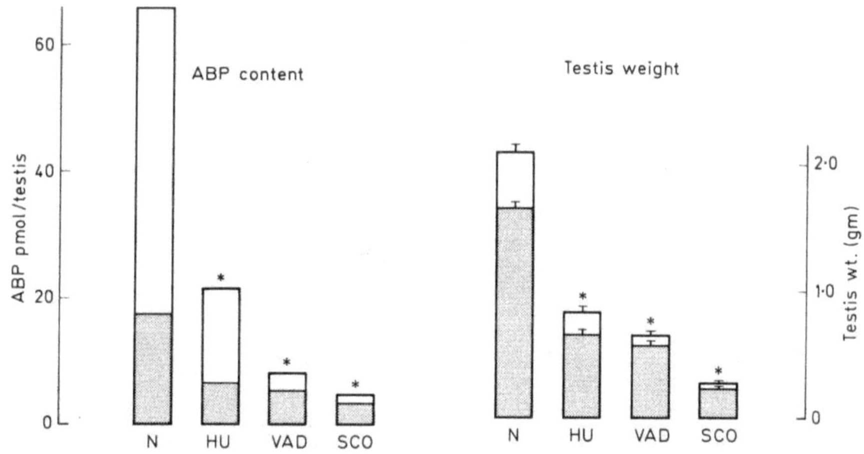

Fig. 7.5. Effect of unilateral efferent duct ligation on testis weight and ABP content in normal *(N)*, hydroxyurea-treated *(HU)*, vitamin A deficient *(VAD)* and fetally irradiated *(SCO)* rats. The *hatched bar* represents the mean testis weight or ABP content of the non-ligated testis and the *clear bar* represents the increase above control after 16 h of efferent duct ligation. ** $P<0.001$. (Rich and de Kretser 1977b)

in rats ABP production by Sertoli cells is impaired. These studies have now been extended (Figs. 7.3, 7.4) and show that within 3 days of inducing cryptorchidism, ABP and fluid production by Sertoli cells are impaired (Jegou and de Kretser 1979). In states of testicular damage induced by fetal irradiation, vitamin A deficiency or hydroxyurea treatment, impaired Sertoli cell function is shown by decreased ABP and fluid production (Fig. 7.5), the degree of impairment being inversely proportional to the levels of FSH (Fig. 7.1) (Rich and de Kretser 1977a). Even the relatively short exposure of the testis to 43 °C for 15 min results in the impairment of ABP secretion by the testis for up to 50 days (Rich and de Kretser 1977b). Impairment of Sertoli cell function has also been shown in naturally occurring models of diminished spermatogenesis. In the H^{re} rat with oligospermia and diminished ABP production, the levels of FSH are elevated (Musto and Bardin 1976; Musto et al. 1978). Furthermore, in rats with the syndrome of testicular feminisation, Hansson et al. (1978) have shown significantly diminished ABP production in vitro. To date, diminished secretory capacity of Sertoli cells has been found in all states of spermatogenic damage studied and emphasises that these cells are also susceptible to noxious agents. From the available data, it is not possible to know whether the agents simultaneously affect both Sertoli and germ cells.

It is of interest that impaired Sertoli cell function is accompanied by structural changes visible by electron microscopy. Accumulation of lipid and dilatation of the smooth endoplasmic reticulum occur within 7 days of cryptorchidism (Figs. 7.6–7.9), and are associated with complex, transient changes in the form of specialised inter-Sertoli cell junctions (Kerr et al. 1979a). Similar changes are also demonstrable in Sertoli cells from rats treated by

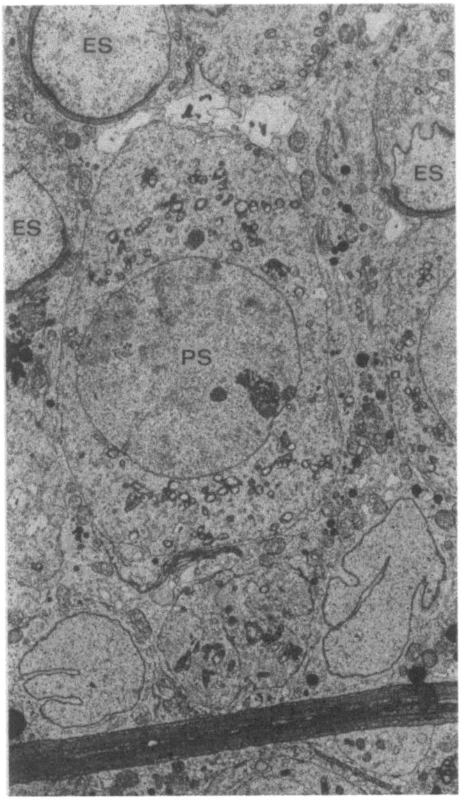

Fig. 7.6. Arrangement of the normal Sertoli cell showing cytoplasmic prolongations between the germ cells. *PS*, primary spermatocytes; *ES*, early spermatids. ×4400

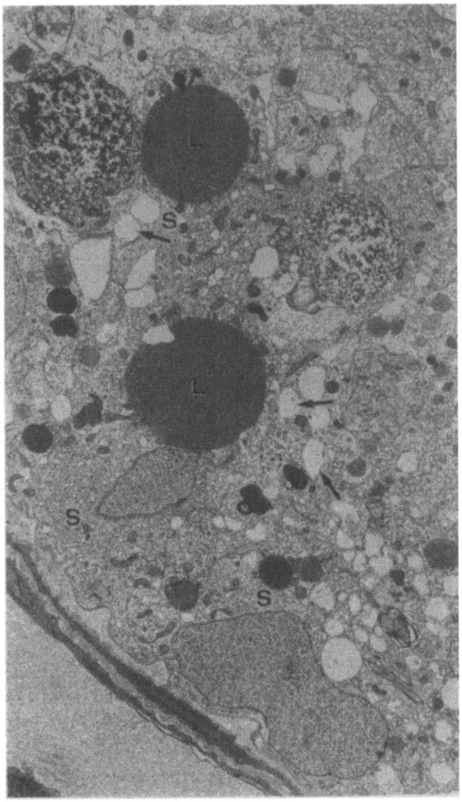

Fig. 7.7. The Sertoli cells *(S)* after 7 days of cryptorchidism show lipid inclusions *(L)* and dilation of cisternae *(arrows)* associated with inter-Sertoli cell junctions. Note degenerating germ cells. ×4500

Fig. 7.9a–d. Diagrammatic representation of a proposed relationship between the appearance of vacuoles and complex membranous bodies associated with inter-Sertoli cell tight junctions. The hypothesis is based upon observations of the Sertoli cells as cryptorchidism persisted. **a** An inter-Sertoli cell junctional complex within a normal testis. The intercellular space between adjacent Sertoli cells is frequently fused at intervals forming tight junctions. Cisternae of endoplasmic reticulum are separated from the cell surface by hexagonal groups of filaments. **b** After 7 days of cryptorchidism, the intercellular junctions expand between the sites of plasma membrane fusion, giving rise to multiple sites of dilation along the pathway of each junctional complex. The sub-surface cisternae expand with the dilated intercellular space, thus usually encompassing each vacuole. **c** With the prompt depletion of germ cells in the sustained cryptorchid state, the Sertoli cells collapse and become compacted. The vacuoles probably undergo compression forces which produce distortion and they behave like a "concertina" mechanism, being squeezed along the pathway of the junctional complex. **d** After 4 weeks of cryptorchidism, the vacuoles are compressed into thin membrane-bound saccules, aggregated in parallel where they form alternate layers with their accompanying smooth cisternae and bundles of filaments. (Kerr et al. 1979a) ▶

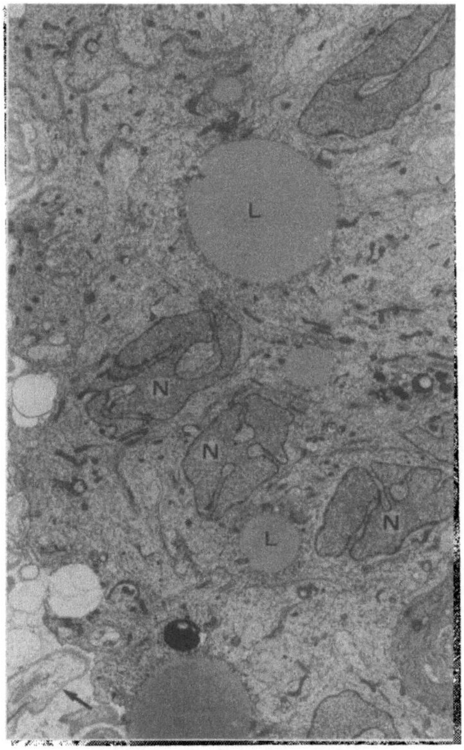

Fig. 7.8. Sertoli cells after 4 weeks of cryptorchidism contain pleomorphic nuclei *(N)* and large lipid inclusions *(L)*. Note infolding of basement membrane *(arrow)*. (Kerr et al. 1979a) × 4300

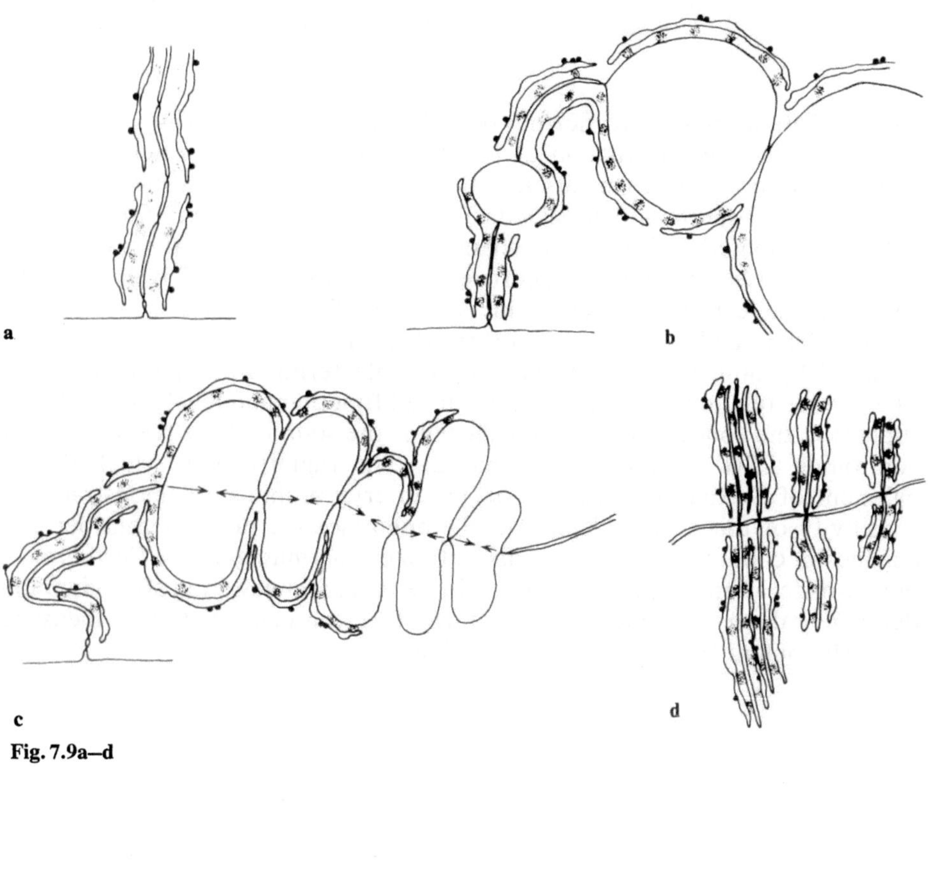

Fig. 7.9a–d

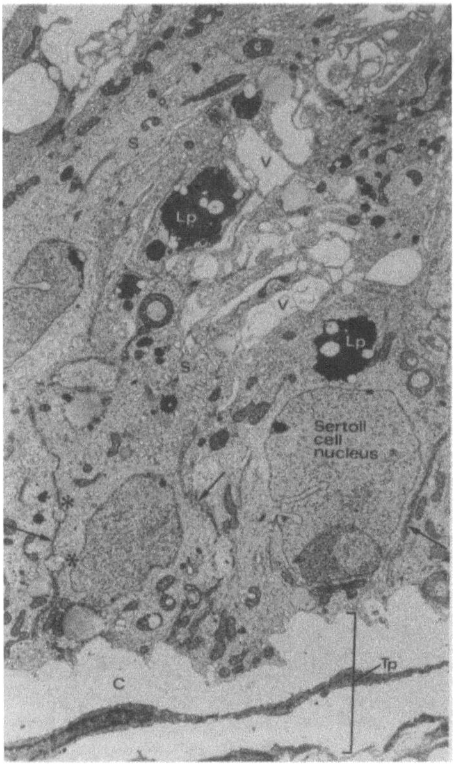

Fig. 7.10. The vacuolated appearance *(V)* of the cytoplasm of Sertoli cells from a rat treated with hydroxyurea is shown. Note dilated smooth endoplasmic reticulum *(S)*, lipofuscin granules *(Lp)* and inter-Sertoli cell junctional complexes *(arrows)*. The sub-surface cisternae which are associated with the junctional complex have been displaced laterally around membrane-bound borders of each vacuole *(asterisks)*. Note widened tunica propria *(Tp)* and collagen fibres *(C)*. × 5500

fetal irradiation, vitamin A dificiency or hydroxyurea treatment (Figs. 7.10–7.12).

Vacuolisation and retraction of the apical extension and ramifications of Sertoli cells occur in association with the early stages of testicular lesions induced by anti-spermatogenic agents, Trininom (Kierszenbaum 1970) and DL-6-N-2-pipecolinomethyl-5-hydroxy-indane maleate (Fang and Anderson 1976), during the onset of vitamin A deficiency (Sobhon et al. 1979) or following ligation of the efferent testicular ducts (Anton 1979).

From the preceding data it is evident that Sertoli cell function can be rapidly impaired by numerous agents capable of interfering with spermatogenesis. The inverse relationship between Sertoli cell function and levels of FSH lends support to the concept that the Sertoli cell is the source of the feedback signal controlling FSH secretion (see Chap. 2). The rapidity with which the impairment of Sertoli cell function occurs in cryptorchidism demonstrates the sensitivity of this cell to damage and emphasises the need to consider such changes in conjunction with any disruption of spermatogenesis. Furthermore, during restoration of spermatogenesis by retinol administration after vitamin A deficiency there is a simultaneous return of Sertoli cell function as measured by ABP content (Rich and de Kretser 1980).

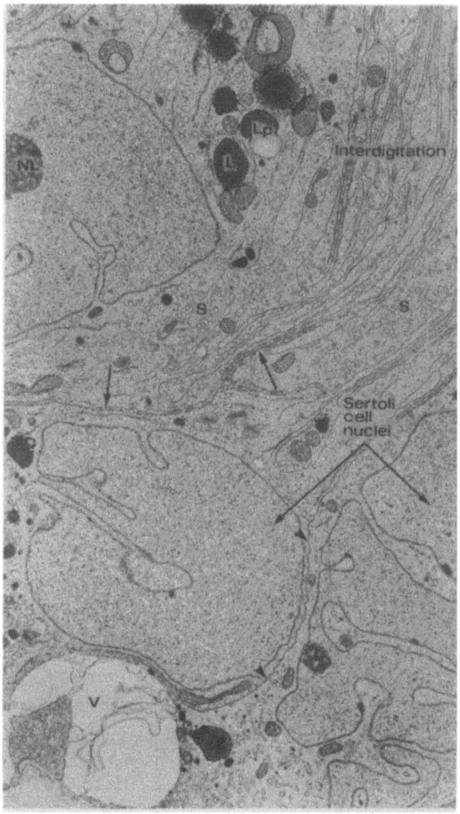

Fig. 7.11

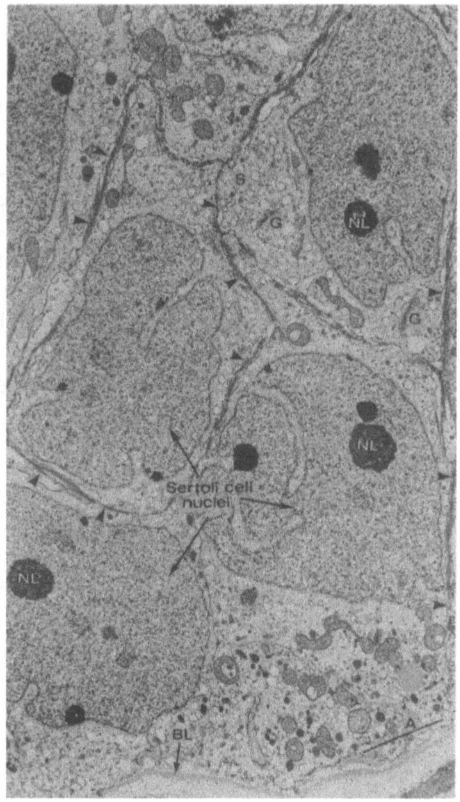

Fig. 7.12

Fig. 7.11. Electron micrograph of the basal aspect of Sertoli cells in chronic vitamin A deficiency. The Sertoli cells contain large vacuoles *(V)* lipofuscin bodies *(Lp)* and lipid inclusions *(L)*. The nuclei are highly pleomorphic and extensively lobulated, and the cytoplasm is filled with numerous small dilated vesicles of smooth endoplasmic reticulum *(S)*. The cytoplasmic surfaces of apposing Sertoli cells form complex interdigitations, at times giving rise to specialised junctional regions *(arrows)*. The passage of an extremely lengthy inter-Sertoli cell junction which appears to lose the adjacent sub-surface endoplasmic reticulum *(arrowheads)* may be traced between the adjacent Sertoli cell nuclei. × 9700

Fig. 7.12. Electron micrograph of the basal aspect of the seminiferous epithelium within the fetal X-irradiated testis, illustrating four closely packed Sertoli cell nuclei, three of which contain a prominent nucleolus *(NL)*. Extremely long lengths of specialised junctional regions can be observed to occur at the apposed surfaces of adjacent Sertoli cells *(arrowheads)*. The cytoplasm contains numerous small dilated vesicles of smooth endoplasmic reticulum *(S)* and extensive Golgi complexes *(G)*. An artefact *(A)* is present in the lower region of the micrograph, near the basal lamina *(BL)* of the seminiferous tubule. × 6500

7.4 Luteinising Hormone, Testosterone and Spermatogenic Damage

For many years the current dogma was that agents which disrupted spermatogenesis did not usually affect Leydig cells. The concept was based on light microscopic observations that Leydig cells often appeared to be more plentiful in such infertile states (Hanes 1911; Nelson 1951; Clegg 1961). Indeed there was some controversy as to whether Leydig cell hyperplasia occurred under conditions of seminiferous epithelial damage, since some investigators suggested that the prominent appearance of Leydig cells was due to the coalescence of existing cells resulting from a decrease in the diameter of the seminiferous tubules.

Using radioimmunoassay techniques in men with testicular damage, a number of early studies claimed that no changes in LH levels were found

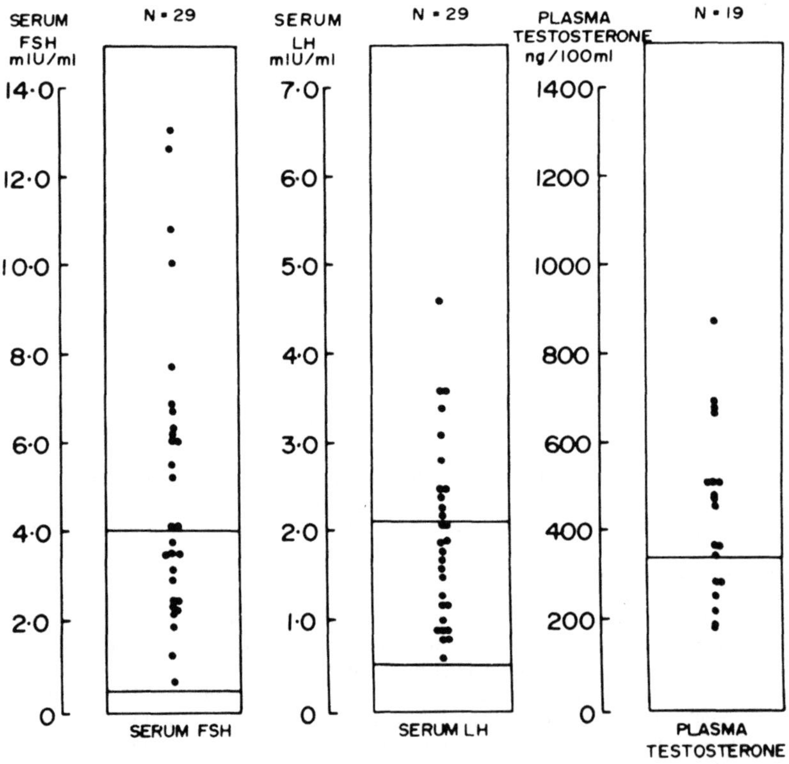

Fig. 7.13. Serum FSH, LH and testosterone levels in men with infertility and the testis biopsy appearance of germ cell arrest

Fig. 7.14. Serum FSH, LH and testosterone levels in men with infertility and the testis biopsy appearance of Sertoli cell only syndrome ▶

Fig. 7.15. Serum FSH, LH and testosterone levels in men with infertility and the testis biopsy appearance of seminiferous tubule hyalinisation ▶

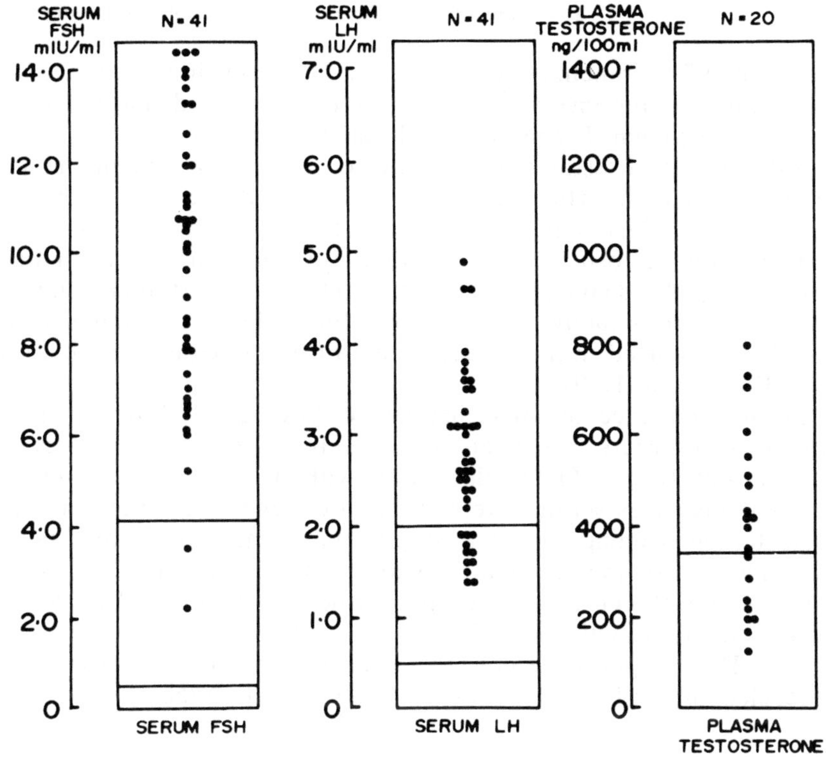

Fig. 7.14

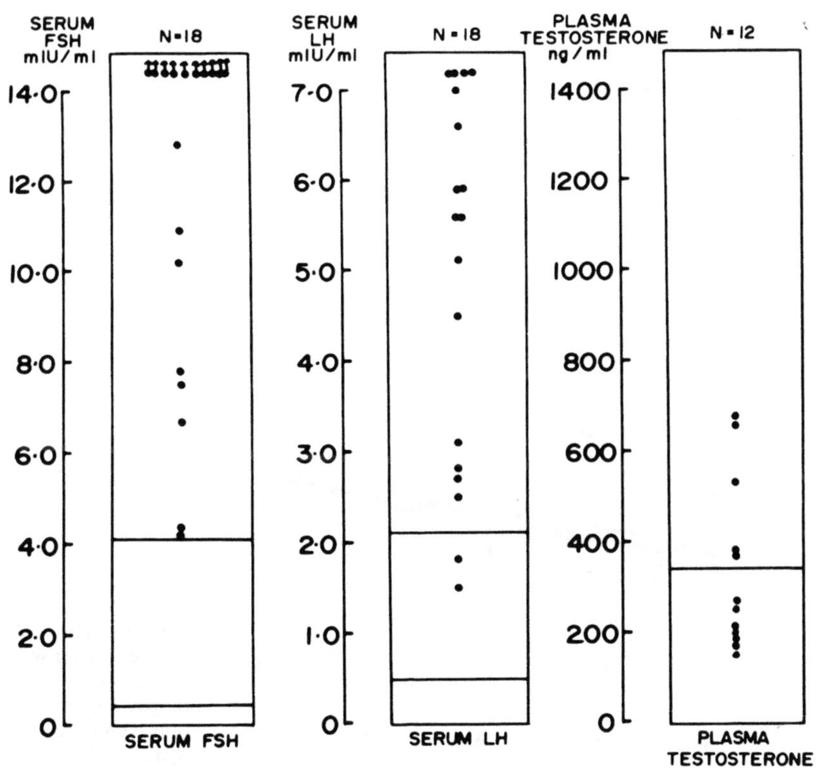

Fig. 7.15

(Johnsen 1970; Franchimont et al. 1972). However, in the study of men with Klinefelter's syndrome who have severe testicular damage, Paulsen et al. (1968) have shown that in nearly all patients the levels of LH are increased and that levels of testosterone are low, or low normal. When LH and testosterone levels of infertile men were analysed with respect to the changes in their testicular histology, de Kretser et al. (1972) have shown that elevated LH and low testosterone levels are present in many of the patients with severe testicular damage, such as germ cell arrest, Sertoli cell only syndrome and seminiferous tubule hyalinisation (Figs. 7.13–7.15). Similar results have also been reported in more recent investigations (Hunter et al. 1974; Rodriguez-Rigau et al. 1980).

Further evidence of abnormalities of Leydig cell function in men with testicular disorders has been adduced from the subnormal response of testosterone (Fig. 7.16) to stimulation with hCG (de Kretser et al. 1975a). In some instances serum levels of LH are elevated despite normal levels of testosterone, leading to the postulate that a state of compensated Leydig cell failure exists in such men. Elevation of the LH response to LHRH in men with the Sertoli cell only syndrome further substantiates these abnormalities in Leydig cell function (Fig. 7.17), since a greater than normal LH rise was found. This supports the concept of decreased feedback from Leydig cells (Mecklenburg and Sherins 1974; de Kretser et al. 1975b).

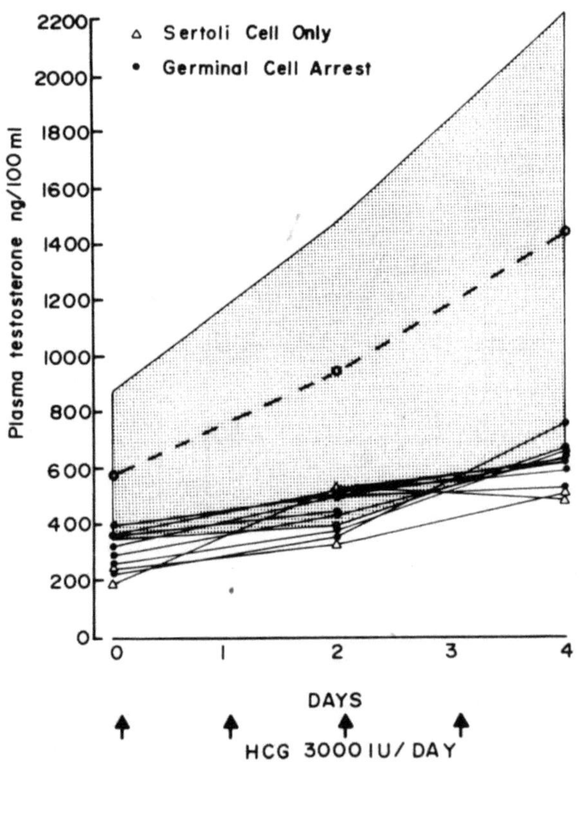

Fig. 7.16. The plasma testosterone response to hCG stimulation in men with the testes biopsy appearance of Sertoli cell only syndrome or germ cell arrest. (de Kretser et al. 1975c)

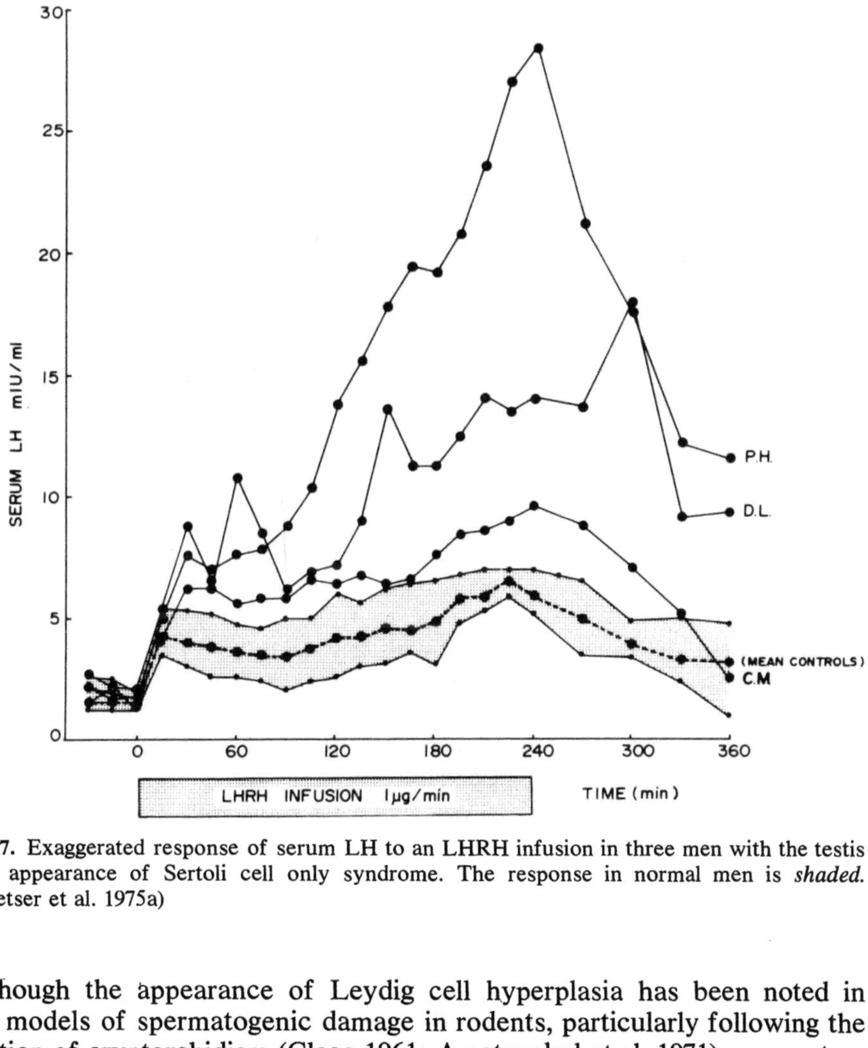

Fig. 7.17. Exaggerated response of serum LH to an LHRH infusion in three men with the testis biopsy appearance of Sertoli cell only syndrome. The response in normal men is *shaded.* (de Kretser et al. 1975a)

Although the appearance of Leydig cell hyperplasia has been noted in some models of spermatogenic damage in rodents, particularly following the induction of cryptorchidism (Clegg 1961; Amatayakul et al. 1971), parameters of Leydig cell function have not been measured until recently. A number of investigators have observed elevated serum levels of LH associated with the induction of cryptorchidism in rats (Amatayakul et al. 1971; Altwein and Gittes 1972; Walsh and Swerdloff 1973a; Steinberger and Chowdhury 1974). In more detailed studies, Kerr et al. (1979b) found that serum levels of LH become elevated at 7 days following cryptorchidism, and continue to rise until 21 days, when a plateau occurs. In this study, testosterone levels were significantly lower between the 7th and 14th days despite a fourfold elevation of serum LH. Furthermore, the changes in testosterone levels to hCG stimulation were less than normal (Kerr et al. 1979b).

Elevated serum levels of LH have now been shown in association with testicular damage induced by vitamin A deficiency, fetal testicular irradiation, and hydroxyurea treatment (Fig. 7.18). This also has been observed

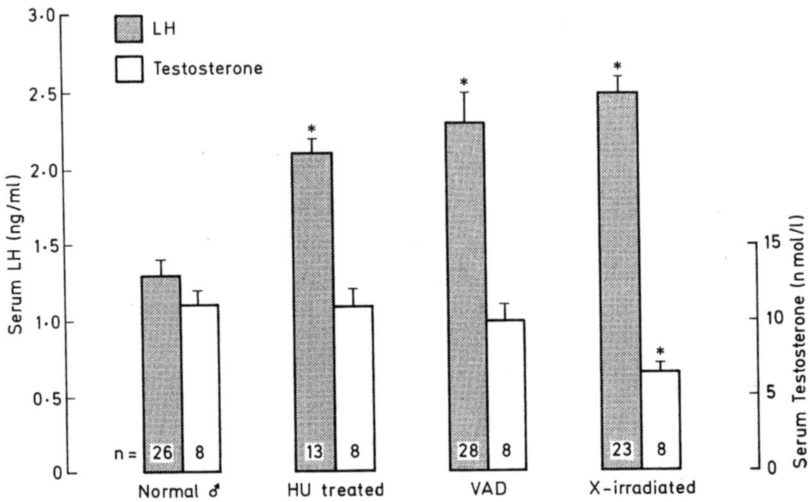

Fig. 7.18. Serum LH and testosterone levels in rats following hydroxyurea treatment *(HU)*, vitamin A deficiency *(VAD)* or fetal irradiation *(X-irradiated)*. * $P < 0.05$

following efferent duct ligation (Collins et al. 1978; Main et al. 1978) and irradiation (Bain and Keene 1975; Hopkinson et al. 1978). In many studies, although testosterone levels are not significantly different from controls, there is certainly no increase in testosterone despite the elevated LH levels—further evidence for the state of compensated Leydig cell failure. Our own studies have demonstrated that testosterone levels are significantly depressed follow-

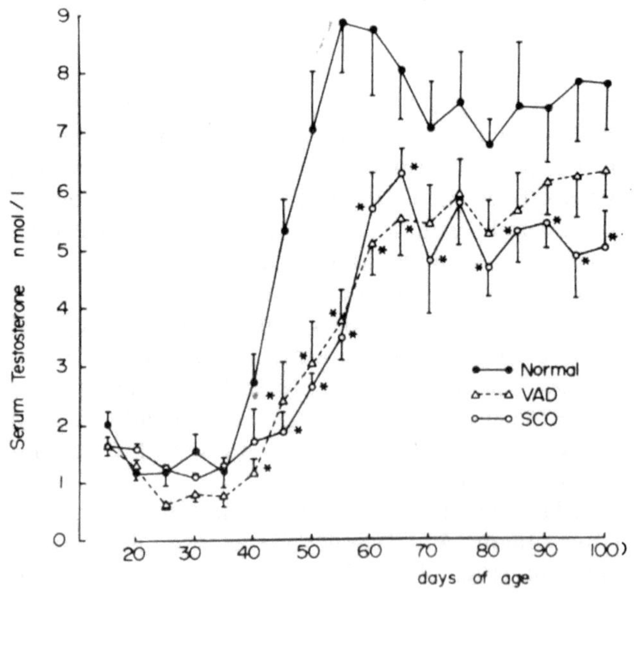

Fig. 7.19. Serum testosterone levels according to the age of normal rats or rats with testicular damage induced by vitamin A deficiency *(VAD)* or fetal irradiation *(SCO)*. * $P < 0.05$

ing severe damage induced by fetal testicular irradiation (Rich and de Kretser 1977a). We have also shown that testosterone response to hCG is impaired in rats with testicular damage induced by hydroxyurea treatment, fetal irradiation or vitamin A deficiency, despite normal basal levels (Rich et al. 1979). It is of interest that basal testosterone levels become progressively lower with increasing duration after testicular damage (Fig. 7.19).

From the preceding review it seems clear that severe testicular damage is associated with Leydig cell dysfunction, as evidenced by elevated serum levels of LH, low levels of testosterone, a poor response of testosterone to hCG, and an exaggerated LH rise following LHRH. This interference with Leydig cell function occurs in rats, rams and men (Lee et al. 1981), and thus would appear to indicate either a common response to the different agents used or to spermatogenic damage. We believe the latter to be the more likely.

7.5 Leydig Cell Structure and Spermatogenic Damage

The cause and nature of the changes in Leydig cell function with spermatogenic damage have not been well understood. The results of a few studies of Leydig cells in the cryptorchid testis have produced conflicting results. Amatayakul et al. (1971) reported that Leydig cells are more granular in appearance when studied by light microscopy following 7 days of cryptorchidism. In ultrastructural studies, Leeson and Leeson, (1970) have noted that the smooth endoplasmic reticulum of Leydig cells is more prominent than normal after 6 weeks of cryptorchidism, whereas Jones et al. (1977) were unable to detect any changes in the electron microscopic appearance of the Leydig cells after 8 weeks of cryptorchidism. The conflicting results reflect the fact that no objective data were obtained to confirm subjective impressions.

Our own studies have utilised morphometric techniques to investigate changes in Leydig cell cytology. In cryptorchid rats measurements of Leydig

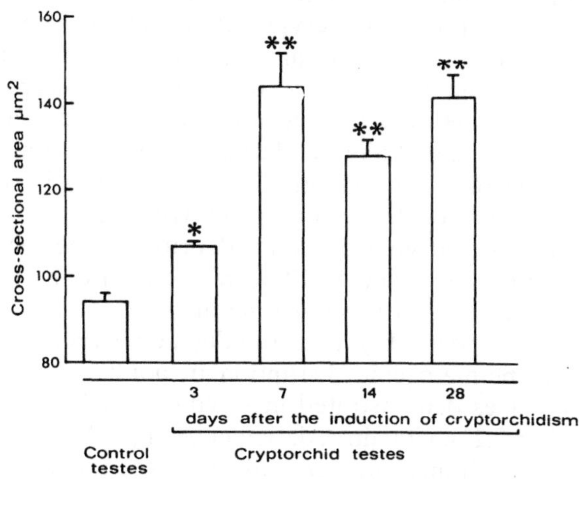

Fig. 7.20. Cross-sectional area of Leydig cells in the rat testis from control and cryptorchid animals. Approximately 50 Leydig cells per animal ($N = 4$ per group) were measured. * $P < 0.05$; ** $P < 0.01$

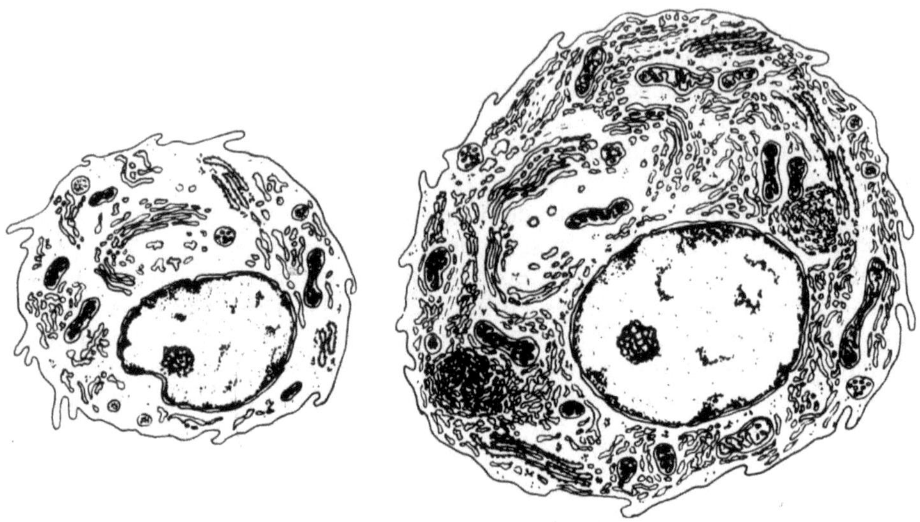

Fig. 7.21. Diagrammatic representation of Leydig cells from normal and cryptorchid rats illustrating the increased size and increment in smooth endoplasmic reticulum, mitochondria and the Golgi complex

cell cross-sectional areas have shown a significant increase which occurs in 7 days and persists thereafter (Fig. 7.20). The increase in cross-sectional area involves both the cytoplasm and nucleus and ultrastructural studies at 4 weeks of cryptorchidism show a marked increase in smooth endoplasmic reticulum and mitochondria (Fig. 7.21). Morphometric analyses have confirmed a significant increase in smooth endoplasmic reticulum, mitochondria, lysosomes and Golgi complex, all of which are involved in steroid biosynthesis (Kerr et al. 1979b).

It would appear that the state of sexual maturation at the time when cryptorchidism is induced influences the subsequent response of the Leydig cell. In rats made cryptorchid shortly after birth by cutting the gubernaculum, Bergh and Damber (1978) were not able to demonstrate Leydig cell hypertrophy; indeed Leydig cells in the cryptorchid testes were significantly smaller. However, in a more recent study rats made bilaterally cryptorchid at birth and studied at 100 days showed some early evidence of Leydig cell hypertrophy (Bergh and Damber 1979). It is possible that the different results represent evidence for alternative mechanisms, since in one group of studies cryptorchidism was induced prior to the establishment of spermatogenesis (Bergh and Damber 1979) whereas in our own studies the cryptorchid state was created after sexual maturity.

The possibility that Leydig cell hypertrophy may occur after any type of spermatogenic disruption in adult animals is supported by the identical changes demonstrated in Leydig cells from rats subjected to fetal irradiation (Fig. 7.22), vitamin A deficiency (Fig. 7.23) or hydroxyurea treatment (Fig. 7.24), in which measurements of cross-sectional area confirmed the ultrastructural

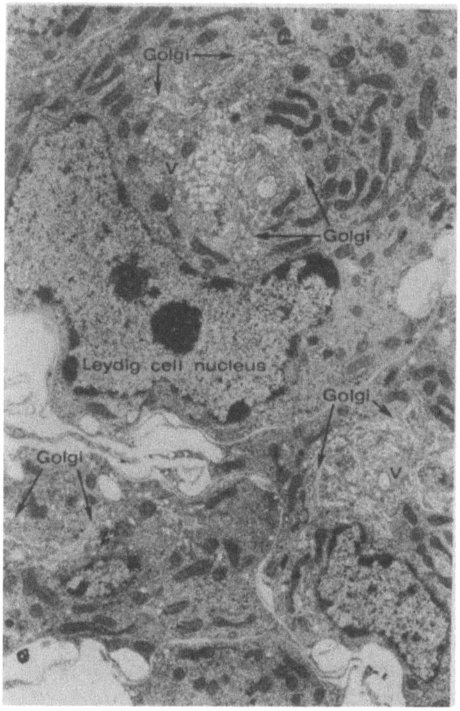

Fig. 7.22

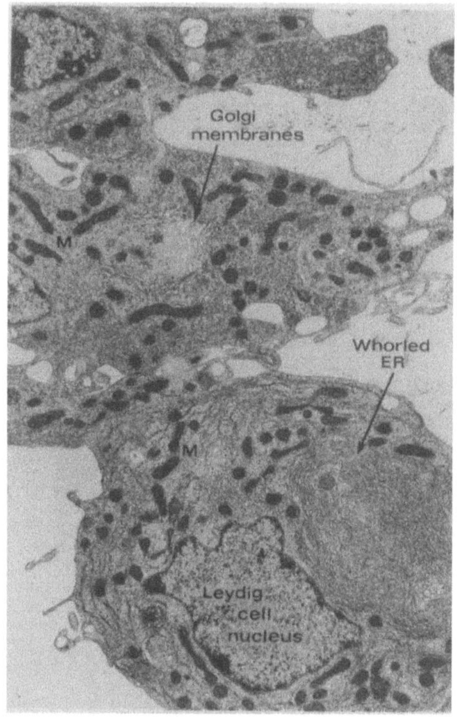

Fig. 7.23

Fig. 7.22. Ultrastructure of Leydig cells typical of those observed within fetal irradiated testes. Each of the three Leydig cells shows a striking proliferation and concentration of the Golgi apparatus arranged into circular configuration and associated with many closely packed vesicles *(V)* × 10800. (Rich et al. 1979)

Fig. 7.23. Electron micrograph of several Leydig cells within the testis of a vitamin A deficient rat. A large part of the cytoplasm of one Leydig cell is occupied by an extensive whorl of fenestrated tubules of smooth endoplasmic reticulum. An adjacent Leydig cell exhibits a prominent area of Golgi membranes within the cytoplasm. Each Leydig cell contains numerous mitochondria *(M)*. (Rich et al. 1979) × 12000

Table 7.1. Effect of treatment on cross-sectional area of Leydig cells. Cytoplasmic area was determined by subtracting the nuclear area from that of the whole cell. Results expressed as means ± SE. (Rich et al. 1979).

	n	Cell size (μm^2)	Nucleus (μm^2)	Cytoplasm (μm^2)
Normal adult male	80	108 ± 6	43 ± 2	65 ± 4
Hydroxyurea treated	126	133 ± 4[a]	51 ± 2[a]	82 ± 3[a]
Vitamin A deficient	93	234 ± 10[a]	75 ± 2[a]	159 ± 8[a]
Sertoli cell only	98	203 ± 9[a]	65 ± 2[a]	138 ± 8[a]

[a] $P < 0.01$

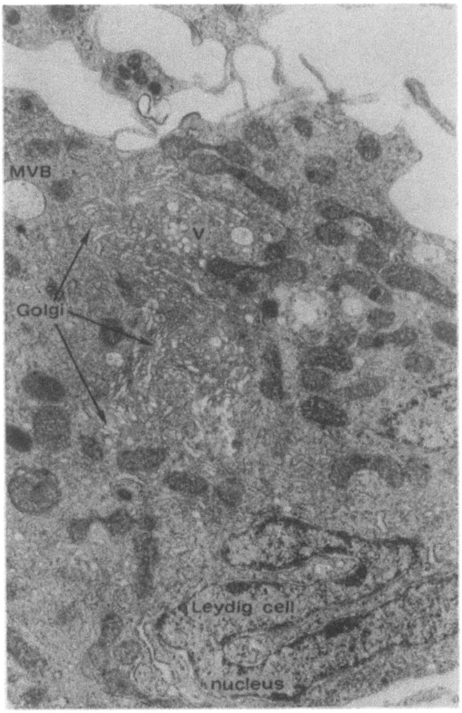

Fig. 7.24. Ultrastructure of a typical Leydig cell from rats treated with hydroxyurea. Note the pleomorphic nucleus and the striking appearance of many Golgi membranes and accompanying vesicles *(V)*. Several large multi-vesicular bodies *(MVB)* are also illustrated. × 21 600

evidence of hypertrophy (Table 7.1) (Rich et al. 1979). The data provided by Aoki and Fawcett (1978), wherein Leydig cell hypertrophy occurred focally around areas of spermatogenic damage induced by silastic implants containing anti-fertility agents, is further evidence for this concept.

7.6 Leydig Cell Function and Testicular Damage

In view of the Leydig cell hypertrophy found in the cryptorchid testis, it seems paradoxical that the function of these cells is subnormal, for instance, the secretory response following hCG is less than normal. This paradox is further compounded by the discovery that when the biosynthetic capacity of Leydig cells from cryptorchid rats is tested in vitro by hCG, the response is two or three times normal (de Kretser et al. 1979). Similar increases in in vitro responsiveness to hCG are also shown by Leydig cells from rats subjected to fetal irradiation (Rich and de Kretser 1979), and dose response data (Fig. 7.25) suggest that the Leydig cells from the damaged testes may be slightly less sensitive to hCG stimulation. This latter change may result from the reduction of LH/hCG receptors in the testes of cryptorchid rats or of rats irradiated in utero (de Kretser et al. 1979; Rich and de Kretser 1979).

It is difficult to explain the contrasting differences in response to hCG stimulation in vitro and in vivo. However, Damber et al. (1978) have shown that testicular blood flow is reduced in cryptorchidism, and have also de-

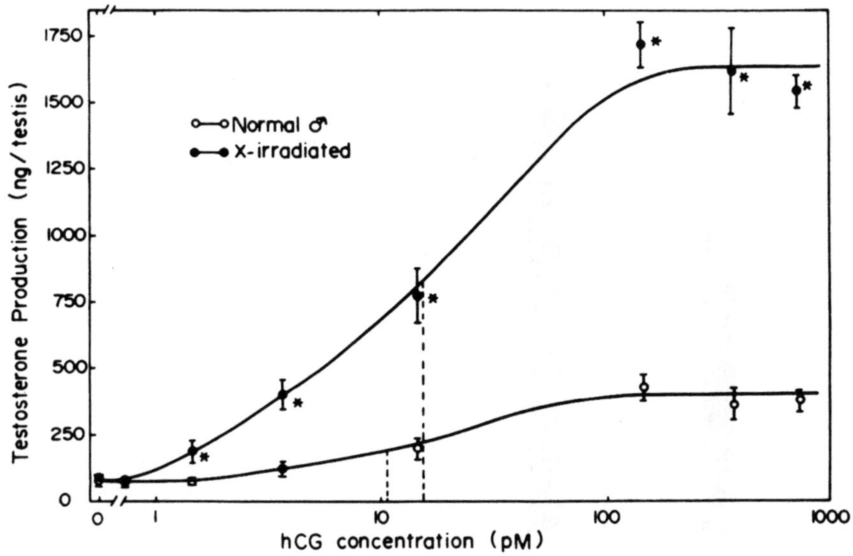

Fig. 7.25. Testosterone production in vitro in response to increasing concentrations of hCG by testes from normal and fetally irradiated male rats. Each *point* with *bar* represents mean ± SE ($N = 5$) * $P < 0.001$. (Rich and de Kretser 1979)

monstrated a positive correlation between blood flow and the secretion of testosterone from the rat testis. Thus, subnormal levels of testosterone after hCG could be a consequence of either reduced delivery of hCG to Leydig cells or decreased outflow of testosterone produced in response to the stimulus. We have shown that the testosterone response of cryptorchid testes to hCG stimulation in vivo is less at low doses or greater than normal at high doses of gonadotrophic stimulation (Table 7.2). This further supports the proposal that blood flow is an important determinant in the testicular response (Risbridger et al. 1981d).

Table 7.2. The dose-response relationship between the levels of serum testosterone and the dose of hCG administered to control and 21-day cryptorchid rats. (Risbridger et al. 1981d)

Dose of hCG	Serum testosterone (ng/ml)	
	Control	21-day cryptorchid
0	2.0 ± 0.2	1.9 ± 0.2
5 IU	16.4 ± 0.9	8.0 ± 1.2[a]
50 IU	18.3 ± 2.2	21.9 ± 2.5
200 IU	17.6 ± 1.5	27.5 ± 3.8[b]

Results are means ± SE ($N = 5$)
Superscripts indicate a significant difference from serum T levels in control rats: [a] $P < 0.001$; [b] $P < 0.05$

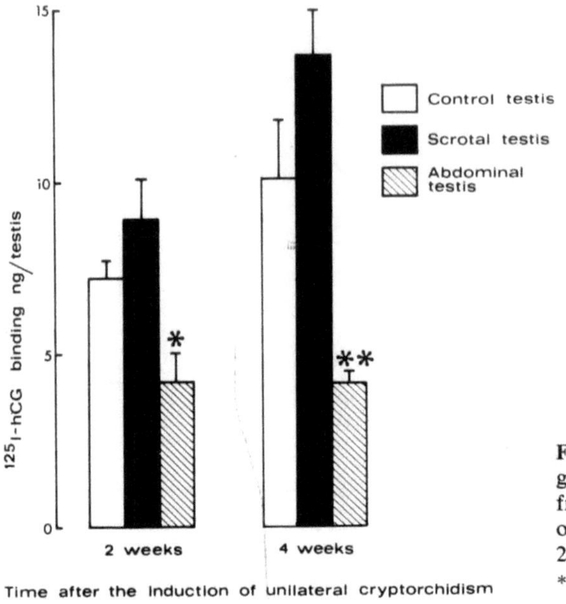

Fig. 7.26. Binding of ^{125}I-hCG to homogenates of testes from control rats and from the scrotal and abdominal testes of rats made unilaterally cryptorchid 2 and 4 weeks earlier. ** $P<0.01$; * $P<0.05$

The cause of the reduction in the number of receptor sites for LH/hCG was initially thought to result from down regulation of receptors, since at 4 weeks after the induction of cryptorchidism serum LH levels are clearly elevated (de Kretser et al. 1979). However, we have shown that receptor loss occurs before LH levels become elevated, and further, that in unilateral cryptorchid rats the cryptorchid testis showed receptor loss, whereas in the

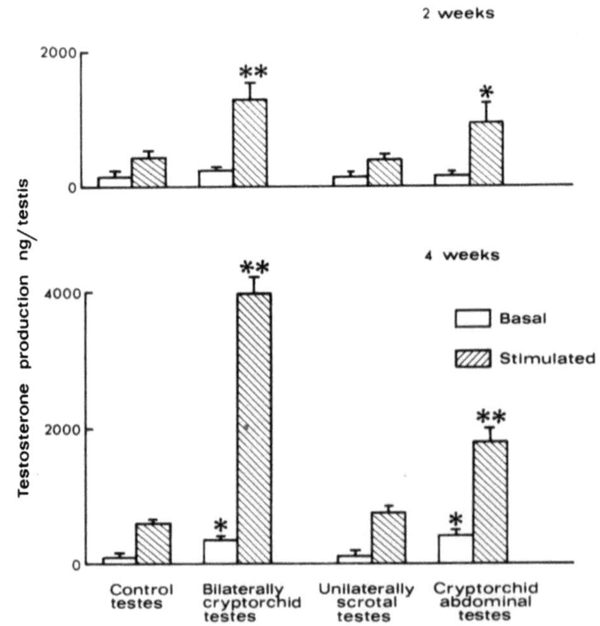

Fig. 7.27. Production of testosterone over 4 h in vitro both basally and following stimulation with hCG (Pregnyl, Organon 700 mIU/ml) for testes from animals made bilaterally or unilaterally cryptorchid 2 and 4 weeks earlier. ** $P<0.01$; * $P<0.05$

scrotal testes receptor numbers were the same as in control rats (Fig. 7.26), which indicates that the receptor loss is not the result of a circulating humoral factor (Risbridger et al. 1981b). Since inhibitors of binding of FSH and LH to their receptors have been identified in extracts of testes and ovaries, it would be of interest to determine whether increases in such factors occur in states of testicular damage (Abou-Issa and Reichert 1976; Reichert and Abou-Issa 1977).

The factors responsible for changes in Leydig cell structure and function are of obvious interest. As with the receptor loss, it was our initial postulate that the Leydig cell changes are the result of increased levels of LH seen in association with testicular damage. However, the relatively rapid hypertrophy of Leydig cells following cryptorchidism is not correlated with the rise in LH (Risbridger et al. 1981d). Furthermore, in experiments using the unilaterally cryptorchid rat, Leydig cell hypertrophy and hyper-responsiveness are limited to the abdominal testes, whereas the scrotal testis of the same rat shows no changes in Leydig cell size or function (Fig. 7.27; Risbridger et al. 1981b). It is therefore most probable that changes in Leydig cell function result from local factors within the testis and since identical changes may be produced unilaterally following efferent duct ligation, agents other than elevated temperature must be involved (Risbridger et al. 1981c). The studies following unilateral efferent duct ligation demonstrate that Leydig cell hypertrophy and increased responsiveness to hCG in vitro (Fig. 7.28) and loss of LH and FSH receptors are found only in the damaged testes, and are not present in the unligated testes of the same rat. Indeed since identical changes in Leydig cell function can be produced by such diverse agents causing seminiferous tubule damage, it is likely that the changes are a response to the tubule damage rather than to each of the agents concerned. It is therefore necessary to postulate that the seminiferous tubules exert a controlling influence on Leydig cells, and that following spermato-

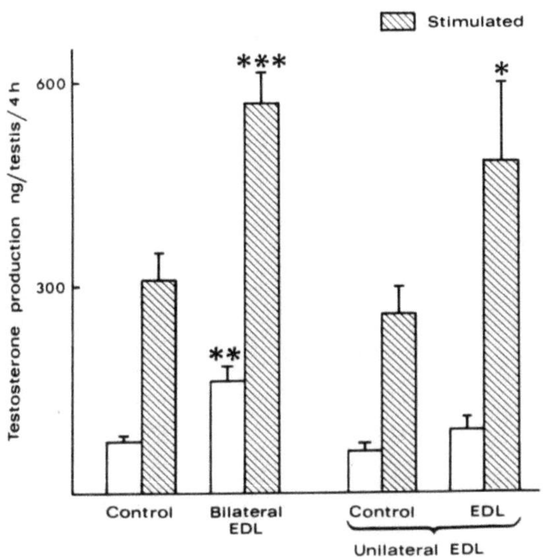

Fig. 7.28. In vitro production of testosterone both basal and stimulated by hCG (700 mIU/ml. Pregnyl, Organon) for testes from rats 4 weeks after either bilateral or unilateral efferent duct ligation (EDL).
*** $P<0.001$; ** $P<0.01$; * $P<0.05$

genic damage, this control is disrupted. Such a concept was postulated by Aoki and Fawcett (1978) following their demonstration that focal spermatogenic damage induced by a variety of agents was associated with Leydig cell hypertrophy only in the vicinity of the tubules showing disruption of spermatogenesis.

The nature of the interaction between the seminiferous tubules and Leydig cells remains unknown. It is not clear whether changes in Leydig cell structure and function in vitro result from the same mechanism that causes the decline of LH and FSH receptors.

The possibility that oestradiol is the link between the two compartments is supported by the presence of oestradiol receptors on Leydig cells (Brinkmann et al. 1972) and of the capacity of immature Sertoli cells to convert testosterone to oestradiol under the influence of FSH (Dorrington and Armstrong 1975; Cannick et al. 1979). However, some investigators have claimed that the site of aromatase activity in the adult rat is in the intertubular compartment and not within the Sertoli cells (Valladares and Payne 1979). Moreover the principal effects of oestradiol on Leydig cells are inhibitory, either directly, or indirectly by decreasing LH levels (van Beurden et al. 1977). It would thus seem difficult to conceive of a mechanism by which oestradiol induces Leydig cell hypertrophy, and increased responsiveness to LH/hCG (Bartke et al. 1977; Dufau et al. 1978).

Alternatively, substances with LHRH-like activity (gonadocrinins), found in the testis and ovary (Ying et al. 1981) may be involved in a link between the tubules and the intertubular tissue. Receptors for LHRH are located on Leydig cells (Clayton et al. 1980) and in a recent study Sharpe et al. (1981) provided data to indicate that the Sertoli cell is a source of a gonadocrinin-like material. Clearly, available data do not permit any definition of the links between the two compartments of the testis. Nevertheless, the results presented in this chapter emphasise that agents which interfere with spermatogenesis also disrupt both Sertoli and Leydig cell function, either directly or by local mechanisms. The data require that the testis be considered as a whole and not as two or more independently functioning compartments.

References

Abou-Issa H, Reichert LE (1976) Properties of follitropin-receptor interaction. J Biol Chem 251:3326–3337

Ahmad N, Haltmeyer GC, Eik-Nes KB (1973) Maintenance of spermatogenesis in rats with intratesticular implants containing testosterone or DHT. Biol Reprod 8:411–419

Aiyer MS, Chiappa S, Fink G (1974) A priming effect of luteinizing hormone releasing factor on the anterior pituitary gland in the female rat. J Endocrinol 62:573–588

Albeau-Fernet M, Bohler CCS-S, Karpas AE (1978) Testicular function in the aging male. In: Greenblatt RB (ed) Geriatric endocrinology, vol. 5, Raven, New York 201–216

Albert A (1956) Human urinary gonadotropin. Recent Prog Horm Res 12:227–301

Albert A, Rosemberg E, Ross GT, Paulsen CA, Ryan RJ (1968) Report of the National Pituitary Agency collaborative study on the radioimmunoassay of FSH and LH. J Clin Endocrinol Metab 28:1214–1219

Alford FP, Baker HWG, Burger HG, de Kretser DM, Hudson B, Johns MW, Masterton JP, Patel YC, Rennie GC (1973a) Temporal patterns of integrated hormone levels during sleep and wakefulness. II. Follicle stimulating hormone, luteinizing hormone, testosterone and estradiol. J Clin Endocrinol Metab 37:848–854

Alford FP, Baker HWG, Patel YC, Rennie GC, Youatt G, Burger HG, Hudson B (1973b) Temporal patterns of circulating hormones as assessed by continuous blood sampling. J Clin Endocrinol Metab 36:108–116

Altwein JE, Gittes RF (1972) Effect of cryptorchidism and castration on FSH and LH levels in the adult rat. Invest Urol 10:167–670

Amatayakul K, Ryan R, Uozumi T, Albert A (1971) A reinvestigation of testicular anterior pituitary relationships in the rat. I. Effects of castration and cryptorchidism. Endocrinology 88:872–880

Amoss M, Burgus R, Blackwell R, Vale W, Fellows R, Guillemin R (1971) Purification, amino acid composition and N-terminus of the hypothalamic LRF of ovine origin. Biochem Biophys Res Commun 44:205–210

Andrew A (1971) The anatomy of aging in man and animals. Grune & Stratton, New York

Anton E (1979) Early ultrastructural changes in the rat testis after ductuli efferentes ligation. Fertil Steril 31:187–194

Aoki A, Fawcett DW (1978) Is there a local feedback from the seminiferous tubules affecting activity of the Leydig cells? Biol Reprod 19:144–158

Aono T, Kurachi K, Mizutani S, Hamanaka Y, Matsumoto K (1972) Influence of major surgical stress on plasma levels of testosterone, luteinizing hormone and follicle stimulating hormone in male patients. J Clin Endocrinol Metab 35:535–542

Aragona C, Friesen HG (1975) Specific prolactin binding sites in the prostate and testis of rats. Endocrinology 97:677–684

Aragona C, Bohnet HG, Friesen HG (1977) Localization of prolactin binding in prostate and testis: the role of serum prolactin concentration on the testicular LH receptors. Acta Endocrinol 84:402–409

Arimura A, Debeljuk L, Shiino M, Rennels EG, Schally AV (1973) Follicular stimulation by chronic treatment with synthetic LH-releasing hormone in hypophysectomized female rats bearing pituitary grafts. Endocrinology 92:1507–1514

Arimura A, Serafini P, Talbot S, Schally AV (1979) Reduction of testicular luteinizing hormone/human chorionic gonadotropin receptors by [D-Trp^6] luteinizing hormone-releasing hormone in hypophysectomized rats. Biochem Biophys Res Commun 90:687–690

Ascoli M, Puett D (1977) Intracellular uptake and catabolism of lutropin by testicular tissue in vitro. FEBS Lett 75:77–82

Ascoli M, Liddle RA, Puett D (1976) Renal and hepatic lysosomal catabolism of luteinizing hormone. Mol Cell Endocrinol 4:297–310

Auclair C, Kelly PA, Labrie F, Coy DH, Schally AV (1977) Inhibition of testicular LH/hCG receptor level by treatment with a potent LHRH agonist or hCG. Biochem Biophys Res Commun 96:855–862.

August GP, Grumbach MM, Kaplan SL (1972) Hormonal changes in puberty. III. Correlation of plasma testosterone, LH, FSH, testicular size and bone age with male pubertal development. J Clin Endocrinol Metab 34:319–26

Baghdassarian A, Guyda H, Johanson A, Migeon CJ, Blizzard RM (1970) Urinary excretion of radioimmunoassayable LH in normal male children and adults according to age and stage of sexual development. J Clin Endocrinol Metab 31:428–35

Bagshawe KD, Wilde CE, Orr AH (1966) Radioimmunoassay for human chorionic gonadotrophin and luteinising hormone. Lancet 1:1118–1121

Bain J, Keene J (1975) Further evidence for inhibin: change in serum luteinizing hormone and follicle-stimulating hormone levels after irradiation of rat testis. J Endocrinol 66:279–280

Baird DT, Galbraith A, Fraser IS, Newsam JE (1973) The concentration of oestrone and oestradiol 17β in spermatic venous blood in men. J Endocrinol 57:285–288

Baker BL (1974) Functional cytology of the hypophysial pars distalis and pars intermedia. In: Knobil E, Sawyer WJ (eds) Handbook of physiology, sec 7, vol 4. Williams & Wilkins, Baltimore, pp 45–80

Baker BL, Pierce JG, Cornell JS (1972) The utility of antiserums to subunits of TSH and LH for immunochemical staining of the rat hypophysis. Am J Anat 135:251–268

Baker HWG (1974) Endocrinology of Liver Disease. Thesis, Monash University

Baker HWG, Bremner WJ, Burger HG, de Kretser DM, Dulmanis Ausma, Eddie LW, Hudson B, Keogh EJ, Lee VWK, Rennie GC (1976a) Testicular control of FSH secretion. Recent Prog Horm Res 32:429–476

Baker HWG, Burger HG, de Kretser DM, Hudson B (1977a) Endocrinology of aging: Pituitary-testicular axis. In: James VHT (ed) Endocrinology. vol 2. International Congress Series No. 403 Excerpta Medica, Amsterdam, pp 479–483

Baker HWG, Burger HG, de Kretser DM, Dulmanis A, Hudson B, O'Connor S, Paulsen CA, Purcell N, Rennie GC, Seah CS, Taft HP, Wang C (1976b) A study of the endocrine manifestations of hepatic cirrhosis. QJ Med 45:145–178

Baker HWG, Burger HG, de Kretser DM, Eddie LW, Higginson RE, Hudson B, Lee VWK (1978) Studies on purification of inhibin from ovine testicular secretions using an in vitro bioassay. Int J Andrology [Suppl 2] 115–124

Baker HWG, Burger HG, de Kretser DM, Hudson B, O'Connor S, Wang C, Mirovics A, Court J, Dunlop M, Rennie GC (1976c) Changes in the pituitary-testicular system with age. Clin Endocrinol (Oxf) 5:349–372

Baker HWG, Burger HG, de Kretser DM, Hudson B, Straffon WGE (1973) Effect of synthetic oral oestrogens in men and patients with prostatic carcinoma: lack of gonadotrophin suppression by chlorotianisene. Clin Endocrinol (Oxf) 2:297–306

Baker HWG, Eddie LW, Higginson RE, Hudson B, Niall HD (1980) Testicular inhibin. In: Cumming IA, Funder JW, Mendelsohn FAO (eds) Endocrinology 1980. Australian Academy of Science, Canberra 251–254

Baker HWG, Santen RJ, Burger HG, de Kretser DM, Hudson B, Pepperell RJ, Bardin CW (1975) Rhythms in the secretion of gonadotropins and gonadal steroids. J Steroid Biochem 6:793–801

Baker HWG, Sonstein FM, Eichner GJ, Santen RJ, Jefferson LS, Bardin CW (1977) Perfusion of rat testis and accessory sex organs: a new method. Endocrinology 100:699–708

Bangham DR, Berryman I, Burger HG, Cotes PM, Furnival BE, Hunter WM, Midgley AR, Mussett MV, Reichert LE, Rosemberg E, Ryan RJ, Wide L (1973) An international collaborative study of 69/104, a reference preparation of human pituitary FSH and LH. J Clin Endocrinol Metab 36:647–60

Bardin CW, Peterson RE (1967) Studies of androgen production by the rat: testosterone and androstenedione content of blood. Endocrinology 80:38–44

Bardin CW, Ross GT, Lipsett MB (1967) Site of action of clomiphene citrate in men: a study of

the pituitary-Leydig cell axis. J Clin Endocrinol Metab 27:1558–1564
Bartke A (1966) Influence of prolactin on male fertility in dwarf mice. J Endocrinol 35:419–420
Bartke A (1971a) Effects of prolactin on spermatogenesis in hypophysectomized mice. J Endocrinol 49:311–316
Bartke A (1971b) Effects of prolactin and luteinizing hormone on the cholesterol stores in the mouse testis. J Endocrinol 49:317–324
Bartke A, Dalterio S (1976) Effects of prolactin on the sensitivity of the testis to LH. Biol Reprod 15:90–93
Bartke A, Lloyd CW (1970) Influence of prolactin and pituitary isografts on spermatogenesis in dwarf mice and hypophysectomized rats. J Endocrinol 46:321–329
Bartke A, Croft BT, Dalterio S (1975) Prolactin restores plasma testosterone levels and stimulates testicular growth in hamsters exposed to short day-length. Endocrinology 97:1601–1604
Bartke A, Williams KIH, Dalterio S (1977) Effects of estrogens on testicular testosterone production in vitro. Biol Reprod 17:645–649
Bayard F, Louvet JP, Thijssens JL, Venot JP, Boulard C (1973) Testosterone and 17β-oestradiol production rate in the ageing man. Acta Endocrinol [Suppl 177] 121
Beale EG, Dedman JR, Means AR (1977) Isolation and regulation of the protein kinase inhibitor and the calcium dependent cyclic nucleotide phosphodiesterase regulator in the Sertoli cell – enriched testis. Endocrinology 101:1621–1634
Beaumont PJV, George GCW, Pimstone BL, Vinik AI (1976) Bodyweight and the pituitary response to hypothalamic releasing hormones in patients with anorexia nervosa. J Clin Endocrinol Metab 43:487–496
Bennett H, Baggenstoss A, Butt H (1950) The testis, breast and prostate of men who died of cirrhosis of the liver. Am J Clin Pathol 20:814–828
Bergada C, Mancini RE, Vilar O, Rivarola MA, Calamera JC, Bianculli C, Schally AV, Kastin AJ (1973) Effect of chronic administration of synthetic LH-RH/FSH-RH on prepubertal boys and in hypogonadotropic hypogonadism. In: Gual C, Rosemberg E (eds) Hypothalamic hypophysiotropic hormones. Excerpta Medica, Amsterdam 299–301
Bergh A, Damber J-E (1978) Morphometric and functional investigation on the Leydig cells in experimental unilateral cryptorchidism in the rat. Int J Andrology 1:549–562
Bergh A, Damber J-E (1979) Morphological and endocrinological differences between the abdominal testes in bilateral and unilateral cryptorchid rats. Int J Andrology 2:319–29
Bermudez JA, Kastin AJ, Schalch DS, Lee-Benitez D, Perez-Pasten E, Gonzalez-Barcena D, Pedro Arzac J, Schally AV (1974) Hormonal response to synthetic LH-releasing hormone (LH-RH) in prepubertal, pubertal and adult human males. Endocrinol Res Commun 1:477–493
Berthezene F, Forest MG, Grimaud JA, Claustrat B, Mornex R (1976) Leydig cell agenesis. A cause of male pseudohermaphroditism. N Engl J Med 295:969–972
Besser GM, McNeilly AS, Anderson DC, Marshall JC, Harsoulis P, Hall R, Ormston BJ, Alexander L, Collins WP (1972) Hormonal responses to synthetic luteinizing hormone and follicle stimulating hormone-releasing hormone in man. Br Med J 3:267–271
Bex FJ, Bartke A (1977) Testicular LH binding in the hamster: modification by photoperiod and prolactin. Endocrinology 100:1223
Biglieri EG, Herron MA, Brust N (1966) 17-hydroxylation deficiency in man. J Clin Invest 45: 1946–1954
Bhalla VK, Reichert LE (1974) Gonadotropin receptors in rat testis. Interaction of an ethanol soluble testicular factor with human follicle stimulating hormone and luteinizing hormone. J Biol Chem 249:7996–8004
Bishop HWH (1970) Aging and reproduction in the male. J Reprod Fertil [Suppl 12] 65–87
Blanc MR, Cahoreau C, Courot M, Dacheux JL, Hochereau de Reviers M-Th, Pisselet Cl (1978) Plasma follicle stimulating hormone (FSH) and luteinizing hormone (LH) suppression in the cryptorchid ram by a non-steroid factor (Inhibin) from ram rete testis fluid. Int J Andrology [Suppl 2] 139–146
Bloch GJ, Masken J, Kragt CL, Ganong WF (1976) Effect of testosterone on plasma LH in male rats of various ages. Endocrinology 94:947–951
Blum V (1936) Das Problem des männlichen Klimakteriums. Wien Klin Wochnschr 2:1133–1140
Bohnet HG, Friesen HG (1976) Effect of prolactin and growth hormone on prolactin and LH receptors in the dwarf mouse. J Reprod Fertil 48:307–311

Bongiovanni AM (1962) Adrenogenital syndrome with deficiency of 3β-hydroxysteroid dehydrogenase. J Clin Invest 41:2086–2092
Boon DA, Keenon RE, Slaunwhite WR Jr, Aceto T Jr (1972) Conjugated and unconjugated plasma androgens in normal children. Pediatr Res 6:111–118
Bouin P, Ancel P (1903) Recherches sur les cellules interstitialles due testicule des mammiferes. Arch Zool Exp Gen 1:437–523
Bowers CY, Currie BL, Johansson KNG, Folkers K (1973) Biological evidence that separate hypothalamic hormones release the follicle stimulating and luteinizing hormones. Biochem Biophys Res Commun 50:20–26
Boyar R, Finkelstein J, Roffwarg H, Kapen S, Weitzman E, Hellman L (1972) Synchronization of augmented luteinizing hormone secretion with sleep during puberty. N Engl J Med 287: 582–586
Boyar RM, Katz J, Finkelstein JW, Kapen S, Weiner H, Weitzman ED, Hellman L (1974) Anorexia nervosa immaturity of the 24-hour luteinizing hormone secretory pattern. N Engl J Med 291:861–865
Boyar RM, Perlow M, Kapen S, Weitzman E, Hellman L (1972) 24 hour pattern of luteinizing hormone secretion in normal men with sleep stage recording. J Clin Endocrinol Metab 35:73–81
Brandtzaeg P, Purvis K, Hansson V (1978) Methodology of immunofluorescence cell surface staining with special reference to LH receptors on Leydig cells and membrane immunoglobulins. Int J Androl [Suppl 2] 287–302
Bremner WJ (1977) Pituitary responses to hypothalamic hormone administration and seasonal effects upon reproduction. Ph. D. Thesis, Monash University
Bremner WJ, Paulsen CA (1974) Two pools of luteinizing hormone in the human pituitary: Evidence from constant administration of luteinizing hormone-releasing hormone. J Clin Endocrinol Metab 39:811–815
Bremner WJ, Paulsen CA (1977) Prolonged intravenous infusions of LH-releasing hormone into normal men. Horm Metab Res 9:r13–16
Bremner WJ, Findlay JK, Cumming IA, Hudson B, de Kretser DM (1976) Pituitary-testicular responses in rams to prolonged infusions of luteinizing hormone-releasing hormone, LHRH. Biol Reprod 15:141–146
Bremner WJ, Fernando NN, Paulsen CA (1977) The effect of luteinizing hormone releasing hormone in hypogonadotrophic eunuchoidism. Acta Endocrinol (Copenh) 86:1–14
Bremner WJ, Burger HG, Abreu RM, de Kretser DM (1978) Patterns of pituitary hormone secretion during prolonged intravenous infusions of LH-RH and TRH in normal subjects and various pituitary-gonadal disorders. In: Gupta D, Voelter W (eds) Hypothalamic hormones, chemistry, physiology and clinical applications. Verlag Chemie, Weinheim New York, pp 529–541
Bremner WJ, Findlay JK, Lee VWK, de Kretser DM, Cumming IA (1980) Feedback effects of the testis on pituitary responsiveness to LHRH infusions in the ram. Endocrinology 106: 329–336
Bricaire H, Luton JP, Laudat P, Legrand JC, Turpin G, Corvol P, Lemner M (1972) A new male pseudohermaphroditism associated with hypertension due to a block of 17α-hydroxylation. J Clin Endocrinol Metab 35:67–72
Brinkman AO, Mulder E, Lamers-Stahlhofen GJM, Michielsen MJ, van der Molen HJ (1972) An oestradiol receptor in rat testis interstitial tissue. FEBS Lett 26:301–305
Brokelmann J (1963) Fine structure of germ cells and Sertoli cells during the cycle of the seminiferous epithelium in the rat. Z Zellforsch 59:820–850
Brown-Grant K, Fink G, Greig F, Murray MAF (1975) Altered sexual development in male rats after oestrogen administration during the neonatal period. J Reprod Fert 44:25–42
Brown-Sequard CE (1889) The effects produced in man by subcutaneous injections of a liquid obtained from the testicles of animals. Lancet 2:105–107
Brown DM, Markland C, Dehner LP (1978) Leydig cell hypoplasia: a cause of male pseudohermaphroditism. J Clin Endocrinol Metab 46:1–7
Bugnon C, Lenys D, Kerdelhue B, Dessy C, Fellman D (1974) Etude cytoimmunologique des cellules gonadotropes du renard roux. C R Soc Biol (Paris) 168:814–818
Burger HG, Baker HWG, Hudson B, Taft HP (1972) Gonadotropic and gonadal function in the normal adult male. In: Saxena BB, Beling CG, Gandy HM (eds) Gonadotropins. Wiley Interscience, New York, pp 569–592

Burger HG, Oliver JR, Davis J, Catt KJ (1968) Radioimmunoassay for human pituitary luteinising hormone using paper chromato-electrophoresis. Aust J Exp Biol Med Sci 46:541–553

Burr IM, Sizonenko PC, Kaplan SL, Grumbach MM (1970) Hormonal changes in puberty. I. Correlation of serum luteinizing hormone and follicle stimulating hormone with stages of puberty testicular size, and bone age in normal boys. Pediatr Res 4:25–35

Butenandt A, Hanisch G (1935) Über Testosteron. Umwandlung des Dehydroandrosterons in Androstenediol und Testosteron: ein Weg zur Darstellung des Testosterons aus Cholesterin. Z Physiol Chem 237:89–97

Byskov AG (1978) Regulation of initiation of meiosis in fetal gonads. Int J Androl [Suppl] 2:29–38

Byskov AG, Saxen L (1976) Induction of meiosis in fetal mouse testis in vitro. Dev Biol 52:193–200

Cannick JA, Makris A, Gunsalus GL, Ryan KJ (1979) Testicular aromatization in immature rats: localization and stimulation after gonadotropin administration in vivo. Endocrinology 104: 285–288

Carmel PW, Araki S, Ferin M (1976) Pituitary stalk portal blood collection in Rhesus monkeys: evidence for pulsatile release of gonadotrophin-releasing hormone (GnRH). Endocrinology 99:243–248

Castro AE, Seiguer AC, Mancini RE (1970) Electron microscopic study of the localization of labelled gonadotropins in the Sertoli and Leydig cells of the rat testis. Proc Soc Exp Biol Med 133:582–586

Castro AE, Alonso A, Mancini RE (1972) Localization of follicle-stimulating hormone and luteinizing hormone in the rat testis using immunohistological tests. J Endocrinol 52:129–136.

Catt KJ, Dufau ML (1978) Gonadotropin receptors and regulation of interstitial cell function in the testis. In: Birnbaumer L, O'Malley BW (eds) Receptors and hormone action, vol III. Academic Press, New York, pp 291–339

Catt KJ, Niall HD, Tregear GW, Burger HG (1968) Disc solid-phase radioimmunoassay of human luteinizing hormone. J Clin Endocrinol Metab 28:121–126

Catt KJ, Dufau ML, Tsuruhara T (1971) Studies on a radioligand-receptor assay system for LH and chorionic gonadotropin. J Clin Endocrinol Metab 32:860–863

Catt KJ, Dufau ML, Tsuruhara T (1972) Gonadotropin binding sites of the rat testis. Biochem Biophys Acta 279:194–201

Catt KJ, Baukal AJ, Davies TF, Dufau ML (1979) Luteinizing hormone-releasing hormone-induced regulation of gonadotropin and prolactin receptors in the rat testis. Endocrinology 104:17–25

Chari S, Duraiswami S, Franchimont P (1976) A convenient and rapid bioassay for inhibin. Horm Res 7:129–137

Chari S, Duraiswami S, Franchimont P (1978) Isolation and characterization of inhibin from bull seminal plasma. Acta Endocrinol (Copenh) 87:434–448

Charreau EH, Attramadal A, Torjesen PA, Purvis K, Calandra R, Hansson V (1977) Prolactin binding in rat testis: specific receptors in interstitial cells. Mol Cell Endocrinol 6:303–307

Chasalow F, Marr H, Haour F, Saez JM (1979) Testicular steroidogenesis after HCG desensitization in rats. J Biol Chem 254:5613–5617

Chen YDI, Payne AH, Kelch RP (1976) FSH stimulation of Leydig cell function in the hypophysectomized immature rat. Proc Soc Exp Biol Med 153:473–475

Chen YDI, Shaw MJ, Payne AH (1977) Steroid and FSH action of LH receptors and LH sensitive testicular responsiveness during sexual maturation of the rat. Mol Cell Endocrinol 8:291–299

Chowdhury AK (1971) Thymidine-^{3}H labeling of spermatogonia in rat and human seminiferous tubules mounted in toto (Abstr) Anat Rec 169:296 (abst)

Chowdhury AK, Steinberger E (1964) A quantitative study of the effects of heat on the germinal epithelium of rat testes. Am J Anat 115:509–524

Chowdhury M, Tcholakian R, Steinberger E (1977) An unexpected effect of oestradiol-17β on luteinizing hormone and testosterone. J Endocrinol 60:375–376

Chowdhury M, Steinberger A, Steinberger E (1978) Inhibition of de novo synthesis of FSH by the Sertoli cell factor (SCF). Endocrinology 103:644–647

Christensen AK (1965) The fine structure of testicular interstitial cells in guinea pigs. J Cell Biol 26:911–935

Christensen AK (1975) Leydig cells. In: Hamilton DW, Greep RO (eds) Handbook of physiology, sect 7, vol 5. Williams & Wilkins, Baltimore, pp 57–94

Christensen AK, Gillim W (1969) The correlation of fine structure and function in steroid-secreting cells, with emphasis on those of the gonads. In: McKern KW (ed) The gonads. Appleton Century Crofts, New York, pp 415–488

Christensen AK, Mason NR (1965) Comparative ability of seminiferous tubules and interstitial tissue of rat testes to synthesize androgens from progesterone-4-^{14}C in vitro. Endocrinology 76:646–656

Christensen AK, Peacock KC (1980) Increase in Leydig cell number in testes of adult rats treated chronically with an excess of human chorionic gonadotropin. Biol Reprod 22:383–391

Cigorraga SB, Dufau ML, Catt KJ (1978) Regulation of luteinizing hormone receptors and steroidogenesis in gonadotropin desensitized Leydig cells. J Biol Chem 253:4297–4304

Cigorraga SB, Sorrell S, Bator J, Catt KJ, Dufau ML (1980) Estrogen dependence of a gonadotropin-induced steroidogenic lesion in rat testicular Leydig cells. J Clin Invest 65:699–705

Clayton RN, Katikineni M, Chan V, Dufau ML, Catt KJ (1980) Direct inhibition of testicular function by gonadotropin-releasing hormone: mediation by specific gonadotropin-releasing hormone receptors on interstitial cells. Proc Natl Acad Sci USA 77:4459–4463

Clegg EJ (1961) Further studies on artificial cryptorchidism: quantitative changes in the interstitial cells of the rat testis. J Endocrinol 21:433–441

Clegg EJ, MacMillan EW (1965) The uptake of vital dyes and particulate matter by the Sertoli cells of the rat testis. J Anat (Lond) 99:219–229

Clermont Y (1963) The cycle of the seminiferous epithelium in man. Am J Anat 112:35–51

Clermont Y (1972) Kinetics of spermatogenesis in mammals: seminiferous epithelium cycle and spermatogonial renewal. Physiol Rev 52:198–236

Clermont Y, Harvey SG (1965) Duration of the cycle of the seminiferous epithelium of normal hypophysectomized and hypophysectomized-hormone treated albino rats. Endocrinology 76:80–89

Clermont Y, Morgentaler H (1955) Quantitative study of spermatogenesis in the hypophysectomized rat. Endocrinology 57:198–236

Clermont Y, Perey B (1957) Quantitative study of the cell population of the seminiferous tubules in immature rats. Am J Anat 100:241–267

Coble YD, Kohler PO, Cargille CH, Ross G (1969) Production rates and metabolic clearance rates of human follicle stimulating hormone in premenopausal and postmenopausal women. J Clin Invest 48:359–363

Collins P, Lacy D (1969) Studies on the structure and function of the mammalian testis. II. Cytological and histochemical observations on the testis of the rat after a single exposure to heat applied for different lengths of time. Proc R Soc [B] 172:17–38

Collins PM, Collins WP, McNeilly AS, Tsang WN (1978) Plasma FSH, LH and testosterone levels in the male rat during degeneration of the germinal epithelium caused by severe heat treatment or ligation of the vasa efferentia. J Reprod Fertil 54:285–291

Conn MP, Tsuruhara T, Dufau ML, Catt KJ (1977) Isolation of highly purified Leydig cells by density gradient centrifugation. Endocrinology 101:639–642

Cooke BA, Lindh ML, Janszen FHA (1976) Correlation of protein kinase activation and testosterone production after stimulation of Leydig cells with luteinizing hormone. Biochem J 160:439–446

Corvol P, Bardin CW (1973) Species distribution of testosterone-binding globulin. Biol Reprod 8:277–282

Courot M (1962) Development du testicule chez l'agneau. Etablissement de la spermatogenese. Ann Biol Anim Bioch Biophys 2:25–41

Courot M (1971) Etablissement de la spermatogenese chez l'agneau (ovis areis). Etude experimentale de son contriole gonadotrope importance des cellules de la lignée Sertolienne. D. Sc. Thesis, University of Paris, CNRS NO. A.O. 6317

Courot M (1974) Blood plasma LH, testosterone and prolactin patterns in the male lamb. In: Forest MG, Bertrand J (eds) Sexual endocrinology of the perinatal period. INSERM v 32: 157–160

Courot M, Hochereau-de-Reviers M-T, Monet-Kuntz C, Locatelli A, Pisselet C, Blanc MR, Dacheux JL (1979) Endocrinology of spermatogenesis in the hypophysectomized ram. J Reprod Fertil [Suppl] 2:165–173

Crim LW, Geschwind II (1972a) Testosterone concentration in spermatic vein plasma of the developing ram. Biol Reprod I:42–46

Crim LW, Geschwind II (1972b) Patterns of FSH and LH secretion in the developing ram: the influence of castration and replacement therapy with testosterone propionate. Biol Reprod 7:47–54

Crowe SJ, Cushing H, Homans J (1910) Experimental hypophysectomy. Bull Johns Hopkins Med J 21:127–169

Cunnigham GR, Tindall D, Huckins C (1975) Serum follicle stimulating hormone, luteinizing hormone and testicular responses during development of normal, Sertoli cell only and hemi castrate rats (abstr). Proceedings 57th Ann Meeting, Endocrine Society, USA 1975: p. 176

Cushing H (1909) The hypophysis cerebri. Clinical aspects of hyperpituitarism and hypopituitarism. JAMA 53:249–255

Cushing H (1910) The functions of the pituitary body. Am J Med Sci 139:473–484

Damber J-E, Janson PO (1978) Testicular blood flow and testosterone concentrations in spermatic venous blood of anaesthetized rats. J Reprod Fertil 52:265–269

Damber J-E, Bergh HA, Janson PO (1978) Testicular blood flow and testosterone concentrations in the spermatic venous blood in rats with experimental cryptorchidism. Acta Endocrinol (Copenh) 88:611–618

Daume E, Chari S, Hopkinson CRN, Sturm G, Hirschhauser C (1978) Nachweis von Inhibin-Aktivität in der Follikelflüssigkeit menschlicher Ovarien. Klin. Wochenschr 56:369–370

David K, Dingemanse E, Freud J, Laquer E (1935) Über krystallinisches männliches Hormon aus Hoden (Testosteron), wirksamer als aus Harn oder aus Cholesterin bereitetes Androsteron. Z Physiol 233:281–282

Davies RV, Main SJ, Setchell BP (1978) Inhibin: evidence for its existence, methods of bioassay and nature of the active material. Int J Andrology [Suppl] 2:102–114

Davies RV, Main SJ, Laurie MS, Setchell BP (1979) The effect of long-term administration of either a crude inhibin preparation or an antiserum to FSH on serum hormone levels, testicular function and fertility of adult male rats. J Reprod Fertil [Suppl] 26:183–191

Davis TE, Lipsett MB, Korenman SG (1965) Suppression of testosterone production by physiologic doses of 2α-methyl dihydrotestosterone propionate. J Clin Endocrinol Metab 25:476–479

Debeljuk L, Arimura A, Schally AV (1973a) Pituitary and serum FSH and LH levels after massive and selective depletion of the germinal epithelium in the rat testis. Endocrinology 92:48–54

Debeljuk L, Arimura A, Shino M, Rennels EG, Schally AV (1973b) Effects of chronic treatment with LH/FSH-RH in hypophysectomized pituitary-grafted male rats. Endocrinology 92:921–930

Decker MH, Loriaux DL, Cutter GB (1981) A seminiferous tubular factor is not obligatory for regulation of plasma follicle-stimulating hormone in the rat. Endocrinology 108:1035–1039

de Duve C, Wattiaux R (1966) Function of lysosomes. Annu Rev Physiol 28:435–92

de Jong FH (1979) Inhibin – Fact or Artifact? Mol Cell Endocrinol 13:1–10

de Jong FH, Sharpe RM (1976) Evidence for inhibin-like activity in bovine follicular fluid. Nature 263:71–72

de Jong FH, Hey AH, von der Molen HJ (1973) Effect of gonadotropins on the secretion of oestradiol-17β and testosterone by the rat testis. J Endocrinol 57:277–284

de Jong FH, Sharpe RM (1977) Gonadotrophins, testosterone and spermatogenesis in neonatally irradiated male rats: evidence for a role of the Sertoli cell in follicle-stimulating hormone feedback. J Endocrinol 75:209–219

de Jong FH, Welschen R, Hermans WP, Smith SD, van der Molen HJ (1978) Effects of testicular and ovarian inhibin-like activity, using in vitro and in vivo systems. Int J Androl [Suppl] 2: 125–138

de Jong FH, Smith SD, van der Molen HJ (1979) Bioassay of inhibin-like activity using pituitary cells in vitro J Endocrinol 80:91–102

de Jong FH, Hermans WP, Jansen EHJM, Steinberger J, van der Molen HJ (1980) Biochemical and physiological aspects of inhibin-like activity. In: Cumming IA, Funder JW, Mendelsohn FAO (eds) Endocrinology 1980, Aust Acad Sci, Canberra, pp 255–258

de Koning J, van Dieten JAMJ, van Rees GP (1976) LHRH-dependent synthesis of protein necessary for LH release from rat pituitary glands in vitro. Mol Cell Endocr 5:151–160

de Kretser DM (1967a) The fine structure of testicular interstitial cells in men of normal androgenic status. Z Zellforsch 80:594–609

de Kretser DM (1976b) Changes in the fine structure of the human testicular interstitial cells after treatment with human gonadotropins. Z Zellforsch 67b 83:344–358

de Kretser DM, Burger HG (1972) Ultrastructural studies of human Sertoli cells in normal men and males with hypogonadotropic hypogonadism before and after gonadotropic treatment. In: Saxena BB, Beling CG, Gandy HM (eds) Gonadotropins. Wiley Interscience, New York, pp 640–656

de Kretser DM, Holstein (1976) Testicular biopsy and abnormal germ cells. In: Hafez ESE (ed) Human semen and fertility regulation in men. Mosby, St Louis, pp 332–343

de Kretser DM, Catt KJ, Burger HG, Smith GC (1969) Radioautographic studies of the localization of ^{125}I-labelled human luteinizing and growth hormone in immature male rats. J Endocrinol 43:105–111

de Kretser DM, Catt KJ, Paulsen CA (1971) Studies on the in vitro testicular binding of iodinated luteinizing hormone in rats. Endocrinology 88:332–337

de Kretser DM, Burger HG, Fortune D, Hudson B, Long AR, Paulsen CA, Taft HP (1972) Hormonal histological and chromosomal studies in adult males with testicular disorders. J Clin Endocrinol Metab 35:392–401

de Kretser DM, Atkins RC, Paulsen CA (1973) The role of the kidney in the metabolism of luteinizing hormone. J Endocrinol 58:425–434

de Kretser DM, Burger HG, Hudson B (1974) The relationship between germinal cells and serum FSH levels in males with infertility. J Clin Endocrinol Metab 38:797–793

de Kretser DM, Burger HG, Dumpys R (1975a) Serum LH and FSH response in four-hour infusions of luteinizing hormone-releasing hormone in normal men, Sertoli cell only syndrome, and Klinefelter's syndrome. J Clin Endocrinol Metab 41:876–886

de Kretser DM, Burger HG, Hudson B, Keogh EJ (1975b) The pituitary-testicular response to luteinizing hormone releasing hormone administration to normal men. Aust NZ J Med 5:227–239

de Kretser DM, Burger HG, Hudson B, Keogh EJ (1975c) The HCG stimulation test in men with testicular disorders. Clin Endocrinol (Oxf) 4:591–596

de Kretser DM, Bremner WJ, Dumpys R, Paulsen CA, Burger HG (1976) Pituitary and gonadal responses to constant infusions of LHRH in normal men and women. In: Anand Kumar TC (ed) Neuroendocrine regulation of fertility. Karger, Basel, pp 294–301

de Kretser DM, Bremner WJ, Burger HG, Hudson B, Irby DC, Kerr JB, Lee VWK (1977) The interaction between the hypothalamus-hypophyseal system and the testis in mammalian species. In: Calaby JH, Tyndale-Biscoe CH (eds) Reproduction and evolution. Aust Acad Sci, Canberra, pp 111–119

de Kretser DM, Burger HG, Dumpys R (1978) Patterns of serum LH and FSH in response to four hour infusions of luteinizing hormone releasing hormone in normal women during menstrual cycle, on oral contraceptives and in the post-menopausal state. J Clin Endocrinol Metab 46:227–235

de Kretser DM, Sharpe RM, Swanston IA (1979) Alterations in steroidogenesis and human chorionic gonadotropin binding in the cryptorchid rat testis. Endocrinology 105: 135–138

de Kretser DM (1982) The Testis In: Austin CR, Short, RV (eds) Reproduction in mammals, vol 3 2nd edn. Cambridge University Press, Cambridge

de Kretser DM, Temple-Smith PD, Kerr JB (1982) Anatomy and histology of the male reproductive tract. Handbook of Urology. Springer, Berlin Heidelberg, New York p 1–131

de Lange WE, Sluiter WJ, van Zanten AK, Doorenbos H (1974) The effect of injection and infusion of LH-RH on serum LH and FSH in normal males and in boys with delayed puberty. Neth J Med 17:196–201

del Castillo EB, Trabucco A, Balze FA (1947) Syndrome produced by absence of the germinal epithelium without impairment of the Sertoli or Leydig cells. J Clin Endocrinol Metab 7:493–502

Döhler K-D, Wuttke W (1974) Gonadotropins, prolactin and progesterone in immature rats. Acta Endocrinol [Suppl] (Copenh) 184:133

Dorrington JH, Armstrong DT (1975) Follicle-stimulating hormone stimulates estradiol-17β synthesis in cultured Sertoli cells. Proc Natl Acad Sci USA 72:2677–2681

Dorrington JH, Fritz IB (1975) Cellular localization of 5α-reductase and 3β-hydroxysteroid dehydrogenase in the seminiferous tubule of the rat testis. Endocrinology 96:879–889

Dorrington JH, Roller NF, Fritz IB (1975) Effects of follicle-stimulating hormone on cultures of Sertoli cell preparations. Mol Cell Endocrinol 3:57–70

Dorrington JH, Fritz IB, Armstrong DT (1978) Control of testicular estrogen synthesis. Biol Reprod 18:55–64

Dragstedt CA (1969) Methusela et al. Perspect Biol Med 12:419–428

Dufau ML, Dulmanis A, Catt KJ, Hudson B (1970) Measurement of plasma estradiol-17β by competitive protein binding assay employing pregnancy plasma. J Clin Endocrinol Metab 30:351–356

Dufau ML, Catt KJ, Tsuruhara T (1971) Gonadotropin stimulation of testosterone production by rat testis in vitro. Biochim Biophys Acta 252:574–579

Dufau ML, Chaneau EH, Catt KJ (1973a) Characteristics of a soluble gonadotropin receptor from the rat testis. J Biol Chem 248:6973–6972

Dufau ML, Watanabe K, Catt KJ (1973b) Stimulation of cyclic AMP production by the rat testis during incubation with hCG in vitro. Endocrinology 92:6–11

Dufau ML, Beitins IZ, McArthur JW, Catt KJ (1976) Effects of luteinizing hormone releasing hormone (LHRH) upon bioactive and immunoreactive serum LH levels in normal subjects. J Clin Endocrinol Metab 43:658–667

Dufau ML, Beitins I, McArthur J, Catt KJ (1977a) Bioassay of serum LH concentrations in normal and LHRH-stimulated human subjects. In: Troen P, Nankin HR (eds) The testis in normal and infertile men. Raven Press, New York, pp 309–325

Dufau ML, Tsuruhara T, Horner KA, Podesta E, Catt KJ (1977b) Intermediate role of adenosine 3′5′-cyclic monophosphate and protein kinase during gonadotropin-induced steroidogenesis in testicular interstitial cells. Proc Natl Acad Sci USA 74:3419–3433

Dufau ML, Hsueh AJ, Cigorraga S, Baukal AJ, Catt KJ (1978) Inhibition of Leydig cell function through hormonal regulatory mechanisms. Int J Androl [Suppl] 2:193–239

Dun RB (1955) Puberty in Merino ram. Aust Vet J 31:104–106

Dym M (1973) The fine structure of the monkey (Macaca) Sertoli cell and its role in maintaining the blood-testis barrier. Anat Rec 175:639–656

Dym M, Cavicchia JC (1977) Further observations on the blood-testis barrier in monkeys. Biol Reprod 17:390–403

Dym M, Fawcett DW (1970) The blood-testis barrier in the rat and the physiological compartmentation of the seminiferous epithelium. Biol Reprod 3:308–326

Dym, M, Raj HGM, Lin YC, Chemes HE, Kotite NJ, Nayfeh SN, French FS (1979) Is FSH required for maintenance of spermatogenesis in adult rats? J Reprod Fertil [Suppl] 26:175–181

Dyrmundsson OR (1973) Puberty and early reproductive performance in sheep. II. Ram lambs (abstr) Anim Breeding Abstracts 41:419–430

Dyrmundsson OR, Lees JL (1972) Pubertal development of Clun Forest ram lambs in relation to time of birth. J Agric Sci 79:83–89

Eddie LW, Baker HWG, Dulmanis A, Higginson RE, Hudson B (1978) Inhibin from cultures of rat seminiferous tubules. J Endocrinol 78:217–224

Eddie LW, Baker HWG, Dulmanis A, Higginson RE, Hudson B (1979) A bioassay for inhibin using pituitary cell cultures. J Endocrinol 81:49–60

Editorial (1975) Hormones and elderly testes. Br Med J 3:2–3

Edwardson JA, Gilbert D (1975) Sensitivity of self-potentiating effect of luteinising hormone-releasing hormone to cycloheximide. Nature 255:71

Eik-Nes KB (1975) Biosynthesis and secretion of testicular steroids. In: Hamilton DW, Greep RO (eds) Handbook of physiology, sect 7, vol 5. Williams & Wilkins, Baltimore, pp 95–115

Elftman H (1950) The Sertoli cell cycle in the mouse. Anat Rec 106:381–393

Elftman H (1963) Sertoli cells and testis structure. Am J Anat 113:25–32

El Safoury S, Bartke A (1974) Effects of follicle stimulating hormone and luteinizing hormone on plasma testosterone levels in hypophysectomized and in intact immature and adult male rats. J Endocrinol 61:193–198

Engle ET, Pincus G (1956) Hormones and the aging process. Academic Press, New York, pp 1–20

Erickson GF, Hsueh AJW (1978) Secretion of "inhibin" by rat granulosa cells in vitro. Endocrinology 103:1960–1963

Evans HM, Long JA (1922) Characteristic effects upon growth, oestrous and ovulation induced by the intraperitoneal administration of fresh anterior hypophyseal substance. Proc Natl Acad Sci USA 8:38–39

Evans JS, Nikitovitch-Winer MB (1969) Functional reactivation and cytological restoration of pituitary grafts by continuous local intravascular infusion of median eminence extracts Neuroendocrinology 4:83–100

Everitt AV (1980) The neuroendocrine system and aging. Gerontology 26:108–119

Ewing L, Zirkin BR, Cochran RC, Kromann N, Peters C (1979) Testosterone secretion by rat, rabbit, guinea pig, dog and hamster testes perfused in vitro: correlation with Leydig cell mass. Endocrinology 105:1135–1142

Fachini G, Toffoli C, Gaudiano A, Marabelli M, Polizzi M, Mangili G (1963) Nemasperm and pituitary inhibition. Nature 199:195–196

Faiman C, Ryan RJ (1967) Radioimmunoassay of human follicle stimulating hormone. J Clin Endocrinol Metab 27:444–447

Fakunding JL, Means AR (1977) Characterization and follicle-stimulating hormone activation of Sertoli cell cyclic AMP-dependent protein kinases. Endocrinology 101:1358–1368

Fakunding JL, Tindall DJ, Dedman JR, Mena C, Means AR (1976) Biochemical actions of fsh in the Sertoli cell of the rat testis. Endocrinology 98:392–402

Fang VS, Anderson WA (1976) Studies on the antitesticular action of d1-6-(n-2-pipecolinomethyl)-5-hydroxy-indane (PHMI) in the rat. Endocrinology 99:358–370

Fawcett DW (1975) Ultrastructure and function of the Sertoli cell. In: Hamilton DW, Greep RO (eds) Handbook of physiology, sect 7, vol 5. Williams & Wilkins, Baltimore, pp:21–55

Fawcett DW, Burgos MH (1956) The fine structure of Sertoli cells in the human testis. Anat Rec 124:401–402

Fawcett DW, Burgos MH (1960) Studies on the fine structure of the mammalian testis. II. The human interstitial tissue. Am J Anat 107:245–269

Fawcett DW, Leak LV, Heidger PM (1970) Electron microscopic observations on the structural components of the blood-testis barrier. J Reprod Fert [Suppl] 10:105–122

Fawcett DW, Neaves WB, Flores MN (1973) Comparative observations on intertubular lymphatics and the organization of the interstitial tissue of the mammalian testis. Biol Reprod 9:500–532

Fink G, Smith GC (1971) Ultrastructural features of the developing hypothalamo-hypophysial axis in the rat. A correlative study. Z Zellforsch 119:208–226

Fjallbrant B (1975) Autoimmune human sperm antibodies and age in males. J Reprod Fertil 43:145–148

Flickinger CJ (1967) The postnatal development of the Sertoli cells of the mouse. Z Zellforsch 78:92–113

Flickinger CJ, Fawcett DW (1967) The junctional specialization of Sertoli cells in the seminiferous epithelium. Anat Rec 158:207–222

Forbes JM, Driver RM, El Shahat AA, Boaz TG, Scanes CG (1975) The effect of daylength and level of feeding on serum prolactin in growing lambs. J Endocrinol 64:549–554

Forest MG, De Peretti E, Bertrand J (1976) Hypothalamic-pituitary-gonadal relationships in man from birth to puberty. Clin Endocrinol 5:551–569

Forest MG, Le Coq A, Saez JM (1979) Kinetics of human chorionic gonadotropin-induced steroidogenic response of the human testis. II. Plasma 17α-hydroxyprogesterone, λ^4-androstenedione, estrone and 17β-estradiol. Evidence for the action of human chorionic gonadotropin on intermediate enzymes implicated in steroid biosynthesis. J Clin Endocrinol Metab 49:284–291

Foster DL, Cook B, Nalbandov AV (1972b) Regulation of LH in the fetal and neonatal lamb: effect of castration during the early postnatal period on levels of LH in sera and pituitaries of neonatal lambs. Biol Reprod 6:253–257

Foster DL, Karsch FJ, Nalbandov AV (1972a) Regulation of luteinizing hormone (LH) in the fetal and neonatal lamb. II. Study of placental transfer of LH in the sheep. Endocrinology 90:589–592

Foster DL, Roach JF, Karsch FJ, Norton HW, Nalbandov AV (1972c) Regulation of LH in the fetal and neonatal lamb. I. LH concentrations in blood and pituitary. Endocrinology 90:102–111

Foster DL, Mickelson IH, Ryan KD, Coon GA, Drongowski RA, Holt JA (1978) Ontogeny of pulsatile luteinizing hormone and testosterone secretion in male lambs. Endocrinology 102: 1137–1146

Franchimont P (1966a) Le dosage des hormones hypophysaires somatotrope et gonadotropes et son application en clinique. Thesis. Arscia S.A., Brussels and Maloine SA. Paris

Franchimont P (1966b) Dosage radioimmunologique des gonadotrophines folliculo-stimulantes et luteinisantes. J Labld Compds 2:R303–322

Franchimont P (1966c) Dosage radioimmunologiques des hormones luteinisantes chorionic et hypophysaire. Ann Endocrinol (Paris) 27:273–280

Franchimont P (1970) Application of radioimmunoassay of gonadotrophins in clinical research.

In: Irvine WJ (ed) Reproductive endocrinology. Livingstone, Edinburgh, pp 1–25
Franchimont P (1972) Human gonadotrophin secretion. J R Coll Physicians Lond 6:283–298
Franchimont P, Burger HG (1975) Human growth hormone and gonadotrophins in health and disease. North Holland/American Elsevier, Amsterdam New York
Franchimont P, Millet D, Vendrely E, Letawe J, Legros JJ, Netter A (1972) Relationship between spermatogenesis and serum gonadotropin levels in azoospermia and oligospermia. J Clin Endocrinol Metab 34:1003–1008
Franchimont P, Chari S, Demoulin A (1975a) Hypothalamus-pituitary-testis interaction. J Reprod Fertil 44:335–350
Franchimont P, Chari S, Hagelstein MT, Duraiswami S (1975b) Existence of a follicle-stimulating hormone inhibiting factor "inhibin" in bull seminal plasma. Nature 257:402–404
Franchimont P, Chari S, Hazee-Hagelstein MT, Debruche ML, Duraiswami S (1977) Evidence for the existence of inhibin. In: Troen P, Nankin HR (eds) The testis in normal and infertile men. Raven Press, New York, pp 253–270
Franchimont P, Demoulin A, Verstraelen-Proyard J, Hazee-Hagelstein MT, Walton JS, Waites GMH (1978) Nature and mechanisms of action of inhibin: perspective in regulation of male fertility. Int J Andrology [Suppl] 2:69–80
Franchimont P, Verstraelen-Proyard J, Hazee-Hagelstein MT, Renard Ch, Demoulin A, Bourguignon JP, Hustin J (1979) Inhibin: from concept to reality Vitam Horm 37:243–302
Freeman H, Parsons OA, Feffer MH, Phillips L, Daneman EA, Elmadjian P, Bloch E, Dorfman RI, Pincus G (1956) Steroid replacement in aged men. J Clin Endocrinol Metab 16:779–789
French FS, Ritzen EM (1973) A high affinity androgen binding protein (ABP) in rat testis: evidence for secretion into efferent duct fluid and absorption by epididymis. Endocrinology 93:88–93
Frick J (1969) Darstellung einer Methode (competitive protein binding) zur Bestimmung des Testosteronspiegels im Plasma und Studie über den Testosteronmetabolismus beim Mann über 60 Jahre. Urol Int 24:481–501
Frick J, Kincl FA (1969) The measurement of plasma testosterone by competitive protein-binding assay. Steroids 13:495–505
Frisch RE (1974) Critical weight at menarche, initiation of the adolescent growth spurt, and control of puberty. In: Grumbach MM, Grave GD, Mayer FE (eds) Control of the onset of puberty. Wiley, New York, pp 403–423
Fritz IB, Dorrington JH (1977) Summary of proceedings of the IVth Testis Workshop, Toronto. Mol Cell Endocrinol 9:121–132
Fritz IB, Kopec B, Lam K, Vernon RG (1974) Effects of FSH on levels of androgen binding protein in the testes. In: Dufau M, Means AR (eds) Hormone binding and target cell activation in the testis. Plenum Press, New York, pp 311–327
Fritz IB, Rommerts FFG, Louis BG, Dorrington JH (1976) Regulation by FSH and cAMP of the formation of ABP in Sertoli cell-enriched cultures. J Reprod Fertil 46:17–24
Fuxe K, Hokfelt T (1969) Catecholamines in the hypothalamus and the pituitary gland. In: Ganong WF, Martini L (eds) Frontiers in neuroendocrinology. Oxford University Press, London, pp 47–95
Galena HJ, Pillai AK, Terner C (1974) Progesterone and androgen receptors in non-flagellate germ cells of the rat testis. J Endocrinol 63:223–237
Garnier F, Saez JM (1980) Response of plasma testosterone to human chorionic gonadotropin stimulation in the ram. Biol Reprod 22:832–836
Geller J, Baron A, Kleinman S (1970) Pituitary luteinizing hormone reserve in elderly men with prostatic disease. J Endocrinol 48:289–290
Gemmell RT, Laychock SG, Rubin RP (1977) Ultrastructural and biochemical evidence for steroid-containing secretory organelle in the perfused cat adrenal gland. J Cell Biol 72:209–215
Gemmell RT, Stacy BD, Thorburn GD (1974) Ultrastructural study of secretory granules in the corpus luteum of the sheep during the estrous cycle. Biol Reprod 11:447–462
Giusti G, Gonnelli P, Borreli D, Fiorelli G, Forti G, Pazzagli M, Serio M (1975) Age-related secretion of androstenedione, testosterone, and dihydrotestosterone by the human testis. Exp Gerontol 10:241–245
Givens JR, Wiser WL, Summitt RL, Kerber IJ, Andersen RN, Pittaway DE, Fish SA (1974) Familial male pseudohermaphroditism without gynecomastia due to deficient testicular 17-ketosteroid reductase activity. N Engl J Med 291:938–944

Glydon RS (1957) The development of the blood supply of the pituitary in the albino rat, with special reference to the portal vessels. J Anat 91:237–244

Goebelsmann U, Horton R, Mestman JH, Arce JJ, Nagata Y, Nakamura RM, Thorneycroft IH, Mishell DR (1973) Male pseudohermaphroditism due to testicular 17β-hydroxysteroid dehydrogenase deficiency. J Clin Endocrinol Metab 36:867–879

Goldman BD, Grazia YR, Kamberi IA, Porter JC (1971) Serum gonadotropin concentrations in intact and castrated neonatal rats. Endocrinology 88:771–776

Gomes WR, Hall RW, Jain SK, Boots LR (1973) Serum gonadotropin and testosterone levels during loss and recovery of spermatogenesis in rats. Endocrinology 93:800–809

Gray GD (1978) Changes in the levels of luteinizing hormone and testosterone in the circulation of ageing male rats. J Endocrinol 76:551–552

Greep RO, Fevold HL, Hisaw PL (1936) Effects of two hypophyseal gonadotropic hormones on the reproductive system of the male rat. Anat Rec 65:261–272

Greenblatt RB, Oettinger M, Bohler CSS (1976) Estrogen-androgen levels in aging men and women: therapeutic considerations. J Am Geriat Soc 24:173–178

Greenwood F (1962) Immunoassay of serum growth hormones in diabetes mellitus. Ciba Found Coll Endocrinol 14, pp. 138–141

Griswold MD, Solari A, Tung PS, Fritz IB (1977) Stimulation by follicle-stimulating hormone of DNA synthesis and of mitosis in cultured Sertoli cells prepared from testes of immature rats. Mol Cell Endocrinol 7:151–165

Grodsky GM (1972) A threshold distribution hypothesis for packet storage of insulin and its mathematical modelling. J Clin Invest 51:2047–2059

Grootegoed JA, Peters MJ, Mulder E, Rommerts FFG, van der Molen HJ (1977) Absence of nuclear androgen receptor in isolated germinal cells of rat testes. Mol Cell Endocrinol 9:159–167

Grota LJ (1971) Effects of age and experience on plasma testosterone. Neuroendocrinology 8:136–143

Grumbach MM, Roth JC, Kaplan SL, Kelch RP (1974) Hypothalamic-pituitary regulation of puberty in man: evidence and concepts derived from clinical research. In: Grumbach MM, Grave GD, Mayer FE (eds) Control of the onset of puberty: Wiley, New York, pp 115–166

Gunsalus GL, Musto NA, Bardin CW (1978b) Factors affecting blood levels of androgen binding protein in the rat. Int J Androl [Suppl] 2:482–492

Gunsalus GL, Musto NA, Bardin CW (1978a) Immunoassay of androgen binding protein in blood: a new approach for study of the seminiferous tubule. Science 200:65–66

Gupta D, Rager K, Zarzycki J, Richner M (1975) Levels of luteinizing hormone, follicle-stimulating hormone, testosterone and dihydrotestosterone in the circulation of sexually maturing intact male rats and after orchidectomy and experimental bilateral cryptorchidism. J Endocrinol 66:183–193

Hafiez AA, Bartke A, Lloyd CW (1972a) The role of prolactin in the regulation of testis function: the synergistic effects of prolactin and luteinizing hormone on the incorporation of (1-^{14}c) acetate into testosterone and cholesterol by testes from hypophysectomized rats in vitro. J Endocrinol 53:223–230

Hafiez AA, Lloyd CW, Bartke A (1972b) The role of prolactin in the regulation of testis function: the effects of prolactin and luteinizing hormone on the plasma levels of testosterone and androstenedione in hypophysectomized rats. J Endocrinol 52:332

Hafiez AA, Philpot JE, Bartke A (1971) The role of prolactin in the regulation of testicular function: the effect of prolactin and luteinizing hormone on 3β-hydroxysteroid dehydrogenase. J Endocrinol 50:619–623

Hagenas L, Ritzen EM (1976) Impaired Sertoli cell function in experimental cryptorchidism in the rat. Mol Cell Endocrinol 4:25–34

Hagenas L, Ritzen EM, Ploen L, Hansson V, French FS, Nayfeh SN (1975) Sertoli cell origin of testicular androgen binding protein (ABP) Mol Cell Endocrinol 2:339–350

Hagenas L, Ritzen EM, Svensson J, Hansson V, Purvis K (1978) Temperature dependence of Sertoli cell function. Int J Androl [Suppl] 2:449–456

Hall PF (1959) Gynaecomastia. Australian Medical Publishing Co, Sydney

Hall PF (1970) Gonadotrophic regulation of testicular function. In: Eik-Nes KB (ed) The androgens of the testis. Marcel Dekker Inc, New York, pp 73–115

Hall PF, Irby DC, de Kretser DM (1969) Conversion of cholesterol to androgens by rat testes:

comparison of interstitial cells and seminiferous tubules. Endocrinology 94:488–496
Hallberg MC, Wieland RG, Zorn EM, Furst BH, Wieland JM (1976) Impaired Leydig cell reserve and altered serum androgen binding in the aging male. Fertil Steril 27:812–814
Hamilton JB (1951) Quantitative measurement of a secondary sex character, axillary hair. Ann NY Acad Sci 53:585–599
Hanes FM (1911) The relation of the interstitial cells of Leydig to the production of an internal secretion by the mammalian testis. J Exp Med 13:338–354
Hansson V, Trygstad O, French FS, McLean WS, Smith AA, Tindall DJ, Weddington SC, Petrusz P, Nayfeh SN, Ritzen EM (1974) Androgen transport and receptor mechanisms in testis and epididymis. Nature 250:387–391
Hansson V, Ritzen EM, French FS, Nayfeh S (1975a) Androgen transport and receptor mechanisms in testis and epididymis. In: Hamilton DW, Greep RO (eds) Handbook of physiology, sect 7, vol 5. Williams & Wilkins, Baltimore, pp 173–201
Hansson V, Weddington SC, McLean NS, Smith AA, Nayfeh SN, French FS, Ritzen EM (1975b) Regulation of seminiferous tubular function by FSH and androgen. J Reprod Fertil 44:363–375
Hansson V, Calandra R, Purvis K, Ritzen EM, French FS (1976) Hormonal regulation of spermatogenesis. Vitam Horm 34:187–214
Hansson V, Purvis K, Attramadal A, Torgesen P, Andersen D, Ritzen EM (1978) Sertoli cell function in the androgen insensitive (Tfm) rat. Int J Andrology 1:96–104
Haour F, Saez JM (1977) HCG-dependent regulation of gonadotropin receptor sites: negative control in testicular Leydig cells. Mol Cell Endocrinol 7:17–24
Harbitz TB (1973) Morphometric studies of the Leydig cells in elderly men with special reference to the histology of the prostate. Acta Pathol Microbiol Scand [A] 81:301–313
Harman SM (1978) Clinical aspects of aging of the male reproductive system. In: Schneider EL (ed) Aging, vol 4, The aging reproductive system, Raven Press, New York, pp 29–58
Harman SM, Tsitouras PD (1980) Reproductive hormones in aging men. I. Measurement of sex steroids, basal luteinizing hormone and Leydig cell response to human chorionic gonadotropin. J Clin Endocrinol Metab 51:35–40
Hashimoto J, Suzuki Y (1966) Androgens in testicular venous blood in the rat, with special reference to pubertal changes in the secretory pattern. Endocrinol Jpn 13:326–337
Hashimoto T, Miyai K, Izumi K, Kumahara Y (1973) Gonadotropin response to synthetic LHRH in normal subjects: correlation between LH and FSH. J Clin Endocrinol Metab 37:910–916
Haug EA, Aakvaag A, Sand T, Torjesen PA (1974) The gonadotrophin response to synthetic gnrh in males in relation to age, dose and basal serum levels of testosterone, oestradiol-17β and gonadotrophins. Acta Endocrinol 77:625–635
Hay MF, Deane HW (1966) Attempts to demonstrate 3β- and 17β-hydroxysteroid dehydrogenases histochemically in the testes of the stallion, boar, ram and bull. J Reprod Fertil 12: 551–560
Healy DL, Pepperell RJ, Stockdale J, Bremner WJ, Burger HG (1977) Pituitary autonomy in hyperprolactinemic secondary amenorrhea: results of hypothalamic-pituitary testing. J Clin Endocrinol Metab 44:809–820
Heller CG, Clermont Y (1964) Kinetics of the germinal epithelium in man. Recent Prog Horm Res 20:545–575
Heller CG, Nelson WO (1945) Hyalinization of the seminiferous tubules associated with normal or failing Leydig cell cell function. Discussion of relationship to eunuchoidism, gynecomastia, elevated gonadotropins, depressed 17-ketosteroids and estrogens. J Clin Endocrinol Metab 5:1–12
Heller CG, Paulsen CA, Mortimore GE, Jungck EC, Nelson WO (1952) Urinary gonadotropins, spermatogenic activity and classification of testicular morphology – their bearing on the utilization hypothesis. Ann NY Acad Sci 55:685–702
Heller CG, Morse HC, Su M, Rowley MJ (1970) The role of FSH, ICSH and endogenous testosterone during testicular suppression by exogenous testosterone in normal men. In: Rosemberg E, Paulsen CA (eds) The human testis. Plenum Press, New York, pp 249–257
Hemsell DL, Grodin JM, Brenner PF, Siiteri PK, MacDonald PC (1974) Plasma precursors of estrogen. II. Correlation of the extent of conversion of plasma androstenedione to estrone with age. J Clin Endocrinol Metab 38:476–479
Henderson WR, Rowlands IW (1938) Gonadotropic activity of anterior pituitary gland in relation to increased intracranial pressure. Br Med J 1:1094–1097

Herbert DC (1975) Localization of antisera to LH-β and FSH-β in the rat pituitary gland. Am J Anat 144:379–385

Herbert DC (1976) Immunocytochemical evidence that luteinizing hormone and follicle stimulating hormone are present in the same cell type in the rhesus monkey pituitary gland. Endocrinology 98:1554–1557

Hilfrich HJ, Konig A (1970) Gonadotropinausscheidung bei in- und subfertilen Mannen. Klin Wochenschr 48:947–948

Hodgen G, Sherins RJ (1973) Enzymes as markers of testicular growth and development in the rat. Endocrinology 93:985–989

Hodgson YM, de Kretser DM (1982) Serum testosterone response to single injections of HCG, ovine-LH and LHRH. Int J Andrology 5:81–91

Hoff JD, Lasley BL, Wang CF, Yen SSC (1977) The two pools of pituitary gonadotropin: regulation during the menstrual cycle. J Clin Endocrinol Metab 44:302–312

Holdsworth S, Atkins RC, de Kretser DM (1977) The pituitary-testicular axis in men with chronic renal failure. N Engl J Med 296:1245–1249

Hollander N; Hollander VP (1958) The microdetermination of testosterone in human spermatic vein blood. J Clin Endocrinol Metab 18:966–971

Hopkins CR (1977) Short term kinetics of luteinizing hormone secretion studied in dissociated pituitary cells attached to manipulable substrates. J Cell Biol 73:685–695

Hopkinson CRN, Daume E, Strum G, Fritze E, Kaiser S, Hirschhauser C (1977) Inhibin-like activity of bovine ovarian extracts in male and female rats. J Reprod Fertil 50:93–96

Hopkinson CRN, Dulisch B, Gauss G, Hilscher W, Hirschhauser C (1978) The effect of local testicular irradiation on testicular histology and plasma hormone levels in the male rat. Acta Endocrinol (Copenh) 87:413–423

Horrobin DF (1973) Prolactin physiology and clinical significance. Eden Press, Montreal

Horton R, Hsieh P, Barberia J, Pages L, Cosgrove M (1975) Altered blood androgens in elderly men with prostate hyperplasia. J Clin Endocrinol Metab 41:793–796

Howard RP, Sniffen RC, Simmons FA, Albright F (1950) Testicular deficiency: a clinical and pathologic study. J Clin Endocrinol Metab 10:121–186

Hseuh AJW, Dufau ML, Catt KJ (1974) Gonadotropin-induced regulation of luteinizing hormone receptors and desensitization of testicular 3′,5′-cyclic AMP and testosterone responses. Proc Natl Acad Sci USA 74:592–595

Hseuh AJW, Dufau ML, Catt KJ (1976a) Regulation of luteinizing hormone receptors in testicular interstitial cells by gonadotropin. Biochem Biophys Res Commun 72:1145–1152

Hseuh AJW, Dufau ML, Katz SI, Catt KJ (1976b) Immunofluorescence labelling of gonadotropin receptors in enzyme dispersed interstitial cells. Nature 261:710–711

Hseuh AJW, Erickson GF (1979) Extrapituitary inhibition of testicular function by luteinizing hormone releasing hormone. Nature 281:66

Hseuh AJW, Schreiber JR, Erickson GF (1981) Inhibitory effect of gonadotropin releasing hormone upon cultured testicular cells. Mol Cell Endocrinol 21:43–49

Hsu AF, Nankin HR, Troen P (1977) Androgen binding protein in human testis: Effect of age. In: Troen P, Nankin HR (eds) The testis in normal and infertile men. Raven Press, New York, p 421

Huang HFS, Hembree WC (1979) Spermatogenic response to vitamin A in vitamin A deficient rats. Biol Reprod 21:891–904

Huckins C (1971) The spermatogonial stem cell population in adult rats. I. Their morphology proliferation and maturation. Anat Rec 169:533–538

Hudson B, Baker HWG, Eddie LW, Higginson RE, Burger HG, de Kretser DM, Dobos M, Lee VWK (1979) Bioassays for inhibin: A critical review. J Reprod Fertil [Suppl] 26:17–29

Huggins C, Moulder PV (1945) Estrogen production by Sertoli cell tumors of the testis. Cancer Res 5:510–514

Hunter WM, Edmond P, Watson GS, McLean N (1974) Plasma LH and FSH levels in subfertile men. J Clin Endocrinol Metab 39:740–749

Isurugi K (1967) Plasma testosterone production rates in patients with prostatic cancer and benign prostatic hypertrophy. J Urol 97:903–908

Isurugi K, Fukutani K, Takayasu H, Wakabayashi K, Tamaoki B-I (1974) Age-related changes in serum luteinizing hormone (LH) and follicle-stimulating hormone (FSH) levels in normal men. J Clin Endocrinol Metab 39:955–957

Iversen J (1971) Secretion of glucagon from the isolated perfused canine pancreas. J Clin Invest 50:2123–2136

Jansen EMH, Steenbergen J, de Jong FH, van der Molen HJ (1981) The use of affinity matrices in the purification of inhibin from bovine follicular fluid. Mol Cell Endocrinol 21:109–117

Jegou B, Risbridger GP, de Kretser DM (to be published): Effects of experimental cryptorchidism on testicular function in adult rats. J Andrology

Johnsen SG (1959) A clinical routine-method for the quantitative determination of gonadotrophins in 24-hour urine samples. II. Normal values for men and women at all age groups from puberty to senescence. Acta Endocrinol 34:209–227

Johnsen SG (1970) Investigations into the feed-back mechanism between spermatogenesis and gonadotropin level in man. In: Rosemberg E, Paulsen CA (eds) The human testis. Plenum Press, New York, pp 231–244

Johnson BH, Ewing LL (1971) Follicle-stimulating hormone and the regulation of testosterone secretion in rabbit testes. Science 173:635–637

Jones TM, Anderson W, Fang VS, Landau RL, Rosenfeld RL (1977) Experimental cryptorchidism in adult male rats: histological and hormonal sequelae. Anat Rec 189:1–27

Jones TM, Fang VS, Landau RL, Rosenfield R (1978) Direct inhibition of Leydig cell function by estradiol. J Clin Endocrinol Metab 47:1368–1373

Josso N, Picard J, Tran D (1977) The antimuellerian hormone. Recent Prog Horm Res 33:117–163

Kaden R (1975) Hodenhistologie beim alternden Mann. Fortschr Med 93:1545–1549

Kalla NR, Nisula BC, Menard R, Loriaux DL (1980) The effect of estradiol on testicular testosterone biosynthesis. Endocrinology 106:35–39

Karacan I, Williams RL, Thornby JI, Salis PJ (1975) Sleep related penile tumescence as a function of age. Am J Psychiatry 132:932–937

Kelch RP, Jenner MR, Weinstein R, Kaplan SL, Grumbach MM (1972) Estradiol and testosterone secretion by human, simian and canine testes, in males with hypogonadism and in male pseudohermaphrodites with the feminizing testis syndrome. J Clin Invest 51:824–830

Kent JR, Acone AB (1966) Plasma testosterme levels and aging in males. In: Vermeulen A, Exley D (eds) Androgens in normal and pathological conditions. Excerpta Medica Foundation International Congress Series No. 101. Amsterdam, pp 31–35

Keogh EJ, Lee VWK, Rennie GC, Burger HG, Hudson B, de Kretser DM (1976) Selective suppression of FSH by testicular extracts. Endocrinology 98:997–1004

Kerr JB, de Kretser DM (1975) Cyclic variations in Sertoli cell lipid content throughout the spermatogenic cycle in the rat. J Reprod Fertil 43:1–8

Kerr JB, Rich KA, de Kretser DM (1979a) Effects of experimental cryptorchidism on the ultrastructure and function of the sertoli cell and peritubular tissue of the rat testis. Biol Reprod 21:823–838

Kerr JB, Rich KA, de Kretser DM (1979b) Alterations of the fine structure and androgen secretion of the interstitial cells in the experimentally cryptorchid rat testis. Biol Reprod 20:409–422

Kerr JB, Irby DC, de Kretser DM (1980) Development of "Reinke-type" crystals within Leydig cells of the Australian bush rat, rattus fuscipes. (abstr 678) Proc. 6th Int Congr Endocr Melb. 1980

Ketelslegers JM, Hetzel WD, Sherins RJ, Catt KJ (1978) Developmental changes in testicular gonadotropin receptors: plasma gonadotropins and plasma testosterone in the rat. Endocrinology 103:212–222

Kierszenbaum AL (1970) Effect of trenimon on the ultrastructure of Sertoli cells in the mouse. Virchows Arch [Cell Pathol] 5:1–12

Kinsey AC, Pomeroy WB, Martin CE (1948) Sexual behaviour in the human male. Saunders, Philadelphia

Kirkland RT, Kirkland JL, Johnson CM, Horning M, Librick L, Clayton GW (1973) Congenital lipoid adrenal hyperplasia in an eight year old phenotypic female. J Clin Endocrinol Metab 36:488–496

Kirschner MA, Coffman GD (1968) Measurement of plasma testosterone and Δ^4-androstenedione using electron capture gas liquid chromatography. J Clin Endocrinol Metab 28:1347–1352

Kjessler B, Wide L (1973) Follicle-stimulating hormone (FSH) and interstitial cell stimulating hormone (ICSH) in relation to gametic output in 643 males. Acta Endocrinol (Copenh) 72:243–256

Kley HK, Nieschlag E, Bidlingmaier F, Kruskemper HL (1974) Possible age dependent influence of estrogens on the binding of testosterone in plasma of adult men. Horm Metab Res 6:213–215

Klinefelter HF, Reifenstein EC, Albright F (1942) Syndrome characterized by gynecomastia, aspermatogenesis without a-Leydigism and increased excretion of follicle-stimulating hormone. J Clin Endocrinol Metab 2:615–627

Knorr DW, Vanha-Perttula T, Lipsett MB (1970) Structure and function of rat testis through pubescence. Endocrinology 86:1298–1304

Kohler PO, Ross GT, Odell WD (1968) Metabolic clearance and production rates of human luteinizing hormone in pre- and postmenopausal women. J Clin Invest 47:38–47

Koninckx P, de Hertogh R, Heyns W, Meulepas E, Brosens I, de Moor P (1976) Secretion rates of LH and FSH during infusion of LH-FSH/RH in normal women and in patients with secondary amenorrhea: suggestive evidence of two pools of LH and FSH. J Clin Endocrinol Metab 43:159–67

Konno M, Hosaka M, Nishimura R (1975) Changes in blood testosterone levels in normal males in relation to age. Clin Endocrinol (Tokyo) 23:1013–1019

Korenchevsky V, Paris SK, Benjamin B (1953) Treatment of senescence in male rats with sex and thyroid hormones and desoxycorticosterone acetate. J Gerontol 8:415–434

Kormano M, Koskimies A, Hunter RL (1971) The presence of specific proteins in the absence of many serum proteins in the rat seminiferous tubule fluid. Experientia 27:1461–1463

Koskimies AI, Kormano M (1973) The proteins in fluids from the seminiferous tubules and rete testis of the rat. J Reprod Fert 34:433–444

Koskimies AI, Kormano M, Alfthan O (1973) Proteins of the seminiferous tubule fluid in man – evidence of a blood-testis barrier. J Reprod Fertil 32:79–86

Kotite NJ, Nayfeh SN, French FS (1978) FSH and androgen regulation of Sertoli cell function in the immature rat. Biol Reprod 18:65–73

Kragt CL, Ganong WF (1968) Pituitary FSH content in male rats at various ages. Proc Soc Exp Biol Med 128:965–957

Kreuger PM, Hodgen GD, Sherins RJ (1974) New evidence for the role of the Sertoli cell and spermatogenic feedback control of FSH secretion in male rats. Endocrinology 95:955–962

Kreutz LE, Rose RM, Jennings JR (1972) Suppression of plasma testosterone levels and psychological stress. Arch Gen Psychiatry 26:479–482

Kulin HE, Reiter EO (1972) Gonadotropin suppression by low dose estrogen in men: Evidence for differential effects upon FSH and LH. J Clin Endocrinol Metab 35:836–839

Kulin HE, Reiter EO (1973) Gonadotropins during childhood and adolescence: A Review. Pediatrics 51:260–271

Kumahara Y, Miyai K, Hashimoto T, Onishi T: Aging and anterior pituitary function – responses of PRL, TSH and gonadotropins to TRH and LH-RH in normal subjects. Jpn J Geriat 12:363–372

Kurosumi K, Oota Y (1968) Electron microscopy of two types of gonadotrophes in the anterior pituitary glands of persistent estrous and diestrous rats. Z Zellforsch 85:34–46

Labhsetwar AP (1970) Age-dependent changes in pituitary-gonadal relationships. III. Changes in pituitary LH and FSH levels in the male rat. J Reprod Fertil 21:407–415

Labrie F, Auclair C, Cusan L, Kelly PA, Pelletier G, Ferland L (1978a) Inhibiting effects of LHRH and its agonists on testicular gonadotropin receptors and spermatogenesis in the rat. Int J Andrology [Suppl] 2:303–318

Labrie F, Lagace L, Ferland L, Kelly PA, Drouin J, Massicotte J, Bonne C, Raynaud JP, Dorrington J (1978b) Interactions between LHRH, sex steroids and "inhibin" in the control of LH and FSH secretion. Int J Andrology [Suppl] 2:81–101

Lacroix M, Smith FE, Fritz IB (1977) Secretion of plasminogen activator by Sertoli cell enriched cultures. Mol Cell Endocrinol 9:227–236

Lacy D (1962) Certain aspects of testis structure and function. Br Med Bull 18:205–208

Le Blond CP, Clermont Y (1952a) Spermiogenesis of rat, mouse, hamster and guinea pig as revealed by the "periodic acid-fuchsin sulphurous acid" technique. Am J Anat 90:167–206

Le Bond CP, Clermont Y (1952b) Definition of the stages of the cycle of the seminiferous epithelium in the rat. Ann NY Acad Sci 55:548–573

Lee PA, Jaffe RB, Midgeley AR, Kohen F, Niswender GD (1972) Regulation of human gonadotropins. VIII. Suppression of serum LH and FSH in adult males following exogenous testosterone administration. J Clin Endocrinol Metab 35:636–641

Lee VWK (1976) Endocrinology of male puberty and the testicular control of FSH. Ph.D. Thesis, Monash University

Lee VWK, Keogh EJ, de Kretser DM, Hudson B (1974) Selective suppression of FSH by testis extracts. IRCS 2:1406

Lee VWK, de Kretser DM, Hudson B, Wang C (1975) Variations in serum FSH, LH and testosterone levels in male rats from birth to sexual maturity. J Reprod Fertil 42:121–126

Lee VWK, Cumming IA, de Kretser DM, Findlay JK, Hudson B, Keogh EJ (1976a) Regulation of gonadotrophin secretion in rams from birth to sexual maturity. I. Plasma LH, FSH and testosterone levels. J Reprod Fertil 46:1–6

Lee VWK, Cumming IA, de Kretser DM, Findlay JK, Hudson B, Keogh EJ (1976b) Regulation of gonadotrophin secretion in rams from birth to sexual maturity. II. Response of the pituitary-testicular axis to LH-RH. J Reprod Fertil 46:7–11

Lee VWK, Keogh EJ, Burger HG, Hudson B, de Kretser DM (1976c) Studies on the relationship between FSH and germ cells: Evidence for selective suppression of FSH by testicular extracts. J Reprod Fertil [Suppl] 24:1–15

Lee VWK, Pearce PT, de Kretser DM (1977) The assessment of rodent models in evaluating the capacity of bovine testes extracts to suppress FSH levels. In: Troen P, Nankin HR (eds) The testis in normal and infertile men. Raven Press, New York, pp 293–303

Lee VWK, Bremner WJ, Cumming IA, de Kretser DM, Findlay JK (1981) Gonadotrophin and testosterone secretion in developing rams: effects of LHRH infusion, castration and cryptorchidism. J Reprod Fertil [Suppl] 30:111–118

Leeson TS, Leeson CR (1970) Experimental cryptorchidism in the rat. A light and electron microscope study. Invest Urol 8:127–144

Lefebvre FA, Reeves JJ, Seguin C, Massicotte J, Labrie F (1980) Specific binding of a potent LHRH agonist in rat testis. Mol Cell Endocrinol 20:127–134

Legros JJ, Demoulin A, Franchimont P (1972) Influence of chlorpromazine on oestrogen induced anterior and posterior pituitary activity in man. Hormones 3:271–272

Leonard JM, Leach RB, Couture M, Paulsen CA (1972) Plasma and urinary follicle stimulating hormone levels in oligospermia. J Clin Endocrinol Metab 34:209–214

Levine N, Marsh DJ (1975) Micropuncture studies of "Sertoli cell only" seminiferous tubules in rats. J Reprod Fertil 43:547–549

Lewis JG, Ghanadian R, Chisholm GD (1976) Serum 5α-dihydrotestosterone and testosterone, changes with age in man. Acta Endocrinol (Copenh) 82:444–449

Lincoln GA (1979) Pituitary control of testicular activity. Br Med Bull 35:167–172

Lindholm J, Korsgaard O, Rasmussen P, Micic S (1976) Luteinising and follicle stimulating hormone and the response to luteinising hormone releasing hormone in relation to sex and age. Eur J Clin Invest 6:249–254

Lindner HR (1961a) Androgens and related compounds in the spermatic vein blood of domestic animals. I. Neutral steroids secreted by the bull testis. J Endocrinol 23:139–159

Lindner HR (1961b) Androgens and related compounds in the spermatic vein blood of domestic animals. IV. Testicular androgens in the ram, boar and stallion. J Endocrinol 23:171–178

Lisk RD (1968) LH in the pituitary gland of the albino rat: concentration and content as a function of sex and age. Neuroendocrinology 3:18–24

Llauraro JP, Dominguez OV (1963) Effect of cryptorchidism on testicular enzymes in involved in androgen biosynthesis. Endocrinology 72:292–295

Longcope C (1973) The effect of human chorionic gonadotropin on plasma steroid levels in young and old men. Steroids 21:583–590

Lording DW, de Kretser DM (1972) Comparative ultrastructural and histochemical studies of the interstitial cells of the rat testis during fetal and postnatal development. J Reprod Fertil 29:261–269

Louis BG, Fritz IB (1977) Stimulation by androgens of the production of androgen binding protein by cultured Sertoli cells. Mol Cell Endocrinol 7:9–16

Louis BG, Fritz IB (1979) FSH and testosterone independently increase the production of ABP by Sertoli cells in culture. Endocrinology 104:454–461

Luborsky-Moore JL, Poliakoff SJ, Worthington WC (1975) Ultrastructural observation of anterior pituitary gonadotrophes following hypophysial portal vessel infusion of luteinizing hormone-releasing hormone. Am J Anat 144:549–555

Ludwig DJ (1950) The effect of androgen on spermatogenesis. Endocrinology 46:453–481

Lugaro G, Giannattasio G, Ciaccolini C, Fachini G, Gianfranceschi G (1969) Biochemical study on the pituitary inhibition of gonadal origin. Experientia 25:147–148
Lugaro G, Carrea G, Casellato MM, Mazzola G, Fachini G (1973) Evidence for a peptidic factor in spermatozoa inhibiting ovarian maturation. Biochem Biophys Acta 304:719–724
Lugaro G, Casellato MM, Mazzola G, Fachini G, Carrea G (1974) Evidence for the existence in spermatozoa of a factor inhibiting follicle stimulating hormone releasing hormone synthesis. Neuroendocrinology 15:62–68
Lynch KM Jr, Scott WW (1950) The lipid content of the Leydig cell and Sertoli cell in the human testis as related to age, benign prostatic hyperplasia, and prostatic growth. J Urol 64:767–776
Lyon MF, Glenister PH, Lamoreux ML (1975) Normal spermatozoa from androgen-resistant germ cells of chimaeric mice and the role of androgen in spermatogenesis. Nature 258:620–622
McCann SM, Ojeda S, Negro-Vilar A (1976) Sex-steroid, pituitary and hypothalamic hormones during puberty in experimental animals. In: Grumbach MM, Grave GD, Mayer FE (eds) Control of onset of puberty. Wiley, New York, pp 1–19
McCullagh DR (1932) Dual endocrine activity of the testis. Science 76:19–20
McCullagh DR, Schneider I (1940) The effect of non-androgenic testis extract on the estrous cycle in rats. Endocrinology 27:899–902
McCullagh EP, Sirridge WT, McIntosh HW (1950) Gametogenic failure with high urinary gonadotrophin (FSH). J Clin Endocrinol Metab 10:1533–1546
MacDonald PC, Grodin JM, Siiteri PK (1971) Dynamics of androgen and oestrogen secretion. In: Baird DT, Strong JA (eds) Control of gonadal steroid secretion. University Press, Edinburgh, pp 158–174
McGee LC (1927) Effect of injections of lipid fraction of bull testicle in capons. Proc Inst Med Chic 6:242
MacKinnon PCB, Puig-Duran E, Laynes R (1978) Reflections on the attainment of puberty in the rat: have circadian signals a role to play in its onset? J Reprod Fertil 52:401–412
MacLeod J, Gold RZ (1953) The male factor in fertility and infertility. VII: Semen quality in relation to age and sexual activity. Fertil Steril 4:194–207
Main SJ, Davies RV, Setchell BP (1978) Feedback control by the testis of gonadotrophin secretion: an examination of the inhibin hypothesis. J Endocrinol 79:255–270
Mancini RE, Vilar O, Lavier JC, Andrada J, Heinrich JJ (1963) Development of Leydig cells in the human testis. A cytological, cytochemical and quantitative study. Amer J Anat 112: 203–214
Mannelli M, Borrelli D, Gonnelli P, Fiorelli G, Forti G, Serio M (1979) 17β-oestradiol concentration in spermatic venous blood with increasing age. Int J Androl 2:131–135
Mantero F, Busnardo B, Riondel A, Veyrat R, Austoni M (1971) Hypertension arterielle alcalose hypokaliemique et pseudohermaphrodisme male par deficit en 17α-hydroxylase. Schweiz Med Wochenschr 101:38–43
Marder ML, Channing CP, Schwartz NB (1977) Suppression of serum follicle stimulating hormone in intact and acutely ovariectomized rats by porcine follicular fluid. Endocrinology 101: 1639–1642
Martin CE (1975) Frequency of male sexual activity in relation to measures of physiologic function and body composition. In: Proceedings of 10th International Congress of Gerontology, vol. 1. Plenary Session, Symposia 1975, pp 183–185
Masters WH, Johnson VE (1966) Human sexual response. Churchill, London
Matsumoto K, Takeyasu K, Mizutani S, Hamanaka Y, Uozumu T (1970) Plasma testosterone levels following surgical stress in male patients. Acta Endocrinol (Copenh) 65:11–17
Maximow A (1899) Die histologischen Vorgänge bei der Heilung von Hodenverletzungen und die Regenerationsfähigkeit des Hodengewebes. Beitr Pathol Anat 26:230–319
Mazzi C, Riva LR, Bernasconi D (1974) Gonadotrophins and plasma testosterone in senescence. In: James VHT, Serio M, Martini, L (eds) The endocrine function of the human testis, vol 2. Academic Press, New York, pp 51–62
Means AR (1975) Biochemical effects of FSH on the testis. In: Greep RO, Hamilton DW (eds) Handbook of physiology, sect 7, vol 5, Williams & Wilkins, Baltimore pp 203–218
Means AR, Dedman JR, Tindall DJ, Welsh MJ (1978) Hormonal regulation of Sertoli cells. Int J Androl [Suppl] 2:403–421
Means AR, Fakunding JL, Huckins C, Tindall DJ, Vitale R (1976) Follicle stimulating hormone, the Sertoli cell and spermatogenesis. Recent Prog Horm Res 32:477–522

Means AR, Vaitukaitis J (1972) Peptide hormone "receptors": specific binding of ^{3}H-FSH to testis. Endocrinology 90:39–46

Mecklenburg RS, Sherins RJ (1974) Gonadotropin response to luteinizing hormone-releasing hormone in men with germinal aplasia. J Clin Endocrinol Metab 38:1005–1008

Mecklenburg RS, Hetzel WD, Gulyas BJ, Lipsett MB (1975) Regulation of FSH secretion: use of hydroxyurea to deplete germinal epithelium. Endocrinology 96:564–570

Melick R, Taft HP (1950) Observations on body hair in old people. J Clin Endocrinol Metab 19:1597–1607

Mendelson C, Dufau M, Catt KJ (1975) Gonadotropin binding and stimulation of cyclic adenosine 3′,5′-monophosphate and testosterone production in isolated Leydig cells. J Biol Chem 250:8818–8823

Midgley AR (1965) Radioimmunoassay of human chorionic gonadotropin (HCG) and human pituitary luteinizing hormone (LH). Fed Proc 24:162–164

Midgley AR (1966) Radioimmunoassay: a method for human chorionic gonadotropin and human luteinizing hormone. Endocrinology 79:10–18

Midgley AR (1967) Radioimmunoassay for human follicle stimulating hormone. J Clin Endocrinol Metab 27:295–299

Mittler JC, Arimura A, Schally AV (1970) Release and synthesis of luteinizing hormone and follicle stimulating hormone in pituitary cultures in response to hypothalamic preparations. Proc Soc Exp Biol Med 133:1321–1325

Miyachi Y, Nieschlag E, Lipsett MB (1973) The secretion of gonadotropins and testosterone by the neonatal male rat. Endocrinology 92:1–5

Moger WH (1976) Serum testosterone response to acute LH treatment in estradiol treated rats. Biol Reprod 14:115–117

Monesi V (1974) Nucleoprotein synthesis in spermatogenesis. In: Mancini RE, Martin L (eds) Male fertility and sterility. Academic Press, New York, pp 59–87

Moore RJ, Gazak JM, Quebbeman JF, Wilson JD (1979) Concentration of dihydrotestosterone and 3α-androstanediol in naturally occurring and androgen induced prostatic hyperplasia in the dog. J Clin Invest 64:1003–1010

Morer-Fargas F, Nowakowski H (1965) Die Testosteronausscheidung im Harn bei männlichen Individuen. Acta Endocrinol (Copenh) 49:443–452

Mori H, Christensen AK (1980) Morphometric analysis of Leydig cells in the normal rat testis. J Cell Biol 84:340–354

Morris ID, Jackson CM (1978) Gonadotrophin response after castration and selective destruction of the testicular interstitium in the normal and aspermatogenic rat. Acta Endocrinol (Copenh) 88:38–47

Mottram JC, Cramer W (1923) On the general effects of exposure to radium on metabolism and tumour growth in the rat and the special effects on testis and pituitary. Q J Exp Physiol 13:209–229

Mulder E, Brinkmann AO, Lamers-Stahlhofen GJ, van der Molen HJ (1973) Binding of oestradiol by nuclear fraction of rat testis interstitial tissue. FEBS Lett 31:131–136

Mulder E, Peters MJ, de Vries J, van der Molen HJ (1975) Characterization of a nuclear receptor for testosterone in seminiferous tubules of mature rat testes. Mol Cell Endocr 2:171–182

Mulder E, van Beurden-Lamers WMO, Brinkmann AO, Mechnielson MJ, van der Molen HJ (1974) High affinity binding of oestradiol by rat testis interstitial tissue and by several other tissues of the male rat. J Steroid Biochem 5:955–959

Murakami T, Yamaji T, Ohsawa N (1976) The effect of ACTH administration on serum estrogens, LH, and FSH in the aged. J Clin Endocrinol Metab 42:88–90

Murphy HD (1965) Intratesticular assay of follicle stimulating hormone in hypophysectomized rats. Proc Soc Exp Biol Med 120:671–675

Murty GSRC, Sheela Rani CS, Moudgal NR, Prasad MRN (1979) Effect of passive immunization with specific antiserum to FSH on the spermatogenic process and fertility of adult male bonnet monkeys (Macaca radiata) J Reprod Fertil [Suppl] 26:147–163

Musto NA, Hafiez AA, Bartke A (1972) Prolactin increases 17β-hydroxysteroid dehydrogenase activity in the testis. Endocrinology 91:1106–1108

Musto NA, Bardin CW (1976) Decreased levels of androgen binding protein in the reproductive tract of the restricted (H^{re}) rat. Steroids 28:1–11

Musto NA, Gunsalus GL, Miljkovic M, Bardin CW (1977) A novel affinity column for isolation

of androgen binding protein from rat epididymis. Endocrinol Res Commun 4:147–157
Musto NA, Gunsalus GL, Bardin CW (1978a) Further characterization of androgen binding protein in epididymis and blood. Int J Androl [Suppl] 2:424–432
Musto NA, Santen RJ, Huckins C, Bardin CW (1978b) Abnormalities of the pituitary-gonadal-axis of H^{re} rats: a study of animals with an inherited disorder of seminiferous tubular and Leydig cell function. Biol Reprod 19:797–806
Muta K, Kato K-I, Akamine Y, Ibayashi H (1981) Age-related changes in the feedback regulation of gonadotrophin secretion by sex steroids in men. Acta Endocrinol (Copenh) 96:154–162
Naftolin F, Ryan KJ, Petro Z (1971a) Aromatization of androstenedione by the diencephalon. J Clin Endocrinol Metab 33:368–370
Naftolin F, Ryan KJ, Petro Z (1971b) Aromatization of androstenedione by limbic system tissue from human foetuses. J Endocrinol 51:795–796
Naftolin F, Yen SSC, Tsai CC (1972) Rapid cycling of plasma gonadotrophins in normal men as demonstrated by frequent sampling. Nature (New Biol) 236:92–93
Naftolin F, Judd HL, Yen SSC (1973) Pulsatile patterns of gonadotropins and testosterone in man. The effects of clomiphene with and without testosterone. J Clin Endocrinol Metab 36:285–288
Nakane PK (1970) Classification of anterior pituitary cell types with immunoenzyme histochemistry. J Histochem Cytochem 18:9–20
Nandini SG, Lipner H, Moudgal NR (1976) A model system for studying inhibin. Endocrinology 98:1460–1465
Nankin HR, Troen P (1971) Repetitive luteinizing hormone elevations in serum of normal men. J Clin Endocrinol Metab 33:558–560
Natoli A, Riondino G, Brancati A (1972) Studio della funzione gonadale ormonica e spermatogenetica nel corso della senescenza maschile. G Gerontol 20:1103–19
Nayfeh S, Barefoot S Jr, Baggett B (1966) Metabolism of progesterone by rat testicular homogenates. II. Changes with age. Endocrinology 78:1041–1048
Nayfeh SN, Coffey JC, Hansson V, French FS (1975) Maturational changes in testicular steroidogenesis: hormonal regulation of 5α-reductase. J Steroid Biochem 6:329–335
Negro-Vilar A, Krulich L, McCann SM (1973) Changes in serum prolactin and gonadotropins during sexual development of the male rat. Endocrinology 93:660–664
Negro-Vilar A, Saad WA, McCann SM (1977) Evidence for a role of prolactin in prostate and seminal vesicle growth in immature male rats. Endocrinology 100:729–737
Nelson WO (1951) Mammalian spermatogenesis: effect of experimental cryptorchidism in the rat and non-descent of the testis in man. Recent Prog Horm Res 6:29–62
Nelson WO (1952) Inter-relations of gonadotropic and gonadal hormones in the regulation of testicular functions. Ciba Found Colloq Endocrinol 4:271–282
New MI (1970) Male pseudohermaphroditism due to 17α-hydroxylase deficiency. J Clin Invest 49:1930–1941
Newman G, Nichols CR (1960) Sexual activities and attitudes in older persons. JAMA 173:33–35
Nicander L (1967) An electron microscopical study of cell contacts in the seminiferous tubules of some mammals. Z Zellforsch 83:375–397
Niemi M, Ikonen M (1962) Cytochemistry of the oxidative enzyme systemes in the Leydig cells of the rat testis and their functional significance. Endocrinology 70:167–174
Niemi M, Ikonen K (1963) Histochemistry of the Leydig cells in the postnatal prepubertal testis of the rat. Endocrinology 72:443–448
Nieschlag E, Kley HK, Wiegelmann W, Solbach H, Kruskemper HL (1973) Lebensalter und endokrine Funktion des Testes des erwachsenen Mannes. Dtsch Med Wochenschr 98:1281–1284
Nieschlag E, Usadel KH, Kley HK (1975) Active immunization with steroids as an approach to investigating testicular and adrenal feed-back control. J Steroid Biochem 6:537–540
Nillius SJ, Wide L (1975) Gonadotrophin-releasing hormone treatment for induction of follicular maturation and ovulation in amenorrhoeic women with anorexia nervosa. Br Med J 2:405–408
Noumura T, Weisz J, Lloyd CW (1966) In vitro conversion of 7-^{3}H-progesterone to androgens by the rat testis during the second half of fetal life. Endocrinology 78:245–253
Nozu K, Dufau ML, Catt KJ (1981) Estradiol receptor-mediated regulation of steroidogenesis in gonadotropin desensitized Leydig cells. J Biol Chem 256:1915–1922
Oakberg EF (1956) Duration of spermatogenesis in the mouse and timing of stages of the cycle of the seminiferous epithelium. Am J Anat 99:507–516

O'Connor S, Baker HWG, Dulmanis A, Hudson B (1973) The measurement of sex steroid binding globulin by differential ammonium sulphate precipitation. J Steroid Biochem 14:331–339

Odell WD, Reichert LE, Swerdloff RS (1968) Correlation between bioassay and immunoassay of human luteinizing hormone. In: Rosemberg E (ed) Gonadotropins. Geron-X Inc., Los Altos, California, pp 401–407

Odell WD, Swerdloff RS (1975) The role of testicular sensitivity to gonadotropins in sexual maturation of the rat. J Steroid Biochem 6:853–857

Odell WD, Swerdloff RS (1976) Etiologies of sexual maturation. A model system based on the sexually maturing rat. Recent Prog Horm Res 32:245–288

Odell WD, Swerdloff RS, Jacobs HS, Hescox MA (1973) FSH induction of sensitivity to LH: on cause of sexual maturation in the male rat. Endocrinology 92:160–165

Ojeda SR, Ramirez VD (1972) Plasma level of LH and FSH in maturing rats: response to hemigonadectomy. Endocrinology 90:466–472

Orth J, Christensen AK (1977) Localization of ^{125}I-labelled FSH in the testes of hypophysectomized rats by autoradiography at the light and electron microscopic levels. Endocrinology 101: 262–278

Orth J, Christensen AK (1978) Autoradiographic localization of specifically bound ^{125}I-labelled follicle stimulating hormone on spermatogonia of the rat testis. Endocrinology 103:1944–1951

Oshima H, Nankin HR, Troen P, Yoshida K-I, Ochi-Ai K-I (1977) Leydig cell number and function in infertile men. In: Troen P, Nankin HR (eds) The testis in normal and infertile men. Raven Press, New York, pp 445–455

Padron RS, Wischusen J, Hudson B, Burger HG, de Kretser DM (1980) Prolonged biphasic response to single intramuscular injections of human chorionic gonadotropin (hCG). J Clin Endocrinol Metab 50:1100–1104

Pahnke VG, Leidenberger FA, Kunzig HJ (1975) Correlation between HCG (LH)-binding capacity, Leydig cell number and secretory activity of rat testis throughout pubescence. Acta Endocrinol (Copenh) 79:610–618

Palmer RL, Crisp AH, Mackinnon PCB, Franklin M, Bonnar J, Wheeler M (1975) Pituitary sensitivity to 50 μg LH/FSH-RH in subjects with anorexia nervosa in acute and recovery stages. Br Med J 1:170–182

Parvinen M, Marana R, Robertson DM, Hansson V, Ritzen EM (1979) Functional cycle of rat Sertoli cells: differential binding and action of FSH at various stages of the spermatogenic cycle. In: Steinberger A, Steinberger E (eds) Testicular development, structure and function. Raven Press, New York, pp 425–432

Parvinen LH, Parvinen M (1978) A "living cell method" for testing the early effect of antispermatogenic compounds: model experiments with two alkylating agents thiotepa and nitrogen mustard. Int J Androl [Suppl] 2:523–536

Paulsen CA (1968) Effect of human chorionic gonadotropin and human menopausal gonadotropin therapy on testicular function. In: Rosemberg E (ed) Gonadotropins. Geron-X Inc, Los Altos, California, pp 491–501

Paulsen CA, Gordon CL, Carpenter RW, Gandy HM, Drucker WD (1968) Klinefelter's syndrome and its variants: a hormonal and chromosomal study. Recent Prog Horm Res 24:321–363

Payne AH, Zipf WB (1978) Regulation of Leydig cell function by prolactin, growth hormone and luteinizing hormone. Int J Androl [Suppl] 2:329–344

Pazzagli M, Forti G, Cappellini A, Serio M (1975) Radioimmunoassay of plasma dihydrotestosterone in normal and hypogonadal men. Clin Endocrinol 4:513–520

Pedersen-Bjergaard K, Tonnesen M (1948) Sex hormone analysis: excretion of sexual hormones by normal males, impotent males, polyarthritics and prostatics. Acta Med Scand [Suppl] 213: 284–291

Pelliniemi LJ, Niemi M (1969) Fine structure of the human foetal testis. I. The Interstitial Tissue. Z Zellforsch 99:507–522

Pelletier G, Leclerc R, Labrie F (1976) Identification of gonadotropic cells in the human pituitary by immunoperoxidase technique. Mol Cell Endocrinol 6:123–128

Pelletier J (1973) Evidence for photoperiodic control of prolactin release in rams. J Reprod Fertil 35:143–147

Pepperell RJ, de Krester DM, Burger HG (1975) Studies on the metabolic clearance rate and production rate of human luteinizing hormone and on the initial half-time of its subunits in man. J Clin Invest 56:118–126

Perey B, Clermont Y, Leblond CP (1961) The wave of the seminiferous epithelium in the rat. Am J Anat 108:47–77

Peterson NT, Midgley AR, Jaffe RB (1968) Regulation of human gonadotropins. III. Luteinizing hormone and follicle stimulating hormone in sera from adult rats. J Clin Endocrinol Metab 28:1473–1478

Peterson RE, Imperato-McGinley J, Gautier T, Sturla E (1977) Male pseudohermaphroditism due to a steroid 5α-reductase deficiency. Am J Med 62:170–191

Pfeiffer E, Davis GC (1972) Determinants of sexual behaviour in middle and old age. Am J Geriatr Soc 20:151–158

Pfeiffer E, Verwoerdt A, Wang HS (1969) The natural history of sexual behaviour in a biologically advantaged group of aged individuals. J Gerontol 24:193–198

Pfeiffer E, Verwoerdt A, Davis GC (1972) Sexual behaviour in middle life. Am J Psychiatry 128:1262–1264

Phifer RF, Midgley AR, Spicer SS (1973) Immunohistologic and histologic evidence that follicle-stimulating hormone and luteinizing hormone are present in the same cell type in the human pars distalis. J Clin Endocrinol Metab 36:125–141

Pickering AJMC, Fink G (1976) Priming effect of luteinizing hormone releasing factor: in vitro and in vivo evidence consistent with its dependence upon protein and RNA synthesis. J Endocrinol 69:373–379

Pirke KM, Doerr P (1973) Age related changes and interrelationships between plasma testosterone, estradiol and testosterone binding globulin in normal males. Acta Endocrinol (Copenh) 74:792–800

Pirke KM, Doerr P (1975a) Age related changes in free plasma testosterone, dihydrotestosterone and oestradiol. Acta Endocrinol (Copenh) 80:171–178

Pirke KM, Doerr P (1975b) Plasma dihydrotestosterone in normal adult males and its relation to testosterone. Acta Endocrinol (Copenh) 79:357–362

Pirke KM, Doerr P, Sintermann R, Vogt HJ (1977) Age dependence of testosterone precursors in plasma of normal adult males. Acta Endocrinol (Copenh) 86:415–429

Plant TM, Hess DL, Hotchkiss J, Knobil E (1978) Testosterone and the control of gonadotropin secretion in the male rhesus monkey (Macaca mulatta). Endocrinology 103:535–541

Podesta EJ, Dufau ML, Catt KJ (1976a) Adenosine 3',5'-monophosphate-dependent protein kinase of Leydig cells: in vitro activation and relationship to gonadotropin action upon cAMP, and steroidogenesis. FEBS Lett 70:212

Podesta EJ, Dufau ML, Catt KJ (1976b) Characterization of two forms of cyclic 3'5'-adenosine monophosphate-dependent protein kinase in rat testicular interstitial cells. Mol Cell Endocrinol 5:109–122

Podesta EJ, Rivarola MA (1974) Concentration of androgens in whole testis, seminiferous tubules and interstitial tissue of rats at different stages of development. Endocrinology 95:455–461

Pomerantz DK (1979) Effects of in vivo gonadotropin treatment on estrogen levels in the testis of the immature rat. Biol Reprod 21:1247–1255

Prader A (1966) Testicular size: assessment and clinical importance. Triangle 7:240–243

Purandare T, Sar M, Stumpf WE (1978) Immunohistochemical localization of FSH and LH in rat pituitary. Mol Cell Endocrinol 10:57–62

Purvis K, Hansson V (1978) Hormonal regulation of Leydig cell function. Mol Cell Endocrinol 12:123–138

Purvis JL, Canick JA, Latif SA, Rosenbaum JH, Hologgitas JH, Menard RH (1973) Lifetime of microsomal cytochrome P-450 and steroidogenic enzymes in rat testis as influenced by human chorionic gonadotropin. Arch Biochem Biophys 159:39–49

Purvis K, Torjesen PA, Haug E, Hansson V (1977) HCG suppression of LH receptors and responsiveness of testicular tissue to HCG. Mol Cell Endocrinol 8:73–80

Purvis K, Calandra R, Sander S, Hansson V (1978) Androgen binding proteins and androgen levels in the human testis and epididymis. Int J Androl 1:531–548

Rajaniemi H, Oksanen A, Vanha-Perttula T (1974) Distribution of ^{125}I-prolactin in mice and rats. Studies with whole-body and microautoradiography. Horm Res 5:6–20

Ramaley JA (1974) Adrenal-gonadal interactions at puberty. Life Sci 14:1623–1633

Ramaley JA (1979) Development of gonadotropin regulation in the prepubertal mammal. Biol Reprod 20:1–31

Ramaley JA, Bunn EL (1972) Seasonal variations in the onset of puberty in rats. Endocrinology 91:611–613

Ramirez VD (1973) Endocrinology of puberty. In: Greep RO, Astwood EB (eds) Handbook of physiology, sect 7, vol 5. Williams & Wilkins, Maryland, pp 1–28
Ravault JP, Courot M (1975) Blood prolactin in the male lamb from birth to puberty. J Reprod Fert 42:563–566
Rebar R, Yen SSC, Vandenberg G, Naftolin F, Ehara Y, Engblom S, Ryan KJ, Rivier J, Amoss M, Guillemin R (1973) Gondatotropin responses to synthetic LRF: dose response relationship in men. J Clin Endocrinol Metab 36:10–16
Reddi AH, Ewing LL, Williams-Ashman HG (1971) Protein phosphokinase reactions in mammalian testis: stimulatory effects of adenosine 3′,5′-cyclic monophosphate on the phosphorylation of basic proteins. Biochem J 122:333–345
Redding TW, Schally AV, Arimura A, Matsuo H (1972) Stimulation of release and synthesis of luteinizing hormone (LH) and follicle stimulating hormone (FSH) in tissue cultures of rat pituitaries in response to natural and synthetic LH and FSH releasing hormone. Endocrinology 90:764–770
Reddy J, Svoboda D (1972) Microbodies (peroxisomes) in the interstitial cells of rodent testes. Lab Invest 26:657–665
Reddy KJ, Svoboda DJ (1967) Alterations in rat testis due to an antispermatogenic agent. Am J Pathol 84:376–392
Reddy VVR, Naftolin F, Ryan KJ (1973) Aromatization in the central nervous system of rabbits: effects of castration and hormone treatment. Endocrinology 92:589–594
Regaud C (1901) Etude sur la structure des tubes seminifères et sur la spermatogenèse chez les mammifères. Arch Anat Microsc Morphol Exp 4:101–156
Reichert LE Jr, Abou-Issa H (1977) Studies on a low molecular weight testicular factor which inhibits binding of FSH to receptor. Biol Reprod 17:614–621
Reitano JF, Caminos-Torres R, Snyder PJ (1975) Serum LH and FSH responses to repetitive administration of gonadotropin-releasing hormone in patients with idiopathic hypogonadotropic hypogonadism. J Clin Endocrinol Metab 41:1035–1042
Reiter EO, Fuldaner VG, Root AW (1976a) Effect of infusion of gonadotropin releasing hormone upon plasma concentrations of sex hormones in prepubertal and pubertal males. Steroids 28:829–835
Reiter EO, Root AW, Duckett GE (1976b) The response of pituitary gonadotropes to a constant infusion of luteinizing hormone-releasing hormone (LHRH) in normal prepubertal and pubertal children and in children with abnormalities of sexual development. J Clin Endocrinol Metab 43:400–411
Reiter T (1963) Testosterone implantation: a clinical study of 240 implantations in aging males. J Am Geriatr Soc 11:540–550
Resko JA, Feder HH, Goy RW (1968) Androgen concentrations in plasma and testis of developing rats. J Endocrinol 40:485–491
Reyes FI, Winter JSD, Faiman C (1976) Gonadotropin-gonadal interrelationships in the fetus. In: Diabetes and other endocrine disorders during pregnancy and in the newborn. Alan R. Liss Inc., New York, pp 83–106
Rich KA, de Kretser DM (1977a) Changes in the levels of FSH and LH in serum and androgen binding protein in the testis and epididymis of the rat following exposure of the testis to local heating (abstr 20). Proceedings Endocrine Soc Aust p 43
Rich KA, de Kretser DM (1977b) Effect of differing degrees of destruction of the rat seminiferous epithelium on levels of serum FSH and androgen binding protein. Endocrinology 101:959–968
Rich KA, de Kretser DM (1978) Altered pubertal development in male rats after neonatal administration of oestradiol benzoate (abstr 62). Proc 21st Annual Meeting, Endocrine Society of Australia, 1978
Rich KA, de Kretser DM (1979) Effect of fetal irradiation on testicular receptors and testosterone response to gonadotrophin stimulation in adult rats. Int J Andrology 2:343–352
Rich KA, de Kretser DM (1980) Recovery of spermatogenesis after retinol administration in chronic Vitamin A deficiency. Proceedings of US Endocrine Soc Abstract 232 p 132
Rich KA, Kerr JB, de Kretser DM (1979) Evidence for Leydig cell dysfunction in rats with seminiferous tubule damage. Mol Cell Endocrinol 13:123–135
Richardson DW, Short RV (1978) Time of onset of sperm production in boys. J Biosoc Sci [Suppl] 5:17–27

Riegle GD, Meites J, Miller AE, Wood SM (1977) Effect of aging on hypothalamic LH-releasing and prolactin inhibiting activities and pituitary responsiveness to LHRH in the male laboratory rat. J Gerontol 32:13–18

Rigaudiere N, Pelardy G, Robert A, Delost P (1976) Changes in the concentrations of testosterone and androstenedione in the plasma and testis of the guinea pig from birth to death. J Reprod Fertil 48:291–300

Rigby MK, Soule SD, Barber W, Rothman D (1964) Sex hormone replacement in the aged. J Gerontol 19:313–316

Rippel RH, Johnson ES, White WF (1974) Effect of consecutive injections of synthetic gonadotropin releasing hormone on LH release in the anestrous and ovariectomized ewe. J Anim Sci 39:907–914

Risbridger GP, Hodgson YM, de Kretser DM (1981a) Mechanism of action of gonadotrophins on the testis. In: Burger HG, de Kretser DM (eds) The testis. Raven Press, New York, pp 195–211

Risbridger GP, Kerr JB, de Kretser DM (1981b) An evaluation of Leydig cell function and gonadotrophin binding in unilateral and bilateral cryptorchidism. Evidence for local control of Leydig cell function by the seminiferous tubule. Biol Reprod 24:534–540

Risbridger GP, Kerr JB, Peake RA, de Kretser DM (1981c) An assessment of Leydig cell function after bilateral or unilateral efferent duct ligation. Further evidence for local control of Leydig cell function. Endocrinology 109:1234–1241

Risbridger GP, Kerr JB, Peake R, Rich KA, de Kretser DM (1981d) The temporal changes in some aspects of Leydig cell function after the induction of bilateral cryptorchidism. J Reprod Fertil 63:415–423

Risbridger GP, Robertson DM, de Kretser DM (1982) Effects of chronic human chorionic gonadotropin treatment on Leydig cell function. Endocrinology 110:138–145

Ritzen EM, French FS (1973) Androgen-receptors in the male gonad. Acta Endocrinol (Copenh) [Suppl] 177:387

Ritzen EM, Hansson V, French FS (1981) The Sertoli cell. In: Burger HG, de Kretser DM (eds) The testis. Raven Press, New York, pp 171–194

Rivarola MA, Podesta EJ, Chemes HE (1972) In vitro testosterone-^{14}C metabolism by rat seminiferous tubules at different stages of development: formation of 5α-androstandiol at meiosis. Endocrinology 91:537–542

Rivier C, Rivier J, Vale W (1979) Chronic effects of [D-Trp^6, Pro^6, NET] luteinizing hormone-releasing factor on reproductive processes in the male rat. Endocrinology 105:1191–1201

Robyn C, Leleux P, Vanhaelst L, Golstein J, Herlant M, Pasteels JL (1973) Immunohistochemical study of the human pituitary with anti-luteinizing hormone, anti-follicle stimulating hormone and anti-thyrotrophin sera. Acta Endocr 72:625–642

Rock J, Robinson D (1965) Effect of intrascrotal hyperthermia on testicular function in man. Am J Obstet Gynecol 93:793–809

Ridriguez-Rigau LJ, Smith KD, Steinberger E (1980) A possible relation between elevated FSH levels and Leydig cell dysfunction in azoospermia and oligospermic men. J Andrology 1:127–132

Rommerts FFG, Grootegoed JA, van der Molen HJ (1976) Physiological role for ABP-steroid complex in testis? Steroids 28:43–49

Rommerts FFG, Kruger-Sewnarian BCH, van Woerkom-Blik A, Grootegoed JA, van der Molen HJ (1978) Secretion of proteins by Sertoli cell enriched cultures: Effects of FSH, dibutyryl cAMP and testosterone and correlation with secretion of oestradiol and androgen binding protein. Mol Cell Endocrinol 10:39–55

Rommerts FFG, Kruger-Sewnarian BCH, Grootegoed JA, de Jong FH van der Molen HJ (1979) Secretion of proteins, androgen binding protein and oestradiol by Sertoli cells in culture: effects of serum. Acta Endocrinol (Copenh) 90:522–561

Roosen-Runge EC (1962) Process of spermatogenesis in mammals. Biol Rev 37:343–377

Roosen-Runge EC, Anderson D (1959) The development of the interstitial cells in the testis of the albino rat. Acta Anat 37:125–137

Root AW (1973) Endocrinology of puberty. I. Normal sexual maturation. J Pediatr 83:1–19

Rose RM, Gordon TP, Bernstein IS (1972) Plasma testosterone levels in the male rhesus: influences of sexual and social stimuli. Science 178:643–645

Rosen SW, Weintraub BD (1971) Monotropic increase of serum FSH correlated with low sperm

count in young men with idiopathic oligospermia and aspermia. J Clin Endocrinol Metab 32:410–416
Rosner WR (1972) A simplified method for the quantitative determination of testosterone-estradiol binding of globulin activity in human plasma. J Clin Endocrinol Metab 34:983–988
Ross MH, Dobler J (1975) The Sertoli cell junctional specializations and their relationship to the germinal epithelium as observed after efferent ductule ligation. Anat Rec 183:267–292
Roth J, Glick SM, Yalow RS, Berson SA (1963) Secretion of human growth hormone: Physiologic and experimental modification. Metabolism 12:577–579
Roth JC, Grumbach MM, Kaplan SL (1973) Effect of synthetic LH-RF on serum testosterone and gonadotropins in prepubertal, pubertal and adult males. J Clin Endocrinol Metab 37:680–686
Roth GS (1974) Changes in hormone binding and responsiveness in target cells and tissues during aging. Adv Exp Med Biol 61:195–208
Roth WD (1965) Metabolic and morphologic studies on the rat pineal organ during puberty. Prog Brain Res 10:552–563
Roy AK, Milin BS, McMinn DM (1974) Androgen receptor in rat liver hormonal and developmental regeneration of the cytoplasmic receptor and its correlation with the androgen-dependent synthesis of alpha-2-globulin. Biochim Biophys Acta 354:213–232
Rubens R, Dhont M, Vermeulen A (1974) Further studies on Leydig cell function in old age. J Clin Endocrinol Metab 39:40–45
Russell LD (1977) Movement of spermatocytes from the basal to the adluminal compartments of the rat testis. Am J Anat 148:313–328
Russell LD (1978) The blood-testis barrier and its formation relative to spermatocyte maturation in the adult rat: a lanthanum tracer study. Anat Rec 190:99–112
Ruzicka L, Wettstein A (1935) Künstliche Herstellung des männlichen Sexualhormones Trans-dehydro-androsten-3, 17-dions. Helv Chim Acta 18:986–994
Ryan RJ, Faiman C (1968) Radioimmunoassay of FSH and LH in human serum: the effects of age and infusion of several polyamines in males. In: Rosemberg E (ed) Gonadotropins. Geron-X Inc, Los Altos, California, pp 333–337
Ryan KJ, Naftolin F, Reddy V, Flores F, Petro Z (1972) Estrogen formation in the brain. Am J Obstet Gynecol 114:454–460
Saez J, Bertrand J (1968) Studies on testicular function in children plasma concentrations of testosterone, dehydroepiandrosterone and its sulfate before and after stimulation with human chorionic gonadotropin. Steroids 12:749–761
Saez JM, Forest MG (1979) Kinetics of human chorionic gonadotropin induced steroidogenic response of the human testis. I. Plasma testosterone; implications for human chorionic gonadotropin stimulation test. J Clin Endocrinol Metab 49:278–283
Saez JM, de Peretti E, Morera AM, David M, Bertrand J (1971) Familial male pseudohermaphroditism with gynecomastia due to a testicular 17-ketosteroid reductase defect. I. Studies in vivo. J Clin Endocrinol Metab 32:604–610
Salamonsen LA, Jonas HA, Burger HG, Buckmaster JM, Chamley WA, Cumming IA, Findlay JK, Goding JR (1973) A heterologous radioimmunoassay for follicle stimulating hormone: application to measurement of FSH in the ovine estrous cycle and in several other species including man. Endocrinology 93:610–618
Samuels LT, Bussmann L, Matsumoto K, Huseby RA (1964) The effect of diethylstilboestrol on testicular 17α-hydroxylase and 17-desmolase activities in BALB/C mice. Acta Endocrinol (Copenh) 45:487–497
Sanborn BM, Steinberger A, Tcholakian RK, Steinberger E (1977) Direct measurement of androgen receptors in cultured Sertoli cells. Steroids 29:493–502
Santen RJ (1975) Is aromatization of testosterone to estradiol required for inhibition of luteinizing hormone secretion in man? J Clin Invest 56:1555–1563
Santen RJ, Bardin CW (1973) Episodic luteinizing hormone secretion in man. J Clin Invest 52:2617–2628
Santen RJ, Leonard JM, Sherins RJ, Gandy HM, Paulsen CA (1971) Short and long-term effects of clomiphene citrate on the pituitary-testicular axis. J Clin Endocrinol Metab 33:970–979
Sarjent JW, McDonald JR (1948) A method for the quantitative estimate of Leydig cells in the human testis. Mayo Clin Proc 23:249–254
Sasano N, Ichigo S (1969) Vascular patterns of the human testis with special reference to its senile changes. Tohuku J Exp Med 99:269–276

Schalch DS, Parlow AF, Boon RC, Reichlin S (1968) Measurement of human luteinizing hormone in plasma by radioimmunoassay. J Clin Invest 47:665–678

Schally AV, Arimura A, Baba Y, Nair RHG, Matsuo H, Redding TW, Debeljuk L, White WF (1971) Isolation and properties of the FSH and LH-releasing hormone. Biochem Biophys Res Commun 43:393–9

Schilsky RL, Lewis BJ, Sherins RJ, Young RC (1980) Gonadal dysfunction in patients receiving chemotherapy for cancer. Ann Intern Med 93:109–114

Schneider HPG, Dahlen HG (1975) Influence of interactive I.V. injection of LHRH in women. In: Franchimont P (ed) Some aspects of hypothalamic regulation of endocrine functions. Schattauer, Stuttgart, pp 163–172

Schwartz NB, Channing CP (1977) Evidence for ovarian "inhibin" suppression of the secondary rise in serum follicle stimulating hormone levels in proestrous rats by injection of porcine follicular fluid. Proc Natl Acad Sci USA 74:5721–5724

Scott RS (1980) Gonadal Control of FSH in Man. Thesis, Monash University

Scott RS, Burger HG (1980) An inverse relationship exists between seminal plasma inhibin and serum follicle-stimulating hormone in man. J Clin Endocrinol Metab 52:796–803

Scott RS, Burger HG (1981) Mechanism of Action of Inhibin. Biol Reprod 24:541–550

Scott RS, Burger HG, Quigg H (1980) A simple and rapid in vitro bioassay for inhibin. Endocrinology 107:1536–1542

Sertoli E (1865) Dell'esistenza di particolari cellule remificate nei canalicoli seminiferi del testicolo umano. Il Morgani 7:31–39

Sertoli E (1878) Sulla struttura dei canalicoli seminiferi dei testicoli studiata in rapporto allo svillupo dei nemaspermi. Arch Sci Med 2:107–146, and 267–295

Setchell BP (1969) Do Sertoli cells secrete fluid into the seminiferous tubules? J Reprod Fertil 19:391–392

Setchell BP (1970) The secretion of fluid by the testis of rats, ram and goats with some observations on the effect of age, cryptorchidism and hypophysectomy. J Reprod Fertil 23:79–85

Setchell BP, Jacks F (1974) Inhibin-like activity in rete testis fluid. J Endocrinol 62:675–676

Setchell BP, Main SJ (1974) Bibliography (with review) on inhibin. Bibliogr Reprod 24:245–252

Setchell BP, Waites GMH (1972) The effects of local heating of the testis on the flow and composition of rete testis fluid in the rat, with some observations on the effects of age and unilateral castration. J Reprod Fertil 30:225–33

Setchell BP, Waites GMH (1975) The blood-testis barrier. In: Hamilton DW, Greep RO (eds) Handbook of physiology, sect 7, vol 5. Williams & Wilkins, Baltimore, pp 143–172

Setchell BP, Sirinathsinghji DJ (1972) Antigonadotrophic activity in rete testis fluid, a possible "inhibin". J Endocrinol 53:lx-lxi.

Setchell BP, Laurie MS, Main SJ, Goats GC (1981) The mechanism of transport of testosterone through the walls of the seminiferous tubules of the rat testis. Int J Androl 1978; Suppl 2:506–10

Shain SA, Boesel RW, Axelrod LR (1975) Aging in the rat prostate. Reduction in detectable ventral prostate androgen receptor content. Arch Biochem Biophys 167:247–263

Sharpe RM (1976) hCG-induced decrease in availability of rat testis receptors. Nature 264:644–666

Sharpe RM, Fraser HM (1980) Inhibition of maturational changes in Leydig cell function by treatment of rats with an agonist of LH-RH. J Reprod Fertil 60:359–368

Sharpe RM, Fraser HM, Sandow J (1981) Effect of treatment with an agonist of luteinizing hormone releasing hormone on early maturational changes in pituitary and testicular function in the rat. J Endocrinol 80:249–257

Shaw MJ, Georgopoulos LE, Payne AH (1979) Synergistic effect of follicle-stimulating hormone and luteinizing hormone on testicular Δ^5-3β-hydroxysteroid dehydrogenase-isomerase: application of a new method for the separation of testicular compartments. Endocrinology 104: 912–918

Sherins RJ, Loriaux DL (1973) Studies on the role of sex steroids in the feedback control of FSH concentrations in men. J Clin Endocrinol Metab 36:886–893

Sherins RJ, Gandy HM, Thorslund TW, Paulsen CA (1971) Pituitary and testicular function studies. I. Experience with a new gonadal inhibitor, 17α-pregn-4-en-20-yno (2,3-d) isoxazol-17-ol (Danazol). J Clin Endocrinol Metab 32:522–531

Sherins RJ, Winters SJ, Wachslicht H (1977) Studies of the roles of HCG and low dose FSH in initiating spermatogenesis in hypogonadotropic men (abstr 312). Proc Am Endocr Soc 59th Ann Meeting.

Sherman BM, Halmi KA, Zamudio R (1975) LH and FSH response to gonadotropin-releasing hormone in anorexia nervosa: effect of nutritional rehabilitation. J Clin Endocrinol Metab 41:135–142

Shino M, Arimura AV, Schally AV, Rennels EG (1972) Ultrastructural observations of granule extrusion from rat anterior pituitary cells after injection of LH-releasing hormone. Z Zellforsch 128:152–161

Siiteri PK, Wilson JD (1970) Dihydrotestosterone in prostatic hypertrophy. I. The function and content of dihydrotestosterone in the hyperplastic prostate of man. J Clin Invest 49:1737–1745

Simpson ME, Li CH, Evans HM (1942) Biological properties of pituitary interstitial-cell-stimulating hormone (ICSH). Endocrinology 30:969–976

Skakkebaek NE, Heller CG (1973) Quantification of human seminiferous epithelium. J Reprod Fertil 32:379–389

Skinner JD (1970) The post-natal development of the male reproductive tract in two indigenous fat-tailed South African sheep, the Fedi and the Namaqua. Proc S Afr Soc Anim Prod 9:195–196

Skinner JD, Booth WD, Rowson LEA, Karg H (1968) The post-natal development of the reproductive tract of the Suffolk ram, and changes in the gonadotrophin content of the pituitary. J Reprod Fertil 16:463–477

Skinner MK, Griswold MD (1980) Sertoli cells synthesize and secrete transferin like protein. J Biol Chem 255:9523–9525

Smith G (1962) The effects of ligation of the vasa efferentia and vasectomy on testicular function in the adult rat. J Endocrinol 23:385–399

Smith GC, Simpson RW (1970) Monoamine fluorescence in the median eminence of foetal, neonatal and adult rats. Z Zellforsch 104:541–556

Smith PE (1930) Hypophysectomy and a replacement therapy in the rat. Am J Anat 45:205–256

Smith SR, Chhetri MK, Johanson AJ, Radfar N, Migeon CJ (1975) The pituitary-gonadal axis in protein-calorie malnutrition. J Clin Endocrinol Metab 41:60–69

Snedecor GW, Cochran WG (1967) Statistical Methods, 6th edn. Iowa State University Press, Ames, Iowa

Sniffen RC (1950) The testis. I. The normal testis. Arch Pathol 50:259–284

Sniffen RC (1952) Histology of the normal and abnormal testis at puberty. Ann N Y Acad Sci 55:609–618

Snyder PJ, Reitano JF, Utiger RD (1975) Serum LH and FSH responses to synthetic gonadotropin releasing hormone in normal men. J Clin Endocrinol Metab 41:938–945

Sobhon P, Mitranond V, Tosukhowong P, Chindaduangrat W (1979) Cytological changes in the testes of Vitamin A-deficient rats. II Ultrastructural study of the seminiferous tubules. Acta Anat 103:169–183

Stearns EL, MacDonnell JA, Kaufman BJ, Padua R, Lucman TS, Winter JSD, Faiman C (1974) Declining testicular function with age: hormonal and clinical correlates. Am J Med 57:761–766

Steinberger A (1975) Initiation of clone cultures of rat anterior pituitary cells which secrete a single gonadotropic hormone. Methods Enzymol 39:128–132

Steinberger A, Heindel JJ, Lindsey JN, Elkington JSH, Sanborn BM, Steinberger E (1975) Isolation and culture of FSH responsive Sertoli cells. Endocr Res Commun 2:261–272

Steinberger A, Hintz M, Heindel JJ (1978) Changes in cyclic AMP responses to FSH in isolated rat Sertoli cells during sexual maturation. Biol Reprod 19:566–572

Steinberger A, Steinberger E (1971) Replication pattern of Sertoli cells in maturing rat testis in vivo and in organ culture. Biol Reprod 4:84–87

Steinberger A, Steinberger E (1976) Secretion of an FSH-inhibiting factor by cultured Sertoli cells. Endocrinology 99:918–921

Steinberger E (1962) A quantitative study of the effect of an alkylating agent (triethylenemelamine) on the seminiferous epithelium of rats. J Reprod Fertil 3:250–259

Steinberger E (1971) Hormonal control of mammalian spermatogenesis. Physiol Rev 51:1–22

Steinberger E, Chowdhury M (1974) Control of pituitary FSH in male rats. Acta Endocrinol 76:235–241

Steinberger E, Duckett GE (1967) Hormonal control of spermatogenesis. J Reprod Fertil [Suppl] 2:75–87

Steinberger E, Tjioe DY (1968) A method for quantitative analysis of human seminiferous epithelium. Fertil Steril 19:860–970

Steinberger E, Root A, Ficher M, Smith KD (1973) The role of androgens in the initiation of spermatogenesis in man. J Clin Endocrinol Metab 37:746–751
Stewart-Bentley M, Odell W, Horton R (1974) The feedback control of luteinizing hormone in normal adult men. J Clin Endocrinol Metab 38:545–553
Stockell-Hartree AM (1966) Separation and partial purification of the protein hormones from human pituitary glands. Biochem J 100:754–761
Sundby A, Farahat A (1978) Plasma testosterone in bulls. Response to various doses of HCG and PMSG. Acta Endocrinol (Copenh) 88:793–800
Suoranta H (1971) Changes in the small blood vessels of the adult human testis in relation to age and some pathological conditions. Virchows Arch Pathol Anat 352:165–181
Swerdloff RS, Odell WD (1968) Some aspects of the control of secretion in LH and FSH in humans. In: Rosemberg E (ed) Gonadotropins. Geron X Inc, Los Altos, California, pp 155–162
Swerdloff RS, Odell WD (1977) Modulating influences of FSH, GH and prolactin on LH-stimulated testosterone secretion. In: Troen P, Nankin HR (eds) The testis in normal and infertile men. Raven Press, New York, pp 395–401
Swerdloff RS, Walsh PC, Jacobs HS, Odell WD (1971) Serum LH and FSH during sexual maturation in the male rat: effect of castration and cryptorchidism. Endocrinology 88:120–128
Swerdloff RS, Grover PK, Jacobs HS, Bain JC (1973) Search for a substance which selectively inhibits FSH-effects of steroids and prostaglandins on serum FSH and LH levels. Steroids 21:703–722
Tait JF (1963) Review: the use of isotopic steroids for the measurement of production rates in vivo. J Clin Endocrinol Metab 23:1285–1297
Taleisnik S, McCann SM (1961) Effects of hypothalamic lesions on the secretion and storage of hypophysial luteinizing hormone. Endocrinology 68:263–272
Tanner JM (1962) Growth at adolescence. Blackwell Scientific, Oxford
Tanoa H, Terada M, Mizutobe K, Aoyama T, Maruta H, Fujita M, Saka T, Kurobatake T, Shiraki K (1975) Endocrine functions of the testis and aging. Clin Endocrinol (Tokyo) 23:431–441
Tcholakian RK, Steinberger A (1978) Progesterone metabolism by cultured Sertoli cells. Endocrinology 103:1335–43
Thieblot L, Blaise S (1963) Influence de la glande pineale sur les gonades. Ann Endocrinol (Paris) 24:270–286
Tillenger GG, Birke G, Franksson C, Plantin LO (1955) The steroid production of the testicles and its relation to number and morphology of Leydig cells. Acta Endocrinol (Copenh) 19:340–348
Tillenger KG (1957) Testicular morphology. Acta Endocrinol (Copenh) 30:28–39
Tindall DJ, Means AR (1976) Concerning the hormonal regulation of androgen binding protein in rat testis. Endocrinology 99:809–818
Tindall DJ, Schrader WT, Means AR (1974) The production of ABP by Sertoli cells. In: Dufau ML, Means AR (eds) Hormone binding and target cell activation in the testis. Plenum Press, New York, pp 167–175
Tindall DJ, Mena CR, Means AR (1978a) Hormonal regulation of androgen binding protein in hypophysectomized rats. Endocrinology 99:809–818
Tindall DJ, Cunningham GR, Means AR (1978b) 5α-dihydrotestosterone binding to androgen binding protein. Effects of testosterone and other compounds in vivo and in vitro on the number of binding sites measured. J Biol Chem 253:166–169
Tougard C, Kerdelhue B, Tixier-Vidal A, Jutisz M (1971) Localisation par cyto-immunoenzymologic de la LH, de ses sous-unites α et β et de la FSH dans l'adenohypophyse de la ratte castrée. CR Acad Sci (Paris) 273:897–900
Toyama Y (1976) Actin-like filaments in the Sertoli cell junctional specializations in the swine and mouse testis. Anat Rec 186:477–91
Tsuruhara T, Dufau ML, Cigorraga S, Catt KJ (1977) Hormonal regulation of testicular luteinizing hormone receptors: effects on cyclic AMP and testosterone responses in isolated Leydig cells. J Biol Chem 252:9002–9009
Tuck RR, Setchell BP, Waites GMH, Young JA (1970) The composition of fluid collected by micropuncture and catheterization from the seminiferous tubules and rete testis of rats. Pfluegers Arch 318:225–243

Utiger R, Parker M, Daughaday WH (1962) Studies on human growth hormone. I. Radioimmunoassay for human growth hormone. J Clin Invest 41:254–261

Valladares LE, Payne AH (1979) Induction of testicular aromatization by luteinizing hormone in mature rats. Endocrinology 105:431–6

Van Beurden WMO, Roodnat B, de Jong FH, Mulder E, van der Molen HJ (1976) Hormonal regulation of LH stimulation of: the effect of hypophysectomy, FSH and estradiol-17β. Steroids 28:847–866

Van Beurden WMO, Roodnat B, de Jong FH, Mulder E, van der Molen HJ (1977) The effect of estrogens on luteinizing hormone plasma levels and on testosterone production in intact and hypophysectomized rats. Endocrinology 101:342–349

Van der Molen HJ, Brinkmann AO, Cooke BA, de Jong FH, Mulder E, Rommerts FFG, van der Vusse GJ (1973) Biochemical functions of isolated interstitial tissue and seminiferous tubules from rat testis. In: James VHT, Serio M, Martini L (eds) The endocrine function of the human testis. Academic Press, New York, pp 533–560

Van der Vusse GJ, Kalkman ML, van der Molen HJ (1975) Endogenous steroid production in cellular and subcellular fractions of rat testis after prolonged treatment with gonadotropins. Biochem Biophys Acta 380:473–485

Van Thiel DH, Sherins RJ, Meyers Jr GH, Devita Jr VT (1972) Evidence for a specific seminiferous tubular factor affecting follicle-stimulating hormone secretion in man. J Clin Invest 51:1009–1019

Vassileva-Popova JG, Yanev TK (1975) Information transfer in ageing: an allosteric model of hormonal regulation. In: Vassileva-Popova JG (ed) Physical and chemical bases of biological information transfer. Plenum Press, New York, pp 63–95

Verjans HL, Eik-Nes KB (1976) Hypothalamic-pituitary-testicular system following testicular X-irradiation. Acta Endocrinol (Copenh) 83:190–200

Vermeulen A (1977) Altered physiology of the senescent testis. In: Troen P, Nankin H (eds) The testis in normal and infertile men. Raven Press, New York, pp 413–420

Vermeulen A, Verdonck L (1968) Studies on the binding of testosterone to human plasma. Steroids 11:609–635

Vermeulen A, Verdonck L, van der Straeten M, Orie N (1969) Capacity of the testosterone-binding globulin in human plasma and influence of specific binding of testosterone on its metabolic clearance rate. J Clin Endocrinol Metab 29:1470–1480

Vermeulen A, Rubens R, Verdonck L (1972) Testosterone secretion and metabolism in male senescence. J Clin Endocrinol Metab 34:730–735

Verwoerdt A, Pfeiffer E, Wang HS (1969) Sexual behaviour in senescence. II. Patterns of sexual activity and interest. Geriatrics 24:137–154

Vigersky RA, Loriaux DL, Howards SS, Hodgen GB, Lipsett MB, Chrambach A (1976) Androgen binding proteins of testis, epididymis and plasma in man and monkey. J Clin Invest 58:1061–1068

Vilchez-Martinex JA, Arimura A, Schally AV (1976) Effect of actinomycin D on the pituitary response to LH-RH. Acta Endocrinol (Copenh) 81:73–81

Vinson GP, Whitehouse BJ, Goddard C, Sibley CP (1979) Steroid profiles formed by rat adrenocortical whole tissue and cell suspensions under different conditions of stimulation. J Steroid Biochem 11:175–183

Vitale R, Fawcett DW, Dym M (1973) The normal development of the blood-testis barrier and the effects of clomiphene and estrogen treatment. Anat Rec 176:333–344

Von Ebner V (1871) Untersuchungen über den Bau der Samenkanälchen und die Entwicklung der Spermatozoiden bei den Säugetieren und beim Menschen. "Rollet's Untersuchungen aus dem Institut für Physiologie und Histologie in Graz". Leipzig pp 200

Waites GMH (1977) Fluid secretion. In: Johnson AD, Gomes WR (eds) The testis, vol IV. Academic Press, New York, pp 91–123

Walton JS, Evins JD, Waites GMH (1978) Feedback control of FSH in pre- and post-pubertal rams as revealed by hemicastration. J Endocrinol 77:75–84

Walsh PC, Swerdloff RS (1973) Experimental cryptorchidism: effect on serum LH and FSH in the rat. Urol Res 1:22–26

Walsh PC, Swerdloff RS, Odell WD (1973) Feedback control of FSH in the male: role of oestrogen. Acta Endocr 74:449–460

Wang C, Burger HG, de Kretser DM, Dulmanis A, Hudson B, Keogh EJ, Suthers MB (1974a)

Effect of mesterolone on serum FSH, LH and plasma testosterone in normal men. Andrologia 6:111–118

Wang C, Youatt G, O'Connor S, Dulmanis A, Hudson B (1974b) A simple radioimmunoassay for plasma testosterone plus 5α-dihydrotestosterone. J Steroid Biochem 5:551–555

Wang C, Chan V, Tse TF, Yeung RTT (1978a) Effect of acute myocardial infarction on pituitary-testicular function. Clin Endocrinol 9:249–253

Wang C, Chan V, Yeung RTT (1978b) Effect of surgical stress on pituitary-testicular function. Clin Endocrinol 9:255–260

Wang C, Baker HWG, Burger HG, de Kretser DM, Hudson B (1975) Hormonal studies in Klinefelter's syndrome. Clin Endocrinol 4:399–411

Wang CF, Lasley BL, Lein A, Yen SSC (1976) The functional changes of the pituitary gonadotrops during the menstrual cycle. J Clin Endocrinol Metab 42:718–728

Warren MP, Jewelewicz R, Dyrenfurth I, Ans R, Khalaf S, Vande Wiele RL (1975) The significance of weight loss in the evaluation of pituitary response to LH-RH in women with secondary amenorrhea. J Clin Endocrinol Metab 40:601–611

Watson RH, Sapsford CS, McCance I (1956) The development of the testis, epididymis and penis in the young Merino ram. Aust J Agricul Res 7:574–590

Weddington SC, Brandtzaeg P, Hansson V, French FS, Petrusz P, Nayfeh SN (1975a) Immunological cross-reactivity between testicular ABP and serum TeBG. Nature 258:257–259

Weddington SC, Brandtzaeg P, Sletten K, Christensen T, Hansson V, French FS, Petrusz P, Nayfeh SN, Ritzen EM (1975b) Purification and characterization of rabbit testicular androgen binding protein (ABP). In: French FS, Hansson V, Ritzen EM, Nayfeh SN (eds) Hormonal regulation of spermatogenesis. Plenum Press, New York, pp 433–451

Weinstein RL, Kelch RP, Jenner MR, Kaplan SL, Grumbach MM (1974) Secretion of unconjugated androgens and estrogens by the normal and abnormal human testis before and after human chorionic gonadotropin. J Clin Invest 53:1–6

Welsh MJ, Wiebe JP (1976) Sertoli cells from immature rats: in vitro stimulation of steroid metabolism. Biochem Biophys Res Commun 1976 69:936–941

Welsh MJ, Wiebe JP (1978) Sertoli cell capacity to metabolize C19 steroids. Variation with age and the effect of FSH. Endocrinology 103:838–844

Wesson MB (1964) The value of testosterone to men past middle age. J Am Geriatr Soc 12:1149–1153

Wide L, Kjessler B (1969) Urinary excretion of interstitial cell stimulating hormone and sperm concentration in 219 males. Acta Endocrinol (Copenh) 62:299–305

Wide L, Nillius SJ, Gemzell C, Roos C (1973) Radioimmunosorbent assay of follicle-stimulating hormone and luteinizing hormone in serum and urine from men and women. Acta Endocrinol (Copenh) 73 [Suppl] 174:1–58

Wilson JD (1975) Metabolism of testicular androgens. In: Hamilton DW, Greep RO (eds) Handbook of physiology, sect 7, vol 5. Williams & Wilkins, Baltimore, pp 491

Winter JSD, Faiman C (1972) Pituitary-gonadal relations in male children and adolescents. Pediatr Res 6:126–135

Wollesen F, Swerdloff RS, Odell WD (1976) LH and FSH responses to luteinizing-releasing hormone in normal, adult, human males. Metabolism 25:845–863

Yaginuma T, Kigawa T, Kobayashi T, Kobayashi T (1969) Further studies on the hypothalamo-pituitary testicular axis of the rat in the neonatal period. J Endocrinol 45:473–474

Ying S-Y, Ling N, Bohlen P, Guillemin R (1981) Gonadocrinins: peptides in ovarian follicular fluid stimulating the secretion of pituitary gonadotropins. Endocrinology 108:1206–1215

Yoshimura F, Harumiya KL (1965) Electron microscopy of the anterior lobe of pituitary in normal and castrated rats. Endocrinol Jpn 12:119–152

Zanisi J, Motta M, Martini L (1973) Inhibitory effect of 5α-reduced metabolites of testosterone on gonadotrophin secretion. J Endocrinol 56:315–316

Zirkin BR, Ewing LL, Kromann N, Cochran RC (1980) Testosterone secretion by rat, rabbit, guinea pig, dog and hamster testes perfused in vitro: correlation with Leydig cell ultrastructure. Endocrinology 107:1867–74

Subject Index

Age
effect on FSH, LH, T 1–3
effect on Leydig cells 20, 21
effect on metabolic clearance rate of sex steroids 76–79
effect on pituitary-testicular axis 71–83
effect on virility and spermatogenesis 74, 75
Androgen binding protein 97–99
in testicular damage 135–137
Anorexia nervosa, effect of LHRH infusions 20, 21
Assay methods for gonadotrophins 1–3

Cirrhosis of liver effect on Leydig cells 131
Cryptorchidism
effect on ABP 135–137
effect on fluid production 135–150
effect on Leydig cells 147–150
effect on Sertoli cell structure 138–141

Episodic secretion of FSH, LH 3–5

Fetal irradiation
effects on Leydig cell 135–137
effects on Sertoli cell 145, 146
Fluid production by seminiferous tubules 136, 137
FSH
action on Sertoli cell 102, 103
changes in fetal life 44, 45
control 12–43
effect of age 75
feedback control 25–43
levels associated with spermatogenic damage 25–27
production rate 9–11
response to LHRH in puberty 48–53, 63–65
site of production 12, 13

Gonadocrinins 154

hCG, stimulation of Leydig cells 122–125
Hydroxyurea, effects on Sertoli cell function 133–141

Hypogonadotrophic hypogonadism, effect of LHRH infusions 20, 21

Inhibin
assays 27, 28
cellular source 38–40, 99
evidence for concept 27, 28
mode for action 41, 42
physiological implications 42, 43
sources 34–38

Klinefelter's Syndrome, effect of LHRH infusions 17

Leydig Cells 107–132
abnormalities in function 128–132
during fetal life 44–57, 108
morphology 108–115
regulation 118–121
role and regulation of LH receptors 121–125
role in spermatogenesis 126, 127
steroid biosynthesis 115–118
LH
effect of age 75, 76
feedback control 23–25
levels in fetal life 44
production rate 6–9
receptors in Leydig cells 121–125
response to LHRH in puberty 48–53, 63–65
role in Leydig cells 118–121
site of production 12, 13
LHRH
influence on FSH and LH 13–23
influence on Leydig cells 125, 126
infusions during puberty 19, 20, 48–53
infusions in Sertoli cell only syndrome 144, 145

Male-pseudo hermaphroditism 128–130
Metabolic clearance rate of FSH and LH 6–11
Metabolic clearance rate of testosterone 76, 77

Oestradiol, metabolic clearance rate 77–79

Plasminogen activator 99
Production rate of FSH 9–11
Production rate of LH 6–9
Prolactin, role in Leydig cell function 120
Puberty
changes in FSH, LH, Testosterone 45–48
changes in rams 60–70
changes in rats 53–60
effect of LHRH infusions 19, 20, 48–53
response to FSH and LH to LHRH 48–53

Reinke crystals 114, 115
Renal disease
effect on FSH, LH production rate 11
effect on Leydig cells 131

Seminiferous tubules
changes during puberty 53, 54, 65, 66
fluid production 96, 97
Sertoli cell
cultures 34, 35
function during testicular damage 135–141
hormonal regulation 101–105
inter-Sertoli cell junctions 93–95
maturation 95, 96
morphology 89–105
secretory products 97–100
steroidogenic activity 100, 101
Sertoli cell only syndrome, effect on FSH, LH, T 142–145
Sex steroid binding globulin, changes with age 76
Spermatogenesis 84–89
kinetics 87, 88
quantitation 88, 89
Spermatogenic damage 133–135
Spermatogenic cycle 85–87
Steroid biosynthesis
organelles involved 111, 112
pathways 115–118
Stress, effect on Leydig cells 130

Testosterone
action on Sertoli cell 103, 104
during puberty in ram 63–70
during puberty in rat 58–60
effect of age 75
levels in fetal life 43, 44
levels in new born 45
levels in puberty 46
secretion into blood 127, 128

Vitamin A deficiency
effects on Leydig cell 146, 147
effects on Sertoli cell 133–141

Volume 12:
Glucocorticoid Hormone Action
Editors: J.D.Baxter, G.G.Rousseau
1979. 176 figures, 58 tables. XIX, 638 pages. ISBN 3-540-08973-X

Volume 11: S.Ohno
Major Sex-Determining Genes
1979. 34 figures, 6 tables. XIII, 140 pages. ISBN 3-540-08965-9

Volume 10: W.I.P.Mainwaring
The Mechanism of Action of Androgens
1977. 12 figures, 17 tables. XI, 178 pages. ISBN 3-540-07941-6

Volume 9: R.E.Mancini
Immunologic Aspects of Testicular Function
1976. 36 figures, 8 tables. IX, 114 pages. ISBN 3-540-07496-1

Volume 8: E.Gurpide
Tracer Methods in Hormone Research
1975. 35 figures. XI, 188 pages. ISBN 3-540-07039-7

Volume 7: E.W.Horton
Prostaglandins
1972. 97 figures. XI, 197 pages. ISBN 3-540-05571-1

Volume 6: K.Federlin
Immunopathology of Insulin
Clinical and Experimental Studies
1971. 53 figures. XIII, 185 pages. ISBN 3-540-05408-1

Volume 5: J.Müller
Regulation of Aldosterone Biosynthesis
1971. 19 figures. VII, 137 pages. ISBN 3-540-05213-5

Volume 4: U.Westphal
Steroid-Protein Interactions
1971. 144 figures. XIII, 567 pages. ISBN 3-540-05313-3

Volume 3: F.G.Sulman
Hypothalamic Control of Lactation
In collaboration with numerous experts.
1970. 58 figures. XII, 235 pages. ISBN 3-540-04973-8

Volume 2: K.B.Eik-Nes, E.C.Horning
Gas Phase Chromatography of Steroids
1968. 85 figures. XV, 382 pages. ISBN 3-540-04277-6

Volume 1: S.Ohno
Sex Chromosomes and Sex-linked Genes
1967. 33 figures. X, 192 pages. ISBN 3-540-03934-1

Springer-Verlag
Berlin
Heidelberg
New York
Tokyo

MIX
Papier aus verantwortungsvollen Quellen
Paper from responsible sources
FSC® C105338

If you have any concerns about our products,
you can contact us on
ProductSafety@springernature.com

In case Publisher is established outside the EU,
the EU authorized representative is:
Springer Nature Customer Service Center GmbH
Europaplatz 3, 69115 Heidelberg, Germany

Printed by Libri Plureos GmbH
in Hamburg, Germany